# PIONEER MEDICINE IN AUSTRALIA

*Editor:* **John Pearn**

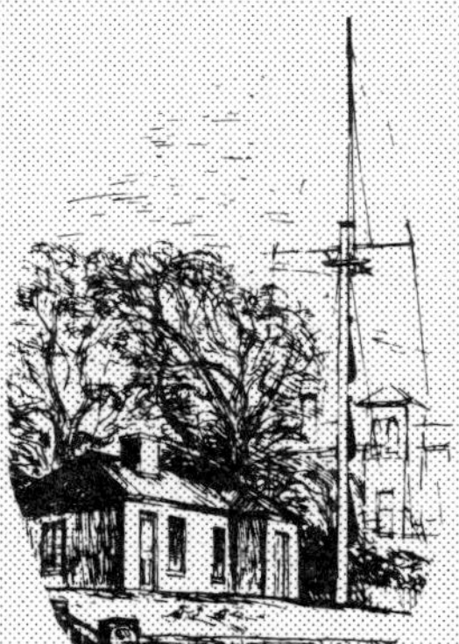

*Amphion Press*
*Brisbane*

# PIONEER MEDICINE IN AUSTRALIA

Bibliography
Illustrations
Notes and References
Tables
Includes Index

1st Edition (English)
First Published 1988



*Editor:* Professor John Pearn

*Typeset and Published by:* Amphion Press, (Department of Child Health Publishing Unit), Department of Child Health, University of Queensland, Royal Children's Hospital, Brisbane, Q. 4029. Australia.

*Printed by:* Merino Lithographics, 18 Baldock Street, Moorooka, Brisbane, Queensland, 4105, Australia.

*Cover by:* Paul Ramsden (Design) and Robert Allen, The Queensland Museum.



CATALOGUING IN PUBLICATION DATA
National Library of Australia
*Editor:* Pearn, John Hemsley

*Pioneer Medicine in Australia*

1. Medicine – Australia – History. 2. Medical care – Australia – History.
3. Aborigines, Australia – Queensland. 4. Convicts. 5. Surgeons. I. Pearn, John.

610.'994

NATIONAL LIBRARY OF AUSTRALIA CARD NUMBER AND ISBN

ISBN 0 86776 268 3.

# *CONTENTS*

Page

# *FOREWORD*

★

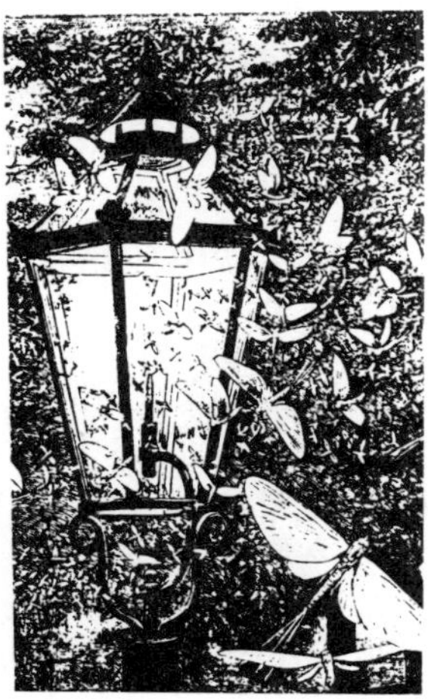

*ACADEMICALLY* speaking, the History of Medicine is still in the main *terra nullius* in this country: land without acknowledged owners or permanent occupants, though adjoining well-defined and assiduously cultivated domains. This is a status not without advantages. Researchers may enter without passport; no work permit is required. Scholars from many fields could do so with every prospect of making a useful contribution, but those who have chosen to do so have mostly been medical doctors. Latterly an increasing number of historians have found themselves there: not always by design, sometimes realising only belatedly that at some indeterminate stage they have passed beyond the accustomed boundary of their discipline.

There are also drawbacks to the present status of the study of medical history. The researcher, whether from the discipline of medicine or from that of history, does not come equipped with all the desirable knowledge and skills. Some have to be acquired on the job. This is not without precedent. The greatest of historians in earlier centuries mastered their craft in that way for want of any alternative; indeed, some writers have done so with distinction in our own day. But the self-taught historian of earlier times had for models the acknowledged masterpieces of the past. The modern writer, in addition, publishes alongside the trained professional historian and is subject to the same critical scrutiny. As things stand, there is no assurance that work in medical history will benefit from either influence. The historian who undertakes research on a medical topic will certainly consult medical reference works, and certainly should seek competent advice to ensure that he or she has selected wisely, and interpreted correctly what has been read therein.

One further means of making up for unavoidable shortcomings in preparation for research into medical history has been neglected too often. The tendency has been for the medical doctor and the historian, having come into medical history from different directions, to return each of them whence he came, to address his findings to his peers, but to interact further scarcely at all.

This book will help communication, interaction and exchange of ideas in this field. In the future, research projects in medical history will require collaboration of researchers from both disciplines from the beginning; collaboration of this nature is not easy and should not be embarked upon lightly. Co-operation and interchange between individual researchers each following his or her own bent, while imposing scarcely any restraint will offer benefits of great value. Not least of these will be some assurance that resulting publications will reach a wide body of readers. There are encouraging signs that co-operation of this nature is already beginning. One is the presence by invitation of papers by historians in symposia arranged as part of medical conferences.

In 1988, the Bicentennial year, heightened interest in all aspects of Australian history is very evident, and the status of Australian studies of all kinds is benefitting. It is not to be expected that the current level of interest will be sustained indefinitely; it may be that some Australians will experience a surfeit of celebration. But it is a reasonable expectation that some lasting benefit will remain: a more general interest in all Australiana, a richer appreciation of the interest and variety of Australian history. The Bicentennial year, we have it on high authority, should be a celebration of Australian achievement combined with candid recognition of what has been less than admirable in our past. Such provides purpose and direction for the future. That spirit seems to me an appropriate one in which to approach the study of medical history.

I am honoured by the invitation to contribute a Foreword to this book. The number and range of the chapters is a credit to the enthusiasm of professional historians, and others with a special secondary interest in this theme. It is an indication of the vigour with which medical history is progressing. Noting with pleasure the presence of historians among the contributors, I hope that this may presage increasing co-operation between medical doctors and historians in pursuing a fascinating area of mutual interest.

B.J. Dalton
Professor of History
James Cook University, Queensland

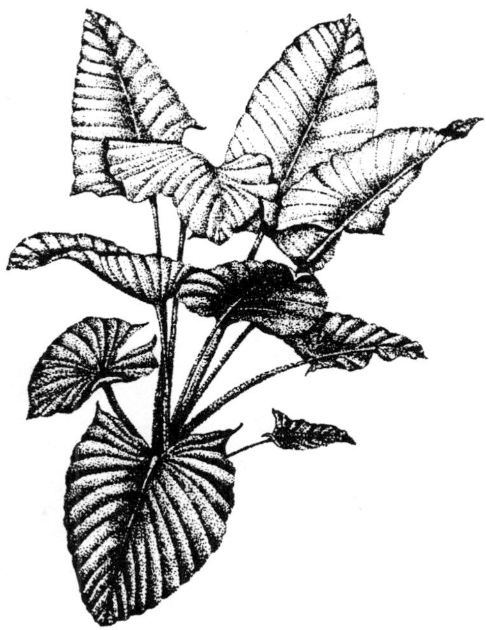

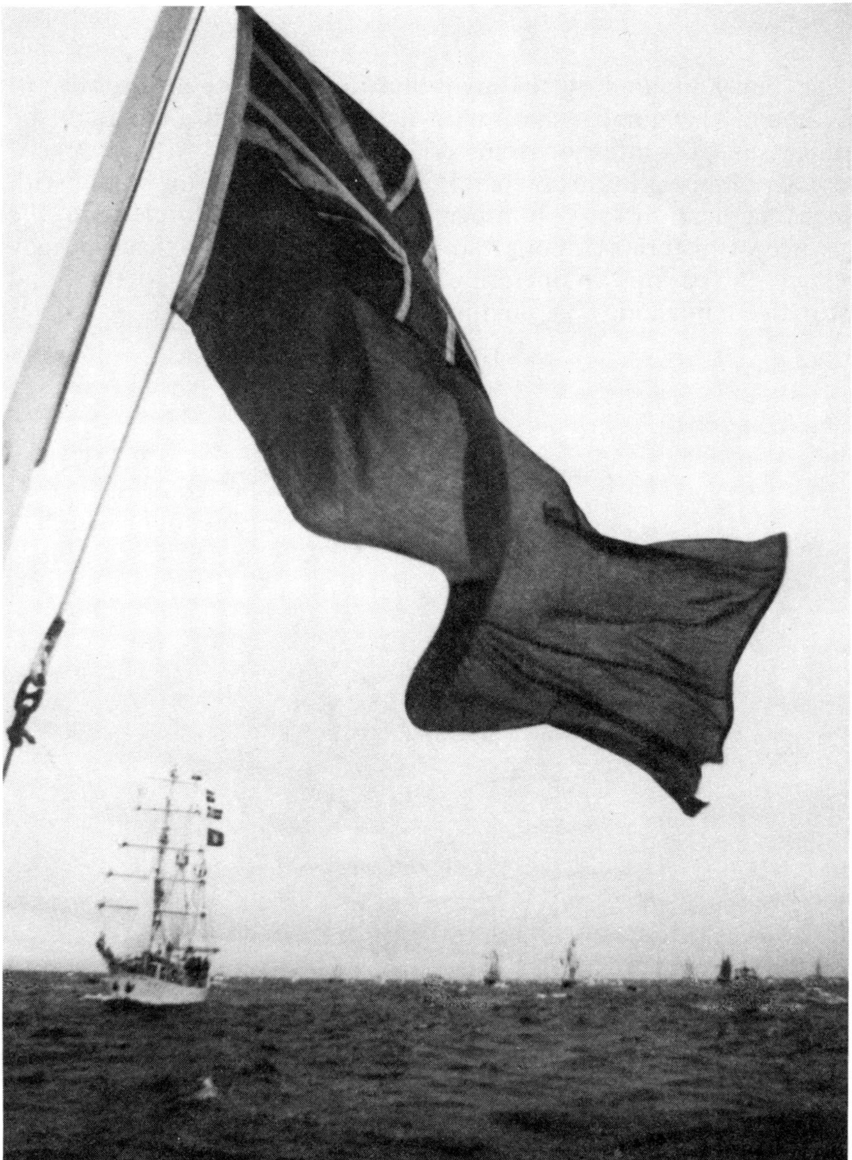

*The First Fleet Re-Enactment Fleet approaches Sydney Heads, Australia Day, 26 January 1988.*

*Photograph by the Fleet Surgeon, Dr Rob Simpson.*

# *CONTRIBUTORS*

★

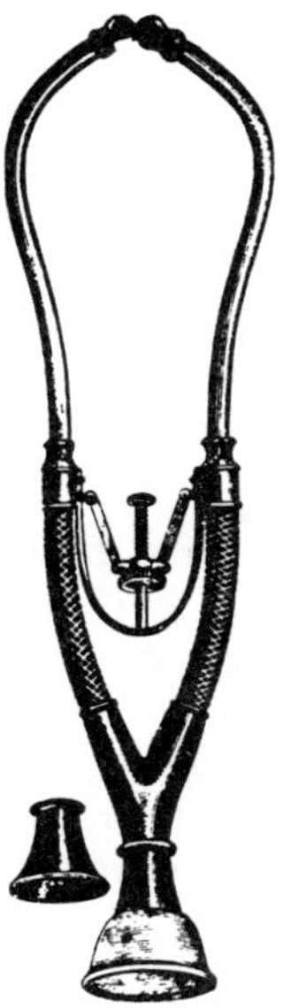

**JOHN CAMPBELL,** MB BS, FRCOG, FRACOG, is the Medical Superintendent, Royal Women's Hospital, Brisbane. As former Senior Lecturer in Obstetrics in the University of Queensland, he has published in the field of caesarean operations and the provision of obstetric services to the wider community; and was formerly an Australian Councillor within the Royal College of Obstetrics and Gynaecology. He has a particular interest in medical history, especially relating to Obstetrics. He founded the Museum of Obstetrics in the Royal Women's Hospital, Brisbane, and is its Curator. His special interests include bookbinding and book collecting.

★

**MERVYN COBCROFT,** MB BS, FFARACS, is a specialist anaesthetist in private practice in Ipswich, Queensland. His historical interests lie with the maritime activities of colonial Australia, especially whaling, sealing, and pearling. His library of original published works relating to these times forms one of the largest private collections in Australia. He has published many articles and two books on these maritime themes of colonial Australian history.

★

**JEANETTE COVACEVICH**, BA, MSc, biologist and scholar, is the Senior Curator (Vertebrates) at The Queensland Museum. She has published extensively on the biogeography of rainforests. Other contributions have included interpretative studies of early navigators' maps, and the documentation and preservation of traditional rainforest Aboriginal lore. A noted conservationist, she is the author of books on some of Australia's unique coastal habitats, and its creatures. She was one of two scientists chosen by the British Broadcasting Commission to feature in the Australian component of *Great Walks of the World*

★

**BRIAN DALTON,** MA(NZ), DPhil (Oxford) is the Foundation Professor, and Head of the Department of History, at James Cook University, Townsville. Born and reared in New Zealand, he has taught History in Australian universities most of his working life. He was appointed Foundation Professor in the new University in Townsville, in 1967, from the University of New England. The regional studies for which the Department of History at James Cook are probably best known have often impinged upon aspects of medical history.

**GEORGE DAVIS/NGANYGABANA** lives in Atherton, North Queensland. A Yidinyji man and retired timber-getter, he is the last surviving fluent speaker of his language. He was a major informant for Professor R.M.W. Dixon's definitive treatise on the Yidinyji language and has mapped one of the major Aboriginal trade routes through the north Queensland rainforest.

★

**ROBERT A. DOUGLAS,** AM, MB BS (Melb), FRCP (Lond), FRACP, Consultant Physician, is Hon. Physician to Townsville General Hospital. He was formerly Visiting Physician to Cairns Base Hospital 1952-1960 and to the Townsville General Hospital 1952-1980. His special interests and contributions have included the promotion of medical history in the North.

★

**CHRISTOPHER GARDNER-THORPE,** MD, FRCP is a consultant neurologist, writer and medical historian of Exeter, Devon UK. He qualified at St Thomas' Hospital in London in 1964. He studied neurology in Southampton, Leeds and Newcastle upon Tyne and was appointed the Consultant Neurologist in Exeter in the South West of England in 1974. He is a Doctor of Medicine and Fellow of the Royal College of Physicians, and is Honorary Tutor in Neurology at the Post-graduate Medical Institute of the University of Exeter. His special interests in clinical neurology include epilepsy and the use of antiepileptic drugs. One of his several books, *James Parkinson*, describes the life, times and contributions of one of the pioneers of modern clinical neurology.

★

**LORI HARLOE** is a Doctorate student in the History Department at James Cook University of North Queensland, Townsville. After graduating from the School of Nursing, Townsville General Hospital, she has nursed in various hospitals in the Eastern States. Special interests include theatre and the arts and currently, she is a full-time historian, researching aspects of health in colonial North Queensland.

★

**ANTHONY IRVINE,** BA (New Engl.) is a biologist with the Tropical Forest Research Unit (CSIRO), at Atherton, Queensland. His special interests include rainforest pollination, and the Aboriginal use of plants as foods and medicines in the rainforests of Northern Australia. He has discovered and described a new genus of palm, and is active in the Society for Growing Australian Plants, and the World Palm Society. Special historical contributions have included interpretation of some of the historical botanical writings of Sir Joseph Banks; and of Christie Palmerston, the adventurer and explorer of the Cairns hinterland.

**GEOFFREY CHARLES TREADGOLD KENNY,** MSc (Melb.), MB BS (Qld) is Senior Lecturer in Anatomy, the University of Melbourne. Anatomist, medical teacher and historian. A Lecturer in Anatomy at the University of Queensland from 1950 to 1959, Geoffrey Kenny is currently Deputy Chairman of the Anatomy Department within the University of Melbourne. He is a Past Chairman of the Medical History Society, AMA (Victorian Branch), co-editor of the newsletter *Medical History Australia* published by that Society and by the Medical History Unit within the University of Melbourne, and Treasurer of The Australian Society of the History of Medicine. He has a particular interest in neurology and neuroanatomy, and for many years has investigated the structure and function of the pineal gland.

★

**BARBARA KINSEY**, BSc (Syd.) is a scientist and writer, at the Sir George Fisher Centre for Tropical Marine Studies at James Cook University of North Queensland, Townsville. After graduation as a microbiologist she has been a consultant on marine environment themes, particularly in the area of public education. She is a Member of the Australian Coral Reef Society and the Australian Marine Science Association. She has collated and interpreted research contributions of the late Dr Jack Barnes, medical practitioner and marine scientist, of North Queensland.

★

**GARY KENNETH LITHERLAND,** MB BS, of Cairns, Queensland. A graduate of the Faculty of Medicine, University of Queensland (1976), he has served as the Royal Flying Doctor at Mt Isa (1982-1984), and at the Cairns Base (1984-current). His special interests include aeromedical evacuation, and obstetric ultrasound diagnosis.

★

**DAWN MAY,** PhD is an historian and Lecturer in Australian History and Politics, at James Cook University, Townsville. She is the author of the book *From Bush to Station – Aboriginal Labour in Nineteenth Century Queensland*, and her research interests have included studies of Aborigines and their contributions to the cattle industry of northern Australia, and aspects of Aboriginal health. She is Treasurer of the National Trust (Townsville), and a Member of the Institute of International Affairs, and the Australian Historical Association.

★

**RODERICK McLEOD,** AO, RFD, ED, MB BS, FRCS (Edin.), FRCS (Eng.), FRACS, Fell Roy Hist Soc Qld, is a Consultant Surgeon of Brisbane. His special professional interests include the prevention, diagnosis and surgery of malignant disease, and he is Head of the Queensland Melanoma Project. He is President of the Queensland Maritime Museum, and the Royal Historical Society of Queensland.

**NEVILLE PARKER,** MD, FRCPsych, forensic psychiatrist, geneticist and historian of Melbourne. The author of over sixty scientific papers and co-editor (with Professor John Pearn) of the medical biography of Ernest Sandford Jackson. His special interests include the study of accident neurosis, malingering, homicide and inherited disorders of the basal ganglia. He lectures extensively and is Consultant to the World Health Organisation on accident prevention in the Western Pacific region.

★

**ROBERT LYONS PEARCE,** OStJ, MB BS, FRCS, FICS, is a Plastic and Reconstructive Surgeon in private practice in Perth, Western Australia, with particular clinical interests in Dupuytren's Disease and Malignant Melanoma. Dr Pearce is a Consultant Surgeon to the Australian Army with the rank of Lt Colonel. He is also the Commissioner (WA) for St John Ambulance (Australia); he has held Committee positions with the Royal Flying Doctor Service, the Surf Life Saving Association and the Child Accident Prevention Foundation (WA). His interests include military and medical history and sailing.

★

**JOHN HEMSLEY PEARN,** AM, RFD, OStJ, MD (Qld), BSc, PhD (Lond.), FRCP (UK), FRACP, DCH, Fell Amer Coll Trop Med, Fell Roy Hist Soc Qld, is Professor and Head of Department of Child Health, University of Queensland. Paediatrician and clinical geneticist, of Brisbane. His professional contributions include clinical research studies of neuromuscular diseases, toxicology and the prevention of child injuries; and works on the medical history of Australia, of which he is the author of several books. Formerly the Consultant Physician to the Australian Force in Vietnam (1970), he is Colonel Consultant (RAAMC), Army Office, Canberra; District Surgeon for Queensland in the St John Ambulance Brigade (1983-1988) and serves on national committees of the Australian Resuscitation Council, and the Child Accident Prevention Foundation of Australia.

★

**JENNIFER ROBERTS,** BSc (Qld) is a high school mathematics teacher, in Brisbane. A Member of both the Queensland Association of Mathematics Teachers and the American Association for the Advancement of Science, she has special interests in educational methods. A former Board Member of the Brisbane Montessori School she is involved professionally with enrichment programmes for talented youth. She was formerly a youthful collaborator with her father, the late Dr Jack Barnes of Cairns, on venom extraction experiments from the box jellyfish.

**MAXWELL BYRON SIMKIN,** CBE, OStJ, is the Chief Executive of the Royal Flying Doctor Service of Australia (Queensland Section), a position he has held since 1977. Brigadier Simkin has been a career Regular Army Officer for thirty-eight years, and commanded the 1st Australian Logistic Support Group in the Vietnam Campaign. A civil and military pilot, he formed the Australian Army Aviation Corps of which he has been the Honorary Colonel for seven years. Instrumental in forming the Parachute School within the Royal Australian Army he is active in aviation affairs. He is currently Chairman of the Queensland Branch of the St. John Ambulance Association.

★

**ROB SIMPSON,** MB BS, BA, FRACS, surgeon and medical administrator, is Deputy Medical Administrator at Prince Henry's Hospital, Melbourne, and National Secretary of the Medical Association for the Prevention of War, Australia. His interest in medical history generally and First Fleet history in particular was born during his time as Fleet Surgeon on the First Fleet Re-Enactment Voyage. He has special interests in photography, particularly as a medium for the communication of living history, and has extensive lecturing commitments.

★

**M. JOHN THEARLE**, MD, FRCP (Edin.), FRACP, DCH (Lond.) is a Senior Lecturer in Child Health, University of Queensland, and a medical historian. He is a co-author of two paediatric textbooks, editor of a medical history book, and has had many papers published on clinical paediatrics and medical history. As an active committee member of the Brisbane History Group, he pursues his interest in local history and the history of paediatrics in Queensland. He is an avid collector of infantilia, the archaeology of the nursery.

★

**JOHN WILSON,** RN, RM, RPN, BAppSc (Adv.Nsg), is Nursing Supervisor at the Mersey General Hospital, Latrobe, Tasmania. A nursing historian and nursing administrator, he has contributed to numerous published works of the development of the profession of nursing. He has written several biographical works, including a biographical account of Sister Elizabeth Kenny.

**RONALD FRANCIS JAMES WOOD**, RFD, MB BS, DO, FRACS, FRACO, Fell Roy Hist Soc Qld. Consultant Ophthalmologist, of Brisbane. Ronald Wood has extensive interests in military ophthalmology, the medico-legal implications of medical practice, and medical history. Since 1961, he has been engaged in private and hospital ophthalmological practice, serving as Ophthalmologist and Honorary Consultant Ophthalmologist (since 1982) to the Royal Brisbane and Princess Alexandra Hospitals, Visiting Ophthalmologist to the Repatriation General Hospital, Greenslopes. As Lieutenant-Colonel, he served as Consultant Ophthalmologist to the First Military District, Royal Australian Army. Since 1975, he has been President of the Medical Defence Society of Queensland, and Chairman (since 1984) of the Confederation of Australian Medical Defence Organisations. The Jackson Lecturer of 1978, he has been a Councillor of the Royal Historical Society of Queensland for eight years, and is currently Vice-President.

★

**HELEN R. WOOLCOCK**, PhD, historian, of Sydney. She is a Post-doctoral Fellow and Part-time Lecturer, School of Science and Technology Studies at the University of New South Wales. As a social historian her research focuses on biography, public health, the medical aspects of nineteenth-century migration to Australia and Canada, and comparative colonial medicine. Her book, *Rights of Passage: Emigration to Australia in the Nineteenth-Century*, is a study of health care on Queensland immigrant vessels.

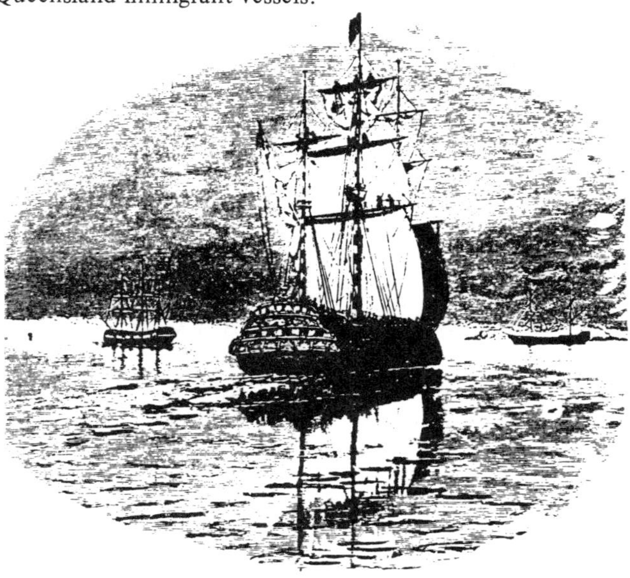

# *ACKNOWLEDGEMENTS*

★

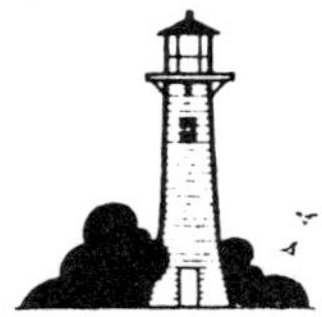

*THE* chapters of this book comprise the papers delivered at the Australian Bicentennial Medical Congress, held in Cairns in August 1988. It is a tribute to the help and co-operation of each of the twenty authors whose works comprise this book, that they have been published as a complete entity on this historic occasion.

The Editor and Authors thank the extended Congress Secretariat of the Australian Bicentennial Medical Congress for their confidence, and for the most generous financial support which has made this volume possible. In particular, we thank Dr Ken Pettit, Dr Max Stewart and Dr Michael McAuliffe for their warm encouragement, both material and personal; and also extend special thanks to Dr Ross Messer, consultant paediatrician of Cairns, whose foresight and support enabled this publication to go ahead.

Further very generous support and encouragement has also been made by the Standing Executive of the North Queensland Medical Conference Coordinating Committee (and, in particular, Dr Graham Cossins) a group which has done so much to promote the high standing of medicine in Northern Australia.

We thank the Federal Council of the Australian Medical Association for their confidence, expressed in most generous support also, which enabled the publication of this book to proceed; and the Director and Staff of The Queensland Museum for much help. In particular, we thank Mr Paul Ramsden and Mr Robert Allen of the Graphics Section, and Jeanette Covacevich for much help and support.

The Editor thanks also Nestlé Australia, Roche Australia, Roussel Australia, and the Queensland Branch of the Australian Medical Association for ongoing and most gracious support.

This work was further made possible by extensive contributions from the Publishing Unit, within the Department of Child Health, University of Queensland, whose terms of reference include the promotion of health perspectives in society through the portal of Australian medical history.

In particular, the Editor thanks Mr Graham Jurott, of the University of Queensland, Mr Charles Scandrett and Staff of Merino Lithographics, and Mrs Peggy Carter, whose special publishing skills have contributed so much to the recording and promotion of medical history in this country.

Professor John Pearn
*Editor:* for The Secretariat,
Australian Bicentennial Medical Congress.
Department of Child Health
Royal Children's Hospital, Brisbane
Queensland, Australia

August 1988

AUSTRALIAN
BI-CENTENNIAL
MEDICAL
CONGRESS
NORTH QUEENSLAND
1988

# PART I

# FIRST DOCTORS

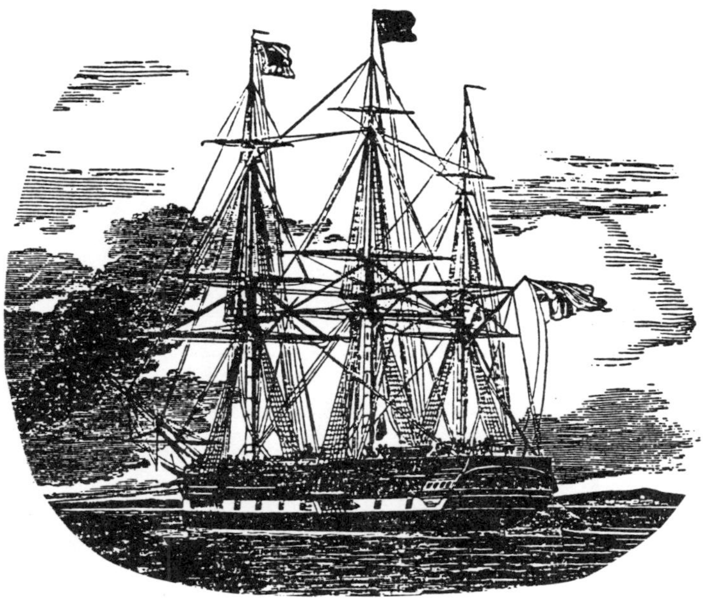

# PIONEER MEDICINE IN AUSTRALIA

# 1

## THE LAND THEY LEFT BEHIND
### England in 1787

**Christopher Gardner-Thorpe**

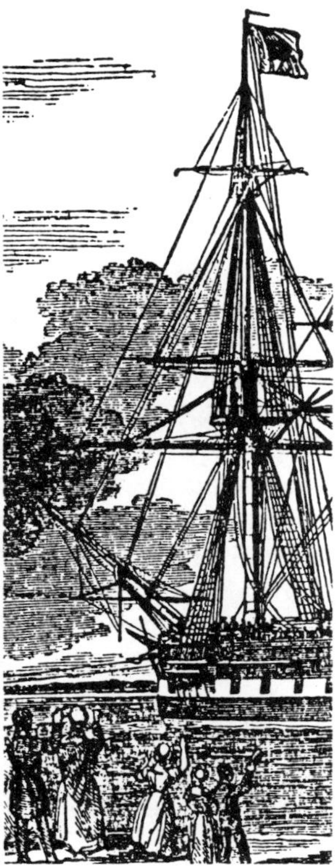

*IN* and around the West Country of England may be found much evidence of early links with Australia. William Dampier in 1688 was the first Englishman to land in Australia. He lived in East Coker in Somerset; those walking in parts of that beautiful village today will see features little changed from those enjoyed by the youthful sailor three hundred years ago (*Figure 1.1*). Voyaging in the *Cygnet*, Dampier sailed beyond the limits of the known world. His grave in London – he died in 1715 – is unmarked and unknown.

Australian colonisation is deemed to have started on 26 January 1788 when the resilient travellers – volunteers, fatalistic sailors, and convicts – who had sailed some fifteen thousand miles proposed the health of their sovereign, King George III, at Sydney Cove. What sort of country had they left behind when they sailed from England on 13 May 1787, seven years after James Cook had landed at Botany Bay?

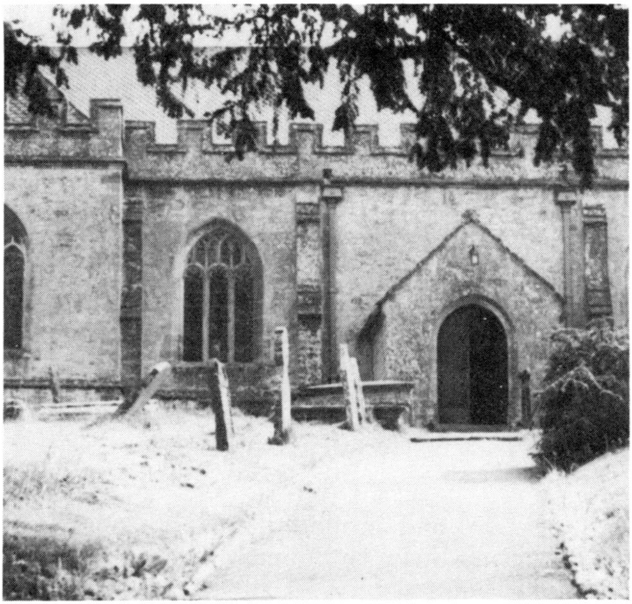

*Figure 1.1:*

***St Michael's Church in East Coker, Somerset. Little changed since Dampier's time, a memorial on its north wall records his travels to Terra Australis in 1688. Photo, by the author, 1988.***

This short account looks at Portsmouth through the eyes of James Parkinson, a doctor of the times; and at Plymouth through the eyes of Devon men of the day – with the perspective of a later Devon doctor after the passage of a further two hundred years.

The First Fleet sailed from near the Square Tower in Old Portsmouth (*Figure 1.2*). Built in 1494, it was the principal magazine for the Portsmouth garrison in the seventeenth and eighteenth centuries. The Fleet assembled in the anchorage at Spithead (*Figures 1.3 and 1.4*), between the Isle of Wight and Portsmouth, within a short distance of where modern discoveries have shown lay Henry VIII's ship *Mary Rose* – in 1787 she had already lain in the silt for two hundred and forty two years. The Fleet was completed by ships from Plymouth, including the *Charlotte* (*Figure 1.5*). Surgeon General John White had been chosen to accompany Captain Arthur Phillip on that historic voyage from the naval anchorage at Spithead.

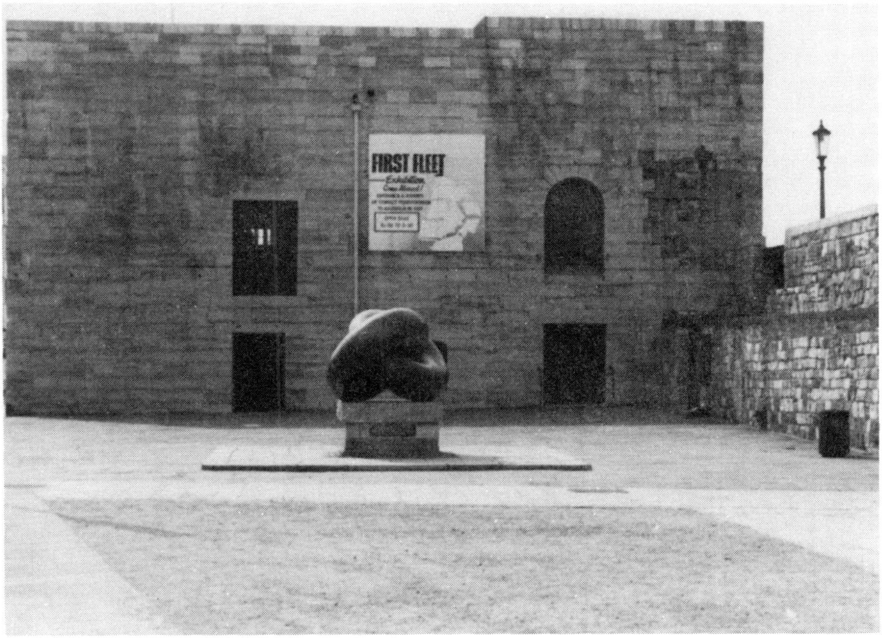
FIRST FLEET

*A*

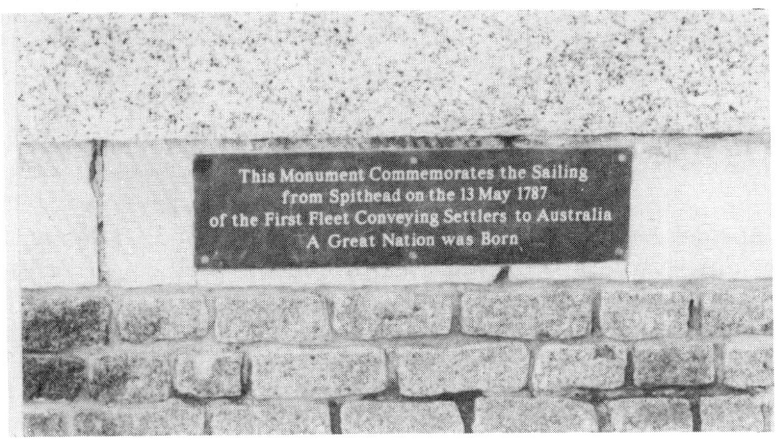
This Monument Commemorates the Sailing
from Spithead on the 13 May 1787
of the First Fleet Conveying Settlers to Australia
A Great Nation was Born

*B*

*Figure 1.2: The origins of Australian colonization; Portsmouth, England.*

*A. The Monument to the departure of the First Fleet, with the square tower behind. At this site, near this former garrison magazine, assembled the eleven ships of the First Fleet.*

*B. Inscription commemorating the departure of the First Fleet, 13 May 1787.*

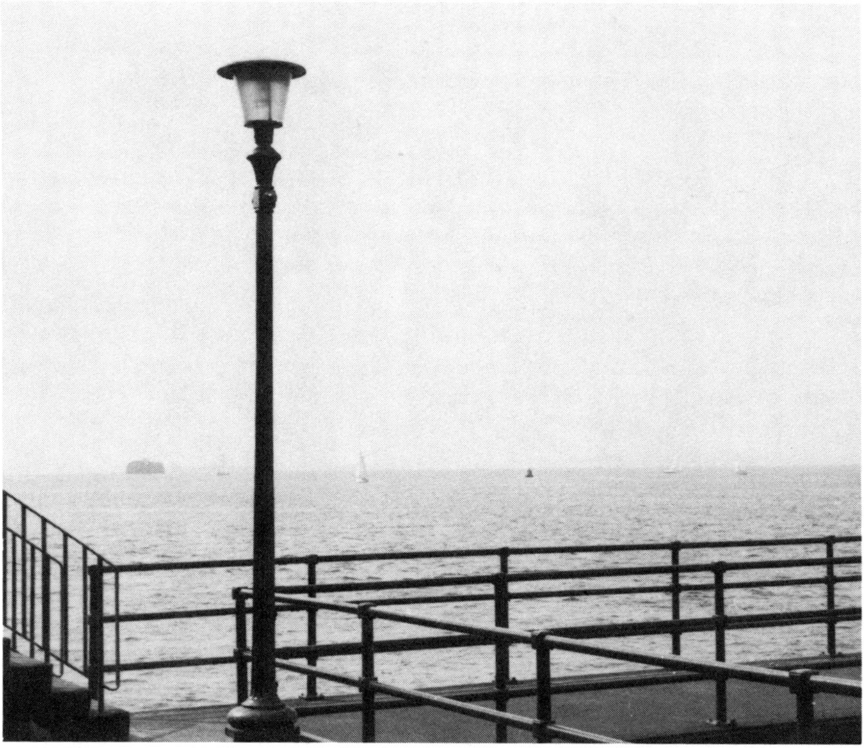

*Figure 1.3: The site of the First Fleet assembly area, 1787, through the camera lens of 1987. The Solent and Spithead at Portsmouth, England, from the gateway site through which passed the naval men, the convicts of both sexes, and the marine garrison who were to be their guards.*

Phillip had been brought back from retirement at Lyndhurst in the New Forest where he farmed. He led the First Fleet in *Sirius*, the name given to the brightest star in the English sky. With the party also went one John Small who was transported from Exeter jail, and who married Mary Parker who bore him seven children. Devon men are long-lived and he was the last known survivor of the First Fleet when he died in October of 1850 at the age of eighty-two.

When the First Fleet sailed in 1787, England was in a state of social change. Medicine, as we know it today, was just beginning to develop. Nelson had been married two months. John Hunter was fifty-nine and had some six years to live; eleven years were to pass before Jenner reported on vaccination and neither Richard Bright nor Thomas Hodgkin was yet born. The music of Mozart was heard for the first time, Wordsworth and Beethoven were seventeen, and the trade bans with France had been lifted only one year before in the Eden Treaty. Pitt was Prime Minister and his government overtook the personal rule of the monarch, King George III, whose episodes of madness probably contributed to the injustices experienced by the populace at that time. William Wilberforce was campaigning against slavery. In America only four years had elapsed since the Boston Tea Party, and the three short years since the American War of Independence still left a feeling of shock among many. Australia was chosen for Colonisation when America closed its ports to the transportation of convicts.

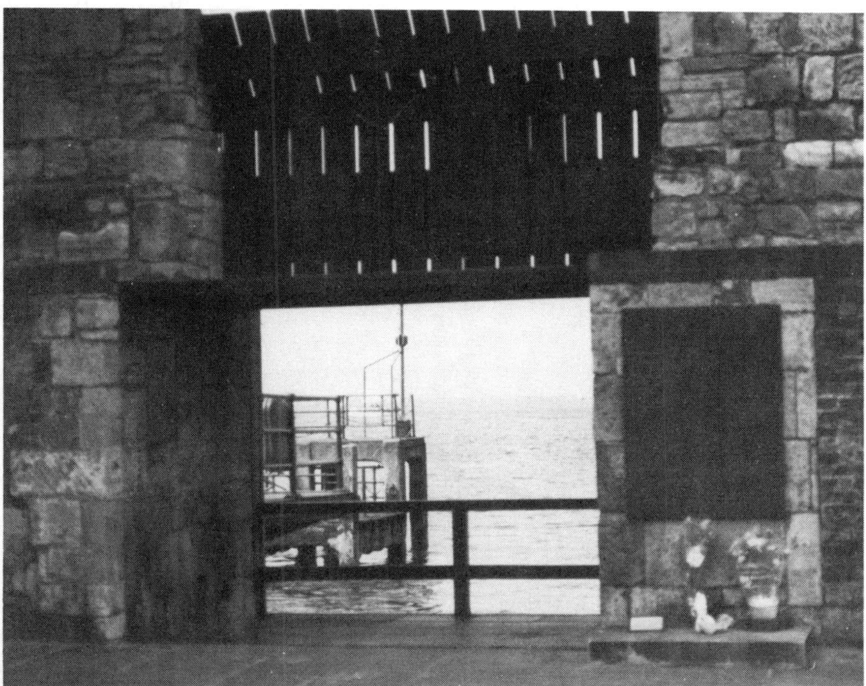

*Figure 1.4: The Gateway, Old Portsmouth, England, through which passed many of the sailors, convicts and marines of the First Fleet, in 1787. Photo, by the author, 1987.*

One man of the day, well known for the disease which bears his name, was to have substantial effects upon English medicine. He was James Parkinson, born in 1755 and thirty-two years old when the First Fleet sailed. He had been born in the old family home in Hoxton Square, an influential area near London where his father had practised medicine. Three generations of doctors were to practise in the family home, close to St Leonard's Church whose chimes are described in the rhyme *Oranges and Lemons* – 'when I grow rich, say the bells of Shoreditch'.

James' father, an apothecary and surgeon, was buried in the churchyard of St Leonard's Church and his headstone can still be seen. In 1824 James was to be buried there too but like so many who have made the greatest contributions to society, the site of his grave is not known. Members of his family were buried in the West of England and his descendants can be traced in the South.

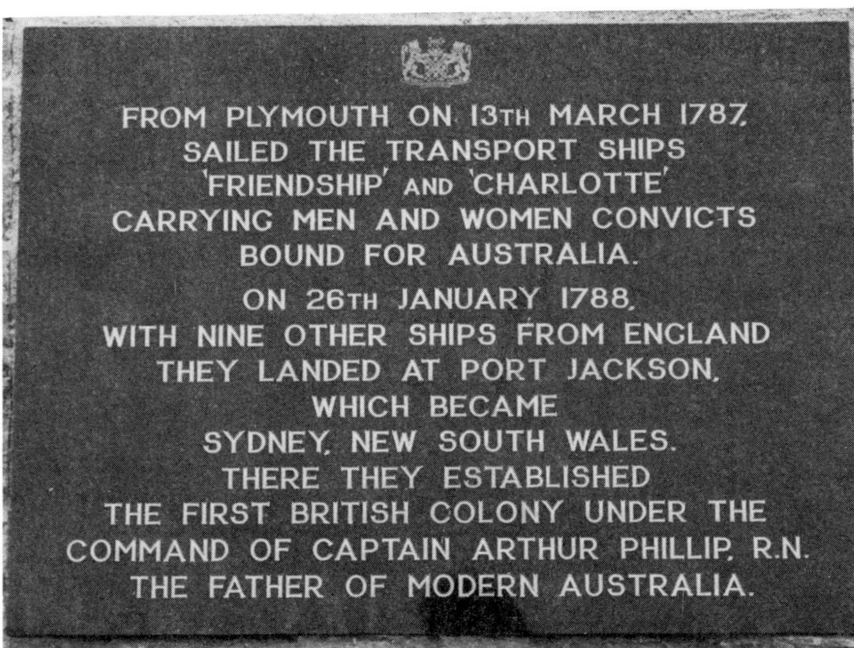


***Figure 1.5:* *Commemorative plaque on the wharf at Plymouth, Devon. Sited near the "Mayflower" steps, it records the contributions of West County folk to the future of the new Colony in Australia. Photo, by the author, 1988.***

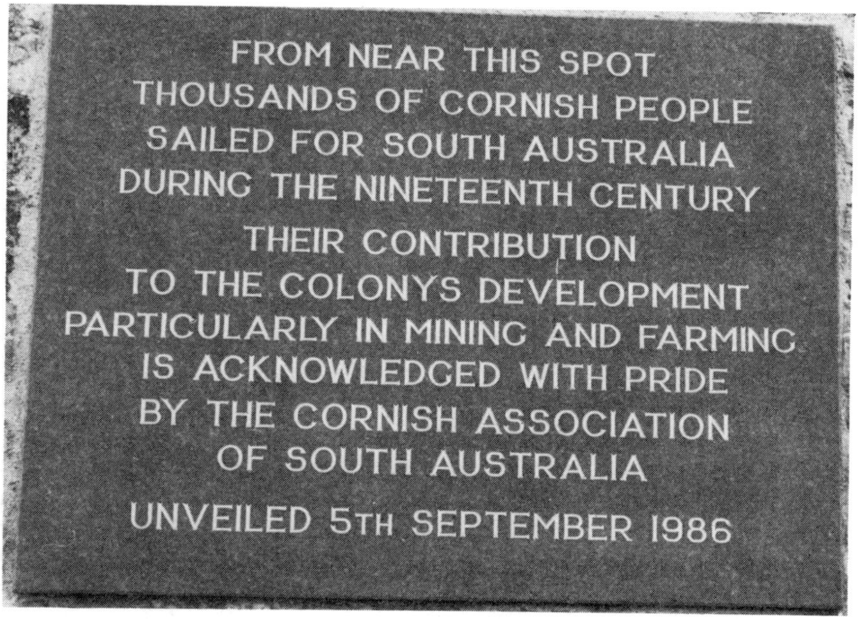


***Figure 1.6:* Plaque from the wharf at Plymouth – the contribution of Western folk to the new Colonies in Australia.**

The area of Hoxton had been developing for a hundred years or so, and had seen much history pass. Ben Johnson had fought a duel in Hogsten Fields *[sic]* and Shakespeare at one time lived in Hoxton, an area where Theological Academies, coffee houses and public houses could be found together with various influential and profitable family businesses in this fashionable outskirt of London. James Parkinson had already been married to Mary Dale for six years when the First Fleet sailed.

Dr James Parkinson, besides his description of the "Shaking Palsy" which bears his name, was not without effect upon the political opinion of his time. In 1787, he was forming his views about the injustices in the world he saw around him; within four years he would start publishing pamphlets. The criticism set forth in these writings caused considerable uproar. The Pop Gun Plot, a plan to kill King George III with an air gun in a theatre some five years later, was a crime planned by members of the London Corresponding Society of which James Parkinson was a prominent member. He was called before the Privy Council to give evidence about this. He described his experiences in the pamphlet 'Assassination of a King'. The link between metabolic disease and behaviour was not understood but it is now known that King George III suffered from porphyria, which may well have accounted for his periods of madness.

Parkinson's views about the world around him were illustrated by his practical work for the poor, the church and the Sunday School near his home. The first Sunday School is thought to have opened in Gloucestershire, near the village where Edward Jenner, famous for his work on vaccination, practised at the time; but it was at Hoxton that James Parkinson became Secretary to the Parish, and a Trustee for the poor. It is for his medicine and in particular his geological works, however, that James is now remembered best.

The young doctor had been qualified for three years when the First Fleet sailed. He was soon to attend the surgical lectures of John Hunter. James distinguished himself in gaining a silver medal from the Royal Humane Society after he had resuscitated a patient. He published papers describing the effects of lightning, and descriptions of rabies and purpura. His ideas flowed into the medical teachings of the day. He described what was needed of a doctor in 'The Hospital Pupil' and for the world at large he published his 'Textbook of Domestic Medicine'. Popular medical texts for the public, mostly described as textbooks of domestic medicine, did not really gain popularity until Victorian times, and are of course still prolific today. Parkinson's more specialised books included a work on trusses and he described gout from which he suffered, like his father before him. James was a founder member of the Medical and Chirurgical Society of London and it may be there that he first met Edward Jenner. Parkinson and Jenner at different times owned the same brass microscope – fortunately preserved today.

James Parkinson was local doctor to the madhouses close to his home. One of his patients was detained in a madhouse on the basis of a history given by the patient's relative and James therefore based his own diagnosis upon the relative's description. He was very severely criticised for this. This episode was one important link which led to changes in the law which subsequently required two medical practitioners to certify insanity. He attempted to distinguish disorders of memory from abnormalities of speech and of true insanity. One of James' medical colleagues was Willis who attended King George III in his first attack of madness in 1788, the year of the Fleet's landing at Sydney Cove.

With his son John, James Parkinson wrote the first account of perforation of the appendix. He became Chairman of the Association of Apothecaries and Surgeon Apothecaries and one year later, in 1817, 'An Essay on the Shaking Palsy' was published. This is Parkinson's most famous publication and the description which it contains can not really be bettered –

> ... *involuntary tremulous motion with lessened muscular power, in parts not in action and even when supported, with a propensity to bend the trunk forwards and to pass from a walking to a running pace: the senses and intellect being uninjured.*

Thus the shaking palsy was first described thirty years after the First Fleet set sail. In 1877 the illness was named after Parkinson by the famous Parisian neurologist, Charcot.

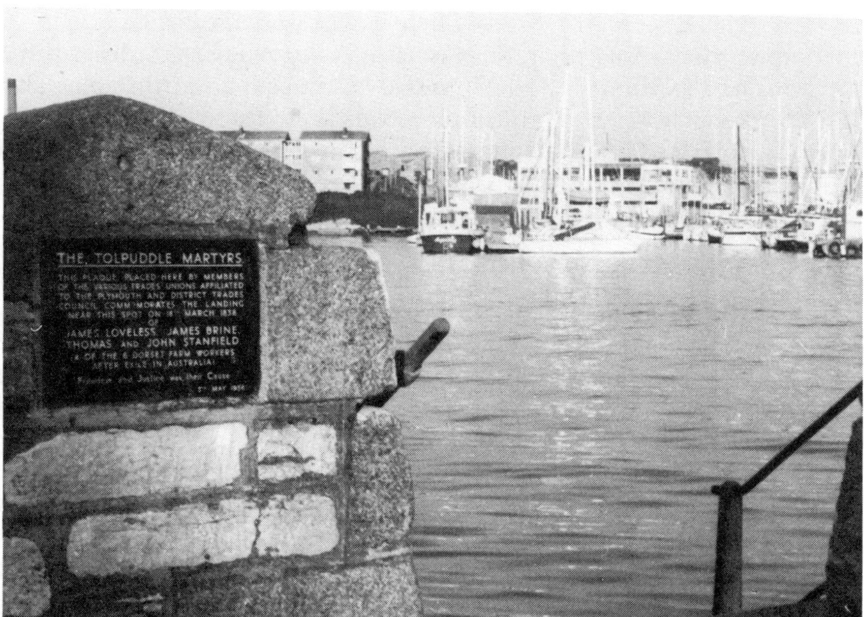


***Figure 1.7:* The steps and wharf at Plymouth, Devon; where stepped ashore, after their transportation to Australia, the Tolpuddle Martyrs, in 1838. Photo, 150 years after their historic return, by the author in 1988.**

James is well remembered for his work on geology and fossils and it was for his discoveries in palaeontology that in 1822 he was the first in a line of distinguished doctors to receive the honorary gold medal of the Royal College of Surgeons. Along with Lamarck, Cuvier and the drawing master William Martin, James has been described as one of the foremost founders of scientific palaeontology in that heroic age of geology. Whilst still a young man, he published his 'Chemical Pocket Book' and in due course his monumental three volume work 'Organic Remains of a Former World'. Later still his 'Outlines of Oryctology' was a smaller and more popular version of the work on fossils. Parkinson was a founder member of the Geological Society along with other medical colleagues including Dr Babbington of Guys Hospital; he published many papers on fossils and geological topics and corresponded by letter with the well-known gentleman scientists of his day such as William Cunnington of Wiltshire and the Reverend William Buckland of Oxford. These were the times when it was possible for one man to encompass the whole breadth of scientific knowledge. At least three surgeons of the First Fleet (White, Bowes Smyth and Considen) also had the broadest scientific outlook in this same tradition.

In his later years James Parkinson moved house nearer to the parish infirmary in the Kingsland Road of London where he was the attending physician. The Infirmary had opened in 1777. He died in his new property which has now been demolished and replaced by a block of flats. His publications and correspondence can still be found and also some of his possessions such as his microscope. He autographed his books. It is in his scientific works and ideas that one finds so many details of the England of 1787 – the writings of an observant doctor of the day, commenting on religion and politics, on medicine and on geological sciences.

The travellers to Australia in the First Fleet would have found better weather on the antipodean shores. They left behind one of the most severe winters on record; in that year in England many people died of starvation. It was the time of the Industrial Revolution and the invention of the spinning mule; and the French Revolution was soon to follow, its seeds simmering at the time.

The West of England contributed a large number of colonists, volunteers and otherwise, to the new country (*Figure 1.6*). One, John Western came from Stepcote Hill, an area of Regency Exeter

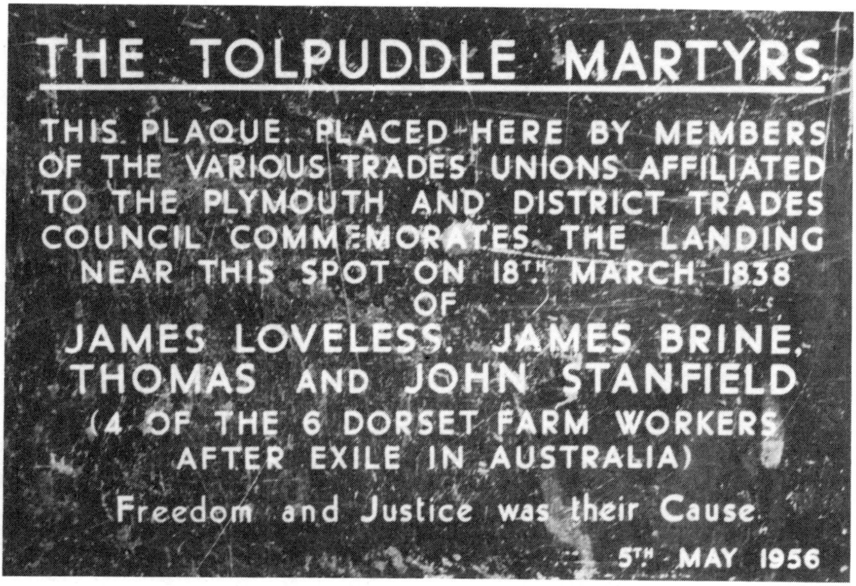


***Figure 1.8:* The origins of the Trade Union Movement. The plaque on the wharf at Plymouth, Devon, commemorating the return from "exile in Australia" of the Dorset men who had the courage to attempt collective bargaining for better working conditions for the labourer.**

now charmingly restored. He was sentenced to transportation for stealing a handkerchief and a snuff box. He left from Topsham, a small port near Exeter, to await transportation from a hulk moored in Plymouth. Labourers and craftsmen were transported or emigrated. Doctors from the South and West also left to start a new life across the world. In November of 1831 Thomas Galloway, a surgeon whose house is now occupied by a firm of chartered accountants, sailed from Portsmouth. Another prominent Portsmouth citizen was Henry Ayers after whom Ayers Rock in the centre of Australia is named. Portsmouth was known to Charles Dickens too who was born there in 1812, in a house in Mile End to which his parents had moved in the summer of 1809. The house is in the shadow of a block of modern flats named *Brisbane House*.

The West of England saw the origins of the Trade Union movement, and in 1787 there were stirrings of worker resentment at the appalling conditions of the common labourer. Devon and Dorset

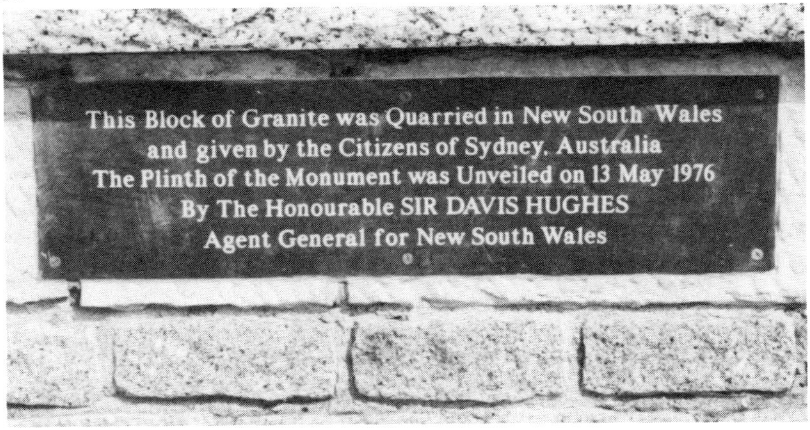


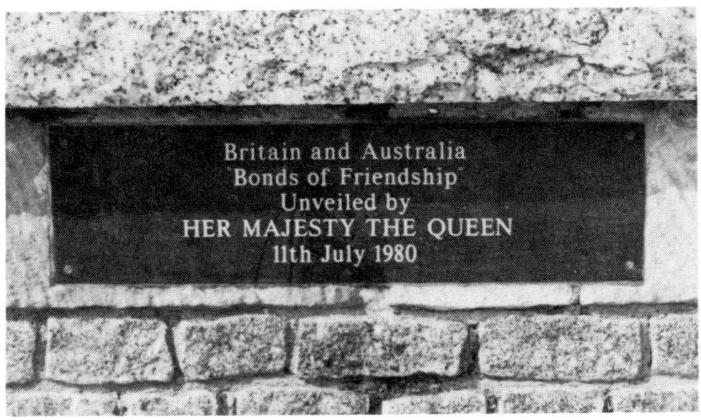
Britain and Australia
'Bonds of Friendship'
Unveiled by
HER MAJESTY THE QUEEN
11th July 1980

***Figure 1.9:***

***The plinth of the Monument — Colonization of Australia — Portsmouth, England. Photo by the author, 1988.***

men have long been noted for their courage, and it was in the village of Tolpuddle that the first men were legally victimized for their attempts, collectively, to seek better working conditions. They were transported as convicts for this felony, the survivors to be hailed as martyrs at Plymouth, on their repatriation from Australia in the *John Barry*, in 1838 (*Figures 1.7 and 1.8*). Their return followed campaigns by Thomas Wakley, Editor of *The Lancet*, and history has rightly termed these courageous men the "Tolpuddle Martyrs".

In the fifty years after the departure of the First Fleet, the wharf at Plymouth saw the departure, never to return, of many who were to give their lives in the new Continent across the world. In the Devon town of Totnes was born on 5 January 1804 to the local surgeon a son, William Wills, who was educated at the grammar school in Ashburton nearby. At the age of sixteen he started medicine.

He accompanied his father in 1852 to Melbourne as Medical Officer on an emigrant ship at the time of the Gold Rush. In 1860 with Burke he set out to cross Australia from South to North, and to survey the unknown interior. It is well known that he perished from thirst and lack of food on the return journey on 28 June 1861. The granite obelisk on The Plains at Totnes was erected in his memory in 1864.

A monument erected to the First Fleet near the Square Tower in Old Portsmouth bears plaques to the memory of the First Fleet. This historic spot saw James Cook return in 1772 when the *Endeavour* berthed nearby, after the discoveries on the east coast of Australia; and has seen in intervening times expressions of the bonds which unite two countries (*Figure 1.9*). The Monument to the First Fleet itself takes the form of two interwoven bronze rings – a symbolic doublet of the bonds of friendship, and the bonds of the convicts which linked the two countries. Set on a granite plinth from New South Wales, it is the twin of a similar memorial in Sydney Cove.

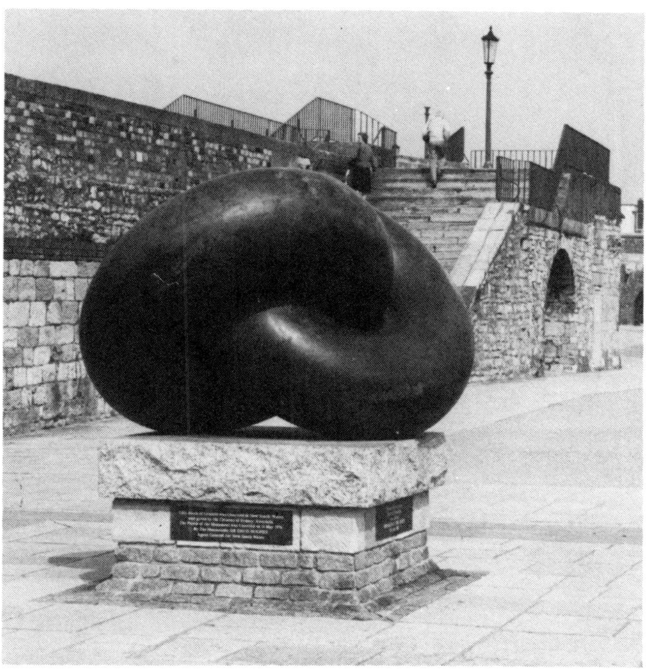

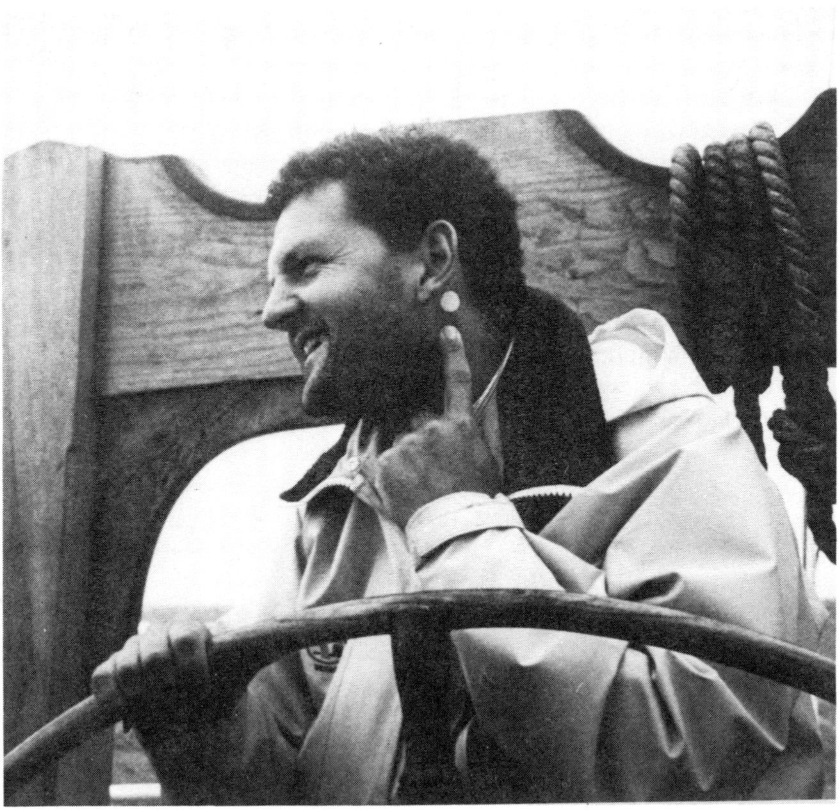

*Figure 2.1: The author, Dr Rob Simpson (Fleet Surgeon of the First Fleet Reenactment Voyage) points to a pledget of hyoscine alkaloids – an effective agent to control seasickness, and the cornerstone of his preventive medicine programme.*

# PIONEER MEDICINE IN AUSTRALIA 2

## *JOHN WHITE MD, RN*
## *Surgeon General to the First Fleet*

**Rob Simpson**

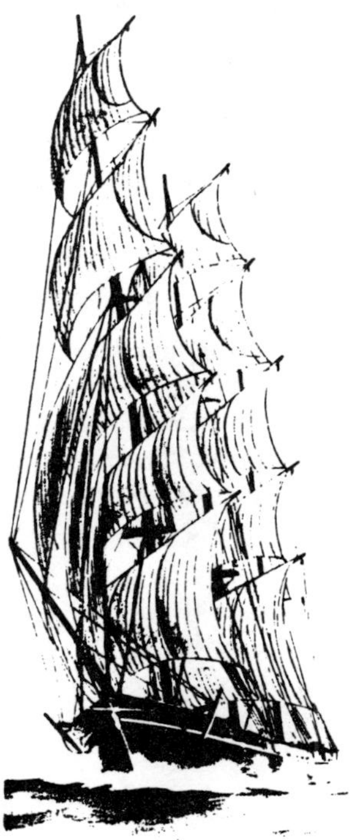

*Lords Commissioners of the Treasury.*

*My Lords.*

*The several goals and places for the confinement of felons in this Kingdom being in so cramped a state that the greatest danger is to be apprehended not only from their escape but from infectious distempers which may hourly be expected to break out amongst them; His Majesty, desirous of preventing by every possible means the ill consequences which might happen from these causes, has been pleased to signify to me his Royal Command that measures should be pursued for sending out of the Kingdom such of the convicts as are under the sentence or order of transportation. His Majesty has thought it advisable to fix upon Botany Bay, as a place likely to answer the purpose.*[1]

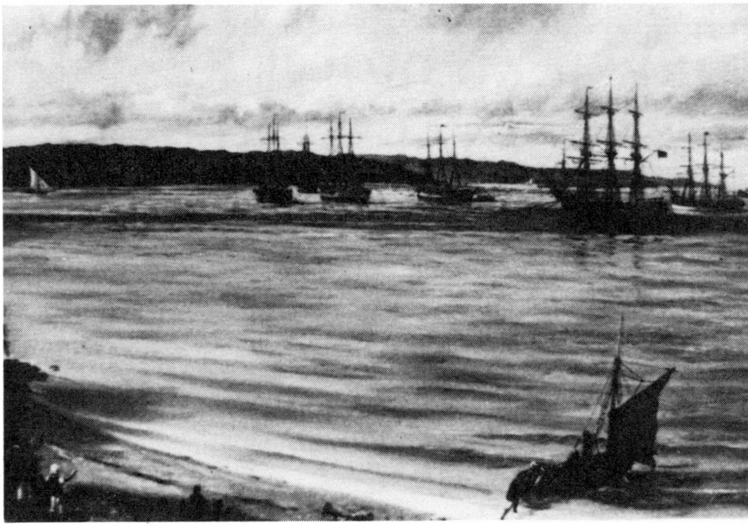

*Figure 2.2: Ships of the First Fleet anchored on the Motherbank in the Solent, near Portsmouth 1787. Reproduced by kind permission of the Australian Heritage Centre, Isle of Wight.*

So wrote Lord Sydney, Secretary for the Home Department on 10th August 1786. And so was created the fleet of square-rigged sailing ships that came to be known as the First Fleet. A fleet whose voyage is so beautifully described by David Collins, Judge Advocate to the colony, on 20th January, 1788 –

> *Thus, under the blessing of God, was happily completed in eight months and one week a voyage which before it was undertaken, the mind hardly dared to contemplate.... we had sailed 5021 leagues; had touched at the American and African continents; and had at last rested within a few days sail of the antipodes of our native country, without meeting any accident in a fleet of 11 sail.*[2]

Seventeen-eighty six was the twenty-sixth year of the sixty year reign of King George III, 'the mad farmer' as he came to be known after his first derangement, which ironically occurred the year he authorised the creation of the First Fleet and hence modern Australia.

Eighteenth Century Europe in general and perhaps London in particular was a mass of contradictions and ambiguities. On the one hand music, literature, art, science, architecture and to a lesser extent medicine were producing some of their most famous sons. On the other hand poverty, malnutrition and disease afflicted large segments of society. In Europe Vivaldi, Johan Sebastian Bach, Haydn, Mozart and Beethoven were all products of the late 17th or 18th Century as were Turner and Constable.

Whence came the convicts and garrison that first peopled the new land across the world? The literature of the day gives some of the answers, much of it written by medical men. What we know as *Gulliver's Travels* appeared in 1726, distanced from its author as *Travels into Several Remote Nations of the World* purportedly written by Lemuel Gulliver. Under the humble disguise of a low church and not overly successful ship's surgeon, Swift addressed the condition of and prognosis for the human race – the result is literature which remains amongst the blackest satire ever written. Tobias Smollett's *The Adventures of Roderick Random* was another classic, written by a surgeon about a surgeon; a surgeon with the unlikely name of Roderick Random.

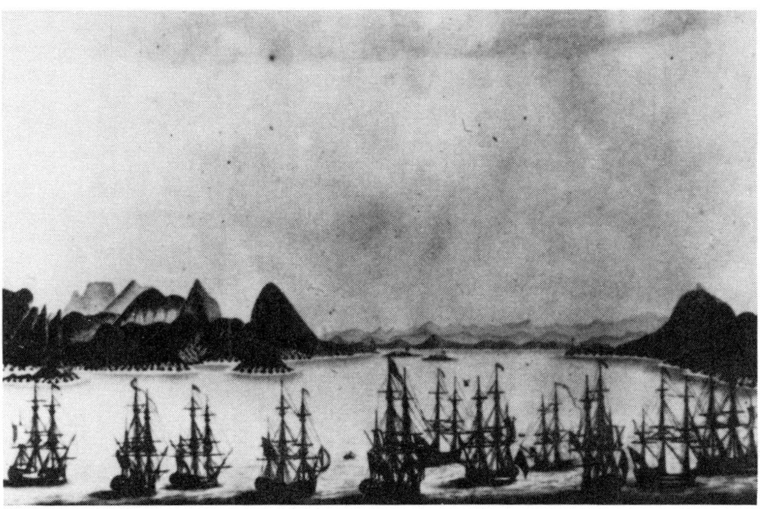

***Figure 2.3: The eleven vessels of the First Fleet waiting to enter the harbour of Rio de Janeiro. Painted by the artist George Raper, this is the only painting made of the whole Fleet. Reproduced by kind permission of the British Museum (Natural History).***

Intellectual literature also blossomed during the 18th Century in the years immediately preceding the First Fleet. Hume's *Treatise on Human Nature,* Bourke's *Thoughts on the Present Discontents*, Gibbon's *Decline and Fall* and Adam Smith's *The Wealth of Nations* were all published during this time. In 1766 Goldsmith published a book the title of which has passed into Australian surgical folklore – *The Vicar of Wakefield.*

However Dorothy George in her book *London life in the 18th Century*[3] paints a very different picture. Although she suggests that living conditions may have improved during the course of the 18th Century they remained, for those who were poverty stricken, essentially appalling. According to George it would hardly be possible to exaggerate the disaster of the cumulative effect of the orgy of spirit drinking between 1720 and 1751. The Rev. James Townley said it more succinctly:

*Gin, cursed fiend with fury fraught*
*Makes human race a prey*
*It enters by a deadly draft*
*And steals our life away.*[4]

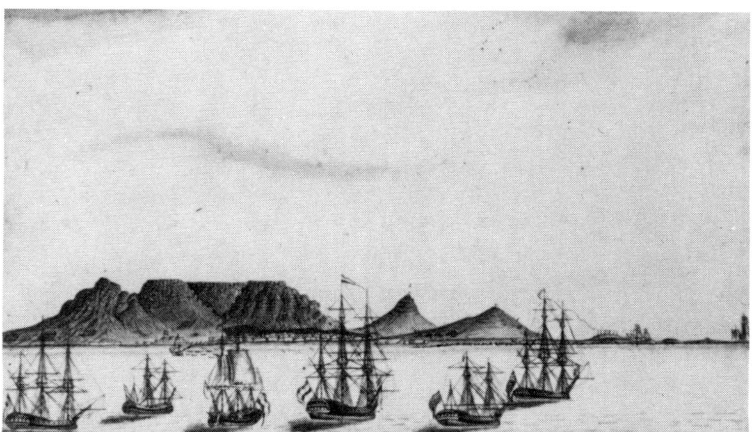

***Figure 2.4: The First Fleet in Table Bay, Cape of Good Hope. The Surgeon-General, John White, climbed to the top of Table Mountain (left of centre) during this visit to Cape Town. From a water-colour by George Raper. Reproduced by kind permission of the British Museum (Natural History).***

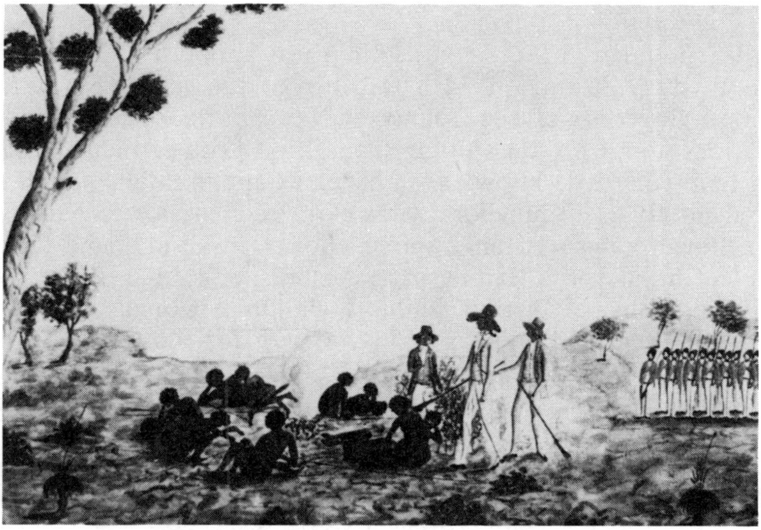

***Figure 2.5: Surgeon General John White (tallest figure, right of centre) visiting Aborigines at Port Jackson. From a water-colour 1788, artist unknown. Reproduced by kind permission of the British Museum (Natural History).***

Not surprisingly such an environment produced criminals. In 1717 a system for transporting convicts to the North American colonies had commenced to deter "wicked and evil disposed persons from committing crimes and to provide labour for the colonies".[5] By 1775 opposition to convicts in America became confounded with opposition to political oppression and convicts were not permitted to land. On 1st April, 1776 Lord North told the House of Commons that –

> *... transportation had been found to be attended with various inconveniences, that in particular it had deprived the Kingdom of many subjects whose labour might be useful to the community and who, indeed, by proper care and attention might be reclaimed from their evil courses. To retain the value of their labour and assist in their reclamation the Government had decided to institute prison hulks.*[6]

In due course however the hulk system also failed. The British Government reinstituted transportation and King George III thought that Botany Bay was "a place likely to answer the purpose".[7]

On 3rd September, 1786 Arthur Phillip was appointed Commodore of the First Fleet and on 12th October of the same year he was appointed Governor of the Colony of New South Wales. Some had reservations about his appointment, the First Lord of the Admiralty saying that "the little knowledge I have of Captain Phillip would not have led me to select him for a service of this complicated nature."[8] Phillip, however, proved an inspired choice. In all planning for the First Fleet he played a leading part. According to Allan Frost in his recent biography of Arthur Phillip,[9] Phillip personally chose his officers and men; and he showed his concern for those in his charge and for the future of the colony by his zealous attention to the needs of the ships and the surgeons, and of the crews, marines and convicts.

On 16th October, 1786 Evan Nepean the Under Secretary of the Home Office, received a letter from Admiral Sir Andrew Snape Hamond recommenending Mr John White as Surgeon General to the First Fleet and to the Colony of New South Wales.

> *Dear Sir, Mr White, the surgeon of the 'Irresistible' is a candidate for Botany Bay. He is a young man of much credit in his profession and of that sort of disposition and temper that render him a very proper person for such an establishment. If no surgeon is yet appointed, and you will do me the favour to recommend him to Lord Sydney, I shall think myself much obliged to you and shall consider myself bound to Government for his good behaviour, I am dear sir your most obedient humble servant, A.S. Hamond.*[10]

The Chief Surgeon was to receive ten shillings per day thereby earning 182 pounds 10 shillings *per annum.* Initially he was to have two assistant surgeons at the cost of five shillings a day. However in due course three assistants were appointed. Dennis Considen as First Assistant, Thomas Arndell as Second Assistant and William Balmain as Third Assistant. There were however ten surgeons or assistant surgeons altogether on the First Fleet.*

The Fleet was made up of eleven ships. The HMS *Sirius* was the flag ship and one of two naval vessels in the Fleet, the other being the HMS *Supply.* The HMS *Sirius* carried Surgeon George Worgan and Surgeon's Mate Thomas Jamison. HMS *Supply* carried Surgeon Callam. The remaining nine ships in the Fleet were chartered from private companies, six being chartered for the transport of convicts and three to act as store ships. All six convict transports carried a surgeon.

*The status of Lowes, Surgeon's Mate of *Sirius*, remains to be clarified (*see page 34*).

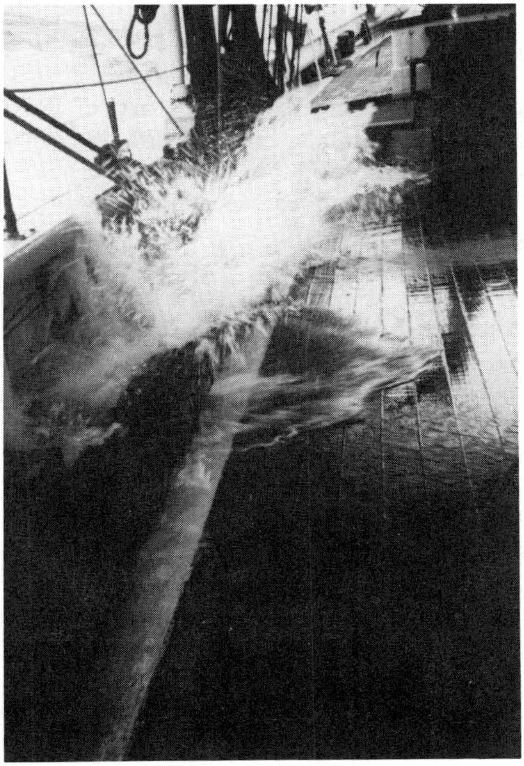

*Figure 2.6:*

***The force of the Sea. Waves aboard the Soren Larsen, Flagship of the First Fleet Reenactment Fleet.***

***Photo by Dr Rob Simpson, 1987.***

There was no surgeon on any of the transport ships. On board *Charlotte* travelled Surgeon General John White. Of his assistants, Dennis Considen was on *Scarborough*, Thomas Arndell on *Friendship* and William Balmain on *Alexander. Lady Penrhyn* carried a volunteer surgeon, John Turnpenny Altree who unfortunately proved unequal to the task. He was replaced by Surgeon Bowes Smyth who was carried as part of the normal crew of the *Lady Penrhyn*. The remaining convict transport, *The Prince of Wales,* was initially without a surgeon. However it transpired that on board *Scarborough* was a convict, John Irving, a surgeon who had unfortunately been convicted of grand larceny. He was transferred to *The Prince of Wales* and performed very creditably as its surgeon. He became the first convict to be emancipated in the Colony of New South Wales.

Much of our knowledge of the events of the First Fleet comes from the journal of John White. He published this work in 1790 in

London under the title of *A Journal of a Voyage to New South Wales*. It became an immediate best seller partly because of its insights into the natural history of Australia. It contains sixty-five plates of "animals, birds, lizards, serpents, curious cones of trees and other natural productions."[11]

It now appears certain that John White was born in Ireland rather than Worthing in Sussex as had previously been supposed, probably either in late 1756 or early 1757. He was born in Drumaran, in County Fermanagh, the son of John and Jane White. He was educated at Royal School, Enniskillen in the same county. In 1778 he entered the navy as Third Surgeon's Mate on HMS *Wasp*. He received his promotion to Surgeon in 1780 by which time he would have been in his early twenties. His Diploma of the Company of Surgeons was issued on 2nd August, 1781. During these years he saw service in the West Indies, where he was stationed for three years, and in India. In 1786 White became Surgeon of HMS *Irresistible* commanded by Captain Sir Andrew Snape Hamond and it was through this association four months later that he was appointed Surgeon General to the First Fleet.

The genesis of John White's training can perhaps be traced back to the court of King Henry VIII. In 1540 the King presented a charter to the Guild of Barber-Surgeons, formed by uniting the previously existing Company of Barbers and the Fellowship of Surgeons. This company survived for two hundred and five years finally collapsing as a result of internecine quarrels. By John White's time the companies had separated, Parliament dissolving the ancient union between barbers and surgeons by an Act dated 25th June, 1745. This Act created the Company of Surgeons. This in turn became the Royal College of Surgeons of London in 1800 and then the Royal College of Surgeons of England in 1848.

During the 18th century the sharp distinction which had existed between physicians and surgeons remained, the physician being a gentleman bound by an ethical code which did not even permit him to sue a defaulting patient for his legitimate fees, whereas the surgeon and the apothecary were regarded as craftsmen. According to Lloyd and Coulter in *Medicine and the Navy*[12] a naval surgeon in the 18th Century was defined as one who was obliged to act in the three capacities of physician, surgeon and apothecary on board a ship of war. His status, though not as transient and embarrassed as in the previous century, was still that of a craftsman. Perhaps his nearest equivalent was the chaplain. Since the conditions under which such men served were so bad, one could hardly blame the surgeon at Forton Prison, for example, for resigning his position in 1797 on the grounds that it was "neither profitable, comfortable nor respectable."[13]

Before a naval surgeon could be appointed to a ship he had to be examined by the Court of Examiners of the Company of Surgeons. It was said however that the examination for second or third surgeon's mates was particularly perfunctory, especially during war. Before being examined by the Surgeons Company, the majority of sea surgeons had taken medical degrees at Glasgow, Edinburgh or Aberdeen. This would not appear to have been the case for our John White. John White's tombstone, situated in St Mary's Church, Broadwater in Worthing, Sussex, shows he had an MD. Evidence now suggests that he received this degree from St Andrews in 1796, after he returned to England.

John White brought with him when he returned from the colony his illegitimate son born to Rachael Turner, a convict of the Second Fleet. In England he married and had a further three children, a son and two daughters. He worked in a variety of naval jobs and was honoured upon retirement with superannuation rather than the usual half pay. He died in 1832 aged seventy-five years and left an estate of £12,000.

Neither the medicine nor the surgery of the 18th Century were particularly sophisticated sciences. Doctors inspected and felt, they did not percuss or auscultate. To make a diagnosis they relied on the sweat, on the temperature of the skin to touch (no clinical thermometer being as yet available), on the presence, sight and severity of pain, and on the appearance of tne excreta. For therapy they relied on empiricals. According to Australian physician and historian Dr John Cobley[14] it would appear that when it came to treatment,

> *...the physicians of the 18th century cashed in on the natural tendency of the human body to recover and their own credulity. In spite of recent advances in physiology, repeated blood letting, purgation, the induction of vomiting, artificial sweating and deliberate restriction of food and water remained the stock in trade of the physician.*

As Voltaire has said the doctor's role was to amuse the patient while nature did the healing.

On the other hand surgical techniques were a function of the time and digital dexterity: the absence of a proper anaesthetic transferred the whole burden of the operative procedure to human fortitude. Surgically speaking however the 18th century was pivotal. Surgery, anatomy and biology swept ahead in the hands of John Hunter; born in 1728 and dying in 1793 he would have read the first reports back from Sydney Cove. Hunter's surgical contributions were immense. One of his surgical colleagues on the occasion of Hunter's death is quoted as saying "he alone made us gentlemen".[15] Arriving in London from Scotland in 1748 he joined his brother William, the most eminent obstetrician of the day. He learned surgery under Cheselden and Pott. His pupils included Jenner, Abernethy Astley Cooper and Cline. Examination of the works of Hunter, Cheselden and Pott shows the general state of surgery in the 18th Century, and gives us insight into the surgery that John White would have practised. Surgery had, with few exceptions, to remain confined more or less to the surface of the body until the advent of

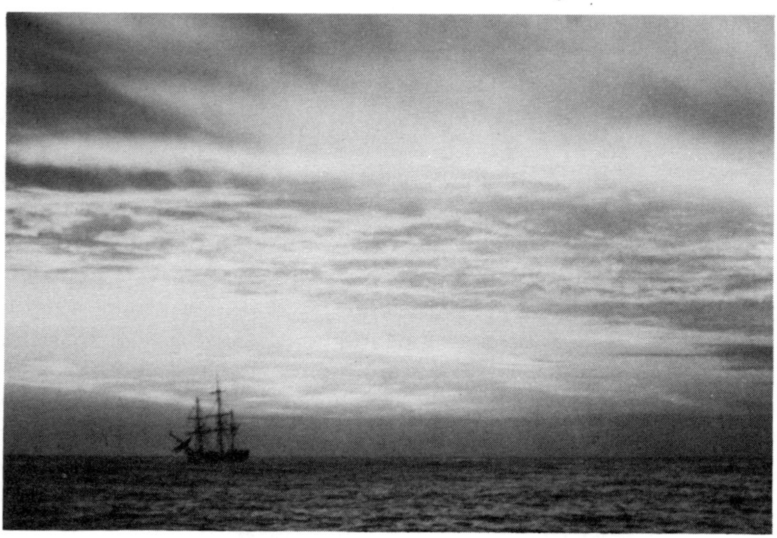

*Figure 2.7: "Like a painted ship on a painted ocean." HMAV Bounty at sunset in the Indian Ocean. Photo, 1987 on the First Fleet Reenactment Voyage (1987-88) by the Fleet Surgeon, Dr Rob Simpson.*

anaesthesia in the mid 19th Century. This is perhaps no more graphically demonstrated than in the writings of ship surgeon John Woodall in 1639.

> *The amputation once resolved upon and all things ready for the work let the surgeon with all his assistants and friends not forget for the beginning of the work heartily to call upon God for a blessing upon their endeavours, and let the patient have notice given him that he may also take time to prepare himself with true resolution of soul and body to undergo the work, as being never performed without danger of death, which done, then let the surgeon prepare also with his helpers namely at least five persons beside himself.*[16]

Such would have been the education of John White, who led the surgeons of the First Fleet.

I would argue, as has done my distinguished colleague Dr John Cobley,[17] that the performance of the surgeons of the First Fleet made a substantial difference to the outcome. The First Fleet carried 1350 people, some 759 of whom were convicts, on a voyage of eight months and one week across 15,000 miles of some of the most isolated parts of our globe. That they did so with the loss of only 48 lives is a tribute both to Arthur Phillip and to his surgeons. The Second Fleet by comparison carrying 1,000 convicts lost 267 during the voyage. John White's attitude to death is perhaps best summarised in a quote from his Journal.

> *So small is our number, and so necessary is every individual who composes it, for one purpose or another, that the loss of even a single man may be truly considered as an irreparable disadvantage.*[18]

This First Fleet mortality rate of only 3.6% is made even more startling by the knowledge that one of the female convicts who died was aged 82 and had been suffering the dropsy for some time. Even more important is the fact that 17 of the convicts who died did so before the Fleet left England!

The reason John White was so successful lay in no small part to the fact that he practised preventive medicine, and perhaps even more remarkably he concentrated his attention on the convicts. Evidence of the high importance he put on adequate clothing, food, fresh air, dryness and cleanliness can clearly be found in his Journal. On the day of his arrival at the Fleet John White said in his Journal:

> *... I would immediately give orders for such as were in want of clothing, to be supplied with what was needful; power delegated to me by Captain Phillip, together with the liberty of giving such other directions as I thought would tend to the recovery or preservation of their health. And, further, as they had been nearly four months on board and during that time had been kept upon salt provisions, I would endeavour to get fresh for them while in port. ... I then pointed out to Lieutenant Johnson, Commanding Officer of the Marines on board, and to the Master of the ship, the necessity there was of admitting the convicts upon the deck, one half at a time, during the course of the day, in order that they might breathe a purer air, as nothing would conduce more to the preservation of their health. To this these gentlemen readily assent; adding that they had no objection to the whole number coming upon deck at once, if I thought it necessary, as they were not apprehensive of any danger from the indulgence.*[19]

Very early in his Journal White mentions the name of Dr Lind, "physician to the Royal Hospital at Haslar, a gentleman as eminently distinguished for his professional abilities as his other amiable qualities."[20] Although some have thought to the contrary, the Dr Lind to whom he refers is almost certainly the son of the great James Lind. James Lind resigned his post at Haslar in 1783 and was succeeded by his son John. James Lind has been called both the father of nautical medicine and the father of preventive medicine. In a dissertation on Fevers and Infection written in 1761 he says "the number of seamen in time of war who die by shipwreck, capture, famine, fire or sword are but inconsiderable in respect of such as are destroyed by the ships' diseases and by the usual maladies of intemperate climates."[21]

Lind's most famous work is his *Treatise on the Scurvy*. In this book he describes the first controlled clinical trial. He divided twelve sufferers of scurvy into six groups of two and treated each group with a product thought to cure scurvy. He found that the two treated with oranges and lemons were cured. The two treated with cider were improved whereas the remaining four groups had worsened during the course of the study. Most unfortunately and no doubt at the cost of many lives the Admiralty took another 42 years to accept Lind's findings. Expressing the frustration that may now be felt by many of his professional successors, Lind said "The province has been mine to deliver precepts; the power is in others to execute."[22]

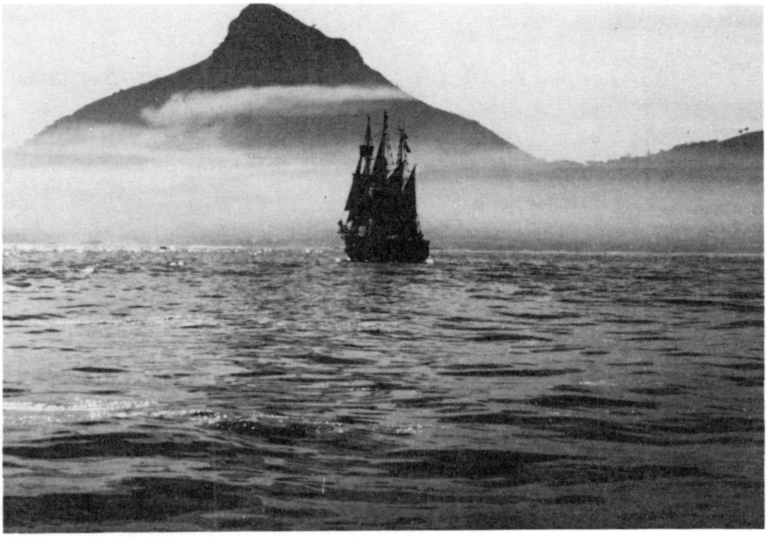

***Figure 2.8:* Our Svanen, Canadian barquentine, approaching the Lion's Head, Cape of Good Hope, on the First Fleet Reenactment Voyage 1987-88.**
***Photo by Dr Rob Simpson, Fleet Surgeon, 1987.***

Neither Arthur Phillip nor John White required any convincing. The First Fleet made stops at Tenerife, Rio de Janeiro and Cape Town and in each place took the opportunity to dine on fresh fruit, vegetables and meat during their time in port and to stock up with such products for the next leg of the voyage.

Although it is difficult to form a complete picture of John White, there is no doubt that he was an adventurer on a major scale and a competent medical practitioner. That he concentrated on preventive measures is clear but his ability as a practitioner is also evident.

His Journal dated 15th May, 1787 only two days after their departure from Motherbank reports –

> *An accident of a singular nature happened today. Corporal Baker of the marines, on laying a loaded musquet* [sic] *down, which he had just taken out of the arms chest was wounded by it in the inner ankle of the right foot. The bones, after being a good deal shattered, turned the ball, which, taking another direction, had still force enough left to go through a harness-cask full of beef at*

> *some distance and to kill two geese which were on the other side of it. The corporal, being a young man, and in good habit of body I had the pleasure, contrary to the general expectation, of seeing him return to his duty in three months, and with the perfect use of the wounded joint.*[23]

In Tenerife John White established a pattern which he was to continue in Rio de Janeiro and Cape Town in that his observations of life in general included a detailed commentary on women of the cities he visited.

> *The women wear veils; those worn by the lower ranks are of black stuff, those of the higher, black silk; and such among the latter as have any claim to beauty, are far from being overcareful in concealing their faces by them ... some of the women are so abandoned and shameless that it would be doing an injustice to the prostitutes met with in the streets of London to say they are like them.*[24]

During the stay of the Fleet in Tenerife John White also comments on:

> *... a sporadic disease which had appeared among the marines and convicts. On its first appearance it resembled the mumps, or swelling of the chaps; and as that distemper sometimes terminates in a translation of the inflammation to the testicles, and so this complaint (after the swelling and induration had subsided) never in one instance failed to fix on those parts; and that in so very obstinant a manner as not to give way to the treatment generally found effectual in similar inflammations. As soon as we got to sea, the motion of the ship acted on all those who were affected to the number of seventeen, in a most surprising and extraordninary manner. Indeed it was so sudden that it was like a placebo. I could never account, with any satisfaction to myself, for the origin of this uncommon disease, though much acquainted with those incident to seamen; nor did I ever see or hear of any that resembled it. The most steady and prudent of the marines, even those who had their wives on board, were equally affected with those who led irregular lives.*[25]

The passage of the First Fleet from Tenerife to Rio de Janeiro was essentially uneventful. Trade-wind sailing dictates that square-rigged sailing ships cross to the western side of the Atlantic hence making a stop at Rio de Janeiro quite logical. During the stop at Rio de Janeiro John White visited a large public hospital attended by Mr Il de Fonso, Surgeon General to the army. His Journal takes up the story:

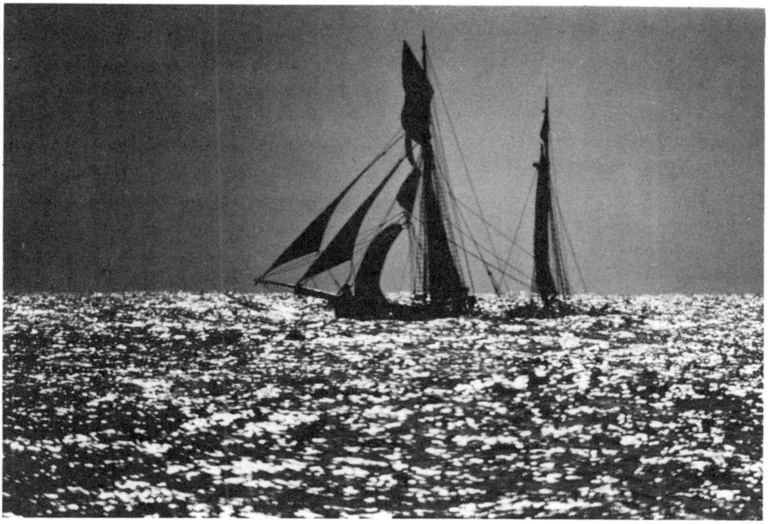

***Figure 2.9: The 100 year old Norwegian galeas Anna Kristina in the Indian Ocean, 1987, during the First Fleet Reenactment Voyage.***
***Photo by Dr Rob Simpson, Fleet Surgeon.***

*While we remained here I prevailed on the surgeon who was about to amputate a limb to allow me to take it off according to Allenson's method. During the operation I could plainly see that he and his pupils did not seem much pleased with it, and he afterwards told me it was impossible it would ever answer. A very short space of time, however, made them of a different opinion; and in eighteen days after, when we sailed, I had the satisfaction to leave the patient with his stump nearly cicatrized, to the no small joy of the surgeon, who said that if the man had died he should have been heavily censured for making him the subject of experiments ... The circumstances of a man's leg being cut off, and almost healed in as many days as it generally takes weeks, soon became known, and added very much to the estimation in which the people of this place held English surgeons. Whenever I visited the hospital afterwards, the objects of pity with which it was filled used to crowd around me in such a manner, and in such numbers, for my advice, that I found it difficult to get from them. And they would now readily have submitted to any operation I should have proposed, but, as I saw the surgeon did not much approve of my interference, I gave up all ideas of it.*[26]

The voyage across the South Atlantic from Rio de Janeiro to Cape Town again is a classic square-rigged sailing ship route, ships swinging down into the Roaring Forties to pick up the westerly winds. During this leg of the voyage the Fleet lost William Brown. In the words of John White –

> *... a very well behaved convict, in bringing some clothing from the bowsprit end, where he had hung them to dry, fell overboard. As soon as the alarm was given of a man being overboard, the ship was instantly hoved to and a boat hoisted out, but to no purpose.*[27]

The First Fleet sighted Table Mountain on 13th October, 1787. White, commenting on the soldiers of the Cape noted that –

> *I could not help observing many of them had either got intoxicated that morning or were not recovered from their overnight's debauch; notwithstanding which they marched to the field and went through their evolutions with a steadiness and regularity that was really astonishing, considering the state they were in: but it is said, and I believe with some truth, that a Dutchman when half drunk is more capable of performing every kind of business than if he were perfectly sober.*[28]

White also noted that:

> *The habits and customs of the women of this place are extremely contrasted with those of the inhabitants of Rio de Janeiro. Among the latter a great deal of reserve and modesty is apparent between the sexes in public. Those who are disposed to say tender and civil things to a lady must do it by stealth, or breathe their soft sighs through the lattice work of a window, or the grates of a convent. But at the Cape, if you wish to be a favourite with the fair, as the custom is, you must in your own defence, if I may use the expression, grapple the lady, and paw her in a manner that does not partake in the least of tenderness.*[29]

The Fleet was ready to leave Cape Town on 11th November but the wind was foul and it was not until 13th that it weighed. While in Cape Town White again revealed his adventurous spirit by climbing to the top of Table Mountain. A strenuous and difficult climb, it was made the more so in White's case by lack of drinking water along the way.

The Fleet was smitten with an epidemic of dysentery during this final leg. The disease broke out on 17th November and according to White –

> *... prevailed with violence and obstinancy until about Christmas when it was got under control by an unremitting attention to cleanliness, and every other method proper and essential to the removal and prevention of contagion. It give me pleasure to add that we only lost one person by this disease, violent and dangerous as it was.*[30]

The passage from Cape Town to Botany Bay and subsequently Port Jackson was certainly the longest, coldest, roughest and wettest of the voyage. John White holds indeed a proud place in the history of medicine in Australia.

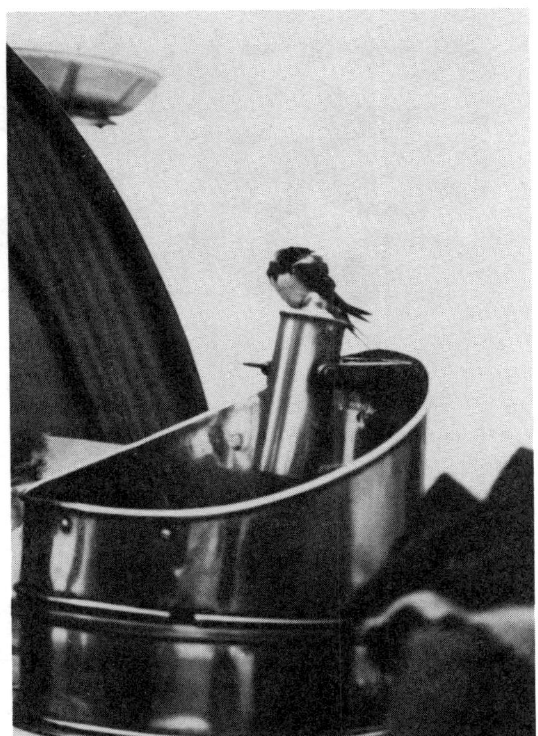

***Figure 2.10:***

***A tired visitor alights on the binnacle of the Soren Larsen, at sea.***

***The Flagship of the First Fleet Reenactment Fleet, and the home also of the author Dr Rob Simpson, Fleet Surgeon.***

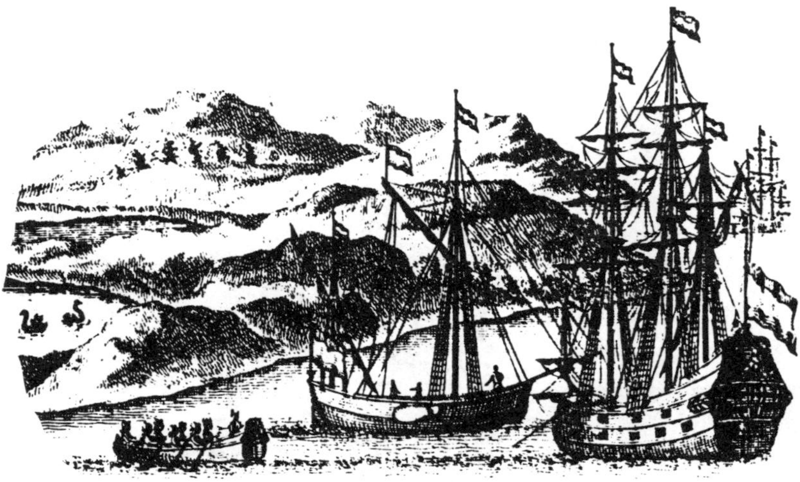

# PIONEER MEDICINE IN AUSTRALIA

# 3

## FIRST FLEET SURGEONS
### A Band of Brothers Disparate

**John Pearn**

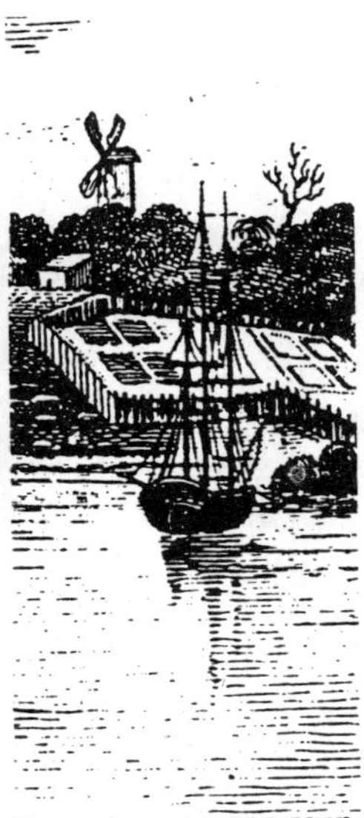

*VARIETY* and diversity make for vigour. An historical perspective of the foundation of medicine in Australia needs look at the range of different attributes brought to these shores by the First Fleet Surgeons.

Geneticists of Darwinian persuasion know that variation in founder stock leads to later survival, richness and vigour; and that uniformity may lead to vulnerability and extinction in later generations. Patients, as consumers, benefit from a choice of practitioners who manifest different attributes, both in personality and in the range of the professional skills they practise. After two hundred years of medicine in Australia, no effort is spared to impose uniformity on the selection of those who would aspire to study medicine; and the training and standards of today's Medical Schools lead to a great uniformity not only in technical skills, but in professional outlook and style.

The two Colonies at Sydney and at Norfolk Island in 1788 comprised, in one sense, two closed communities in which a group of doctors practised. A study of their differences in background, training, style and personalities is revealing in terms of policy about the training of medical graduates today. Do variety and differences in a society's doctors enrich and serve, collectively, that society better? Alternatively, is the uncertainty and disruption that professional disparity brings, something which should be reduced by the imposition of more uniform codes of selection? The First Fleet Surgeons and the two microsocieties in which they worked offer some answers to this question.

Biographies of the majority of the First Fleet Surgeons have not yet been written. The Bicentenary vigour, indeed passion, with which family histories have been compiled has done something to redress this regrettable omission in Australian medical history. Two recent biographies of Surgeon Thomas Arndell[1,2] have revealed much of the personal life of at least one of the First Fleet Surgeons.

There were nine surgeons appointed to the eleven ships of the First Fleet (*Table 1*). To these must be added the names of two further medical men. The prisoner John Irving – the first of some sixteen doctors who were transported to Australia as convicts[3] – was appointed as Assistant Surgeon on the *Lady Penrhyn* when the Fleet was eighteen days "out of Portsmouth". The eleventh "medical man of the First Fleet"[4] was Lowes,* whose elevation to surgical respectability two hundred years later still awaits even the discovery of his Christian name.

The First Fleet Surgeons could not have been more varied. Their personalities varied from that of the hopeless Altree, to the dominant Jamison; from those who sought out a life in the rigid and in some ways protected service existence of the Navy,[5-12] to those who by contrast (such as Bowes Smyth) left maritime service for later independence. Some, such as Worgan[12] who was both a Naval Surgeon and a pianist, gave much service to the Navy, but retired early to an independent and isolated life of farming in Cornwall.

No band of medical brothers could have been more varied, and in a sense their grouping in history as the founders of medicine in the new Colony is an artificiality. The perspective of two hundred

*The status of Lowes remains uncertain. He was not listed in the First Fleet manifests, and appears first in Tench's ***Complete Account*** as Surgeon's Mate of the ***Sirius*** in June 1789. Some of ***Sirius*** complement were not listed, and a number of the marines in particular are not formally listed. In addition, certain crew who left for Norfolk Island also have been omitted from several of the primary sources used to compile the First Fleet muster rolls. It is probable that Lowes was on the 1787-88 voyage, but he may have joined the ***Sirius*** complement after January 1788. The ***Sirius*** left Sydney on 2 Oct 1788, on a desperate trip (in fact a circumnavigation of the globe in southern latitudes, sailing east) to reprovision the Convict colony. She called at Cape Town (February 1789); it is possible Lowes joined ***Sirius*** there, or was transferred from another Royal Navy ship.

years sees them linked by their arrival together at Sydney Cove; yet, viewed as individuals it is their differences rather than any similarities that gave a very real vigour to the medicine of Sydney and Norfolk Island in 1788.

Modern military campaigns (those of the First and Second World Wars, and the Vietnam Campaign as examples) have seen Australia's medical support supplied by a mixture of career Service medical officers, and volunteers who have joined campaigns temporarily to aid the wounded and sick. Such was the case also in 1787 when several surgeons 'joined up' for the specific 'First Fleet Campaign'. Like their successors in later times, their motives varied enormously. Surgeon Thomas Arndell, originally a London apothecary,[2] had fled his family once already as Surgeon's Mate on

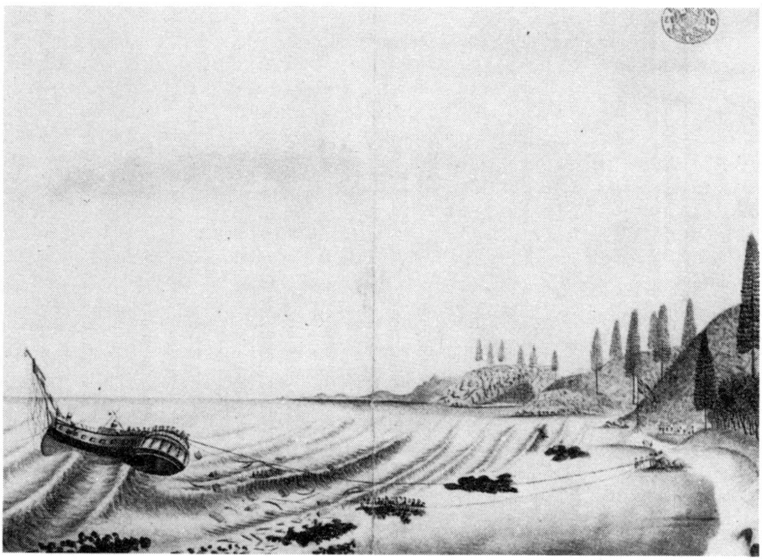

***Figure 3.1:* Disasters of various kinds affected the infant colony. This contemporary water-colour painting shows the wreck of the Flagship, HMS Sirius, at Norfolk Island in 1790. The Sydney Cove colony was facing potential starvation, and Phillip had transferred convicts and Surgeon Irving to Norfolk Island on this voyage. 'A View of the west side of Norfolk Island and the manner in which the crew and provisions were saved out of His Majesty's Ship the Sirius.' By kind permission, and with acknowledgement to the British Museum (Natural History)***

| SHIP | SIZE | COMPLEMENT | SURGEONS | APPOINTMENT IN N.S.W. 1788 | BIOGRAPHICAL NOTE |
|---|---|---|---|---|---|
| HMS SIRIUS | Flagship 540 tons (20 guns) | 128 marines; seamen | George Bouchier Worgan | Surgeon | b. 1757, London d. 1838, Liskeard (Cornwall) aged 80 years. |
| 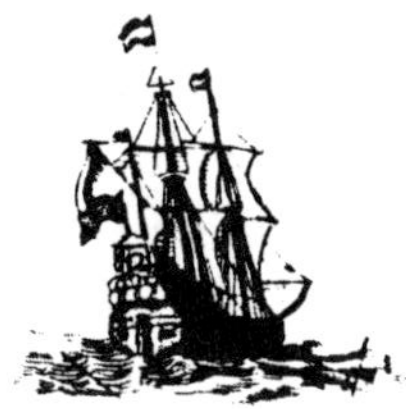 | | | Thomas Jamison | Surgeon's Mate | b. 1745, Egremont (Lake District). d. 1811, London, aged 65 years. |
| | | | Lowes | Acted as Assistant Surgeon's Mate; or appointed in Sydney after landing | Details unknown. |
| ALEXANDER | Transport 450 tons | 240 marines; seamen, convicts | William Balmain | Assistant Surgeon | b. 1762, Rhynd (Scotland). d. 1803, London aged 41 years. |
| SCARBOROUGH | Transport 450 tons | 241 marines; seamen, male convicts | Dennis Considen | First Assistant Surgeon | b. –, Ireland. d. 1815, United Kingdom |
| CHARLOTTE | Transport 340 tons | 131 marines; seamen, convicts | John White | Surgeon-General | b. c. 1756 – probably Ireland. d. 1832 Worthing (W.Sussex) aged 75 years. |

| | | | | | |
|---|---|---|---|---|---|
| **LADY PENRHYN** | Transport<br>335 tons | 171<br>Including 109<br>women & children | Arthur Bowes<br>Smyth | Surgeon | b. 1750, Tolleshurst D'arcy (Suffolk); d. 1790, England (probably Suffolk). |
| 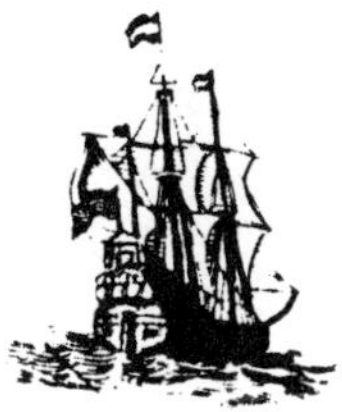 | | | John Turnpenny<br>Altree | Assistant Surgeon | Details unknown. |
| | | | John Irving | A convict, transported for larceny. Acted as Surgeon's Assistant | b. –. Convicted at Lincoln Assizes, March 1784.<br>d. 1795, Parramatta, NSW. |
| **FRIENDSHIP** | Transport<br>275 tons | 133<br>(including 98 male and female convicts and three children) | Thomas Arndell | Second Assistant<br>Surgeon | b. 1753 (son of Anthony and Elizabeth Arndell; born at the Village of Kingston (Herefordshire). d. 1821, Caddie Park, near Windsor NSW |
| **HMS SUPPLY**<br>(Brig) | Armed Tender<br>170 tons | 25<br>(including 14 seamen, 1 convict and 2 marines) | James Callam | Surgeon | Details unknown. |

**TABLE 1:** *First Fleet Ships, which carried doctors, with their listed Surgeons aboard. Appointments, and biographical notes.*

a year's service with the East India Company. Arndell may have joined to escape scandal, or perhaps to defuse a situation where both his wife and his mistress each delivered a daughter to him within four months of each other (in 1781), in two hospitals in London three hundred metres apart.[13]

For the career Naval Surgeons (White, Jamison, Worgan and Callam) a posting to the limits of the known world was part of that fatalistic duty borne by so many of their predecessors and successors in the medical services of many nations. By contrast, one of the surgeons, John Irving[3,4,14] was a convict. It is now known that he was the only medical convict on the First Fleet manifest. Recent research[3] has revealed that he was the first of sixteen doctors who were transported before the Transportation System finally ceased (in Western Australia) in 1868.[15]

Formal biographies, and even the most extensive research after two hundred years can never fully document all the subtleties of the personalities of the First Fleet Surgeons. It is known that their technical skills were reasonably competent; it is their personalities, however, that would have brought either comfort and confidence, or hurt and a feeling of helplessness, to their patients. As clinicians, the First Fleet Surgeons administered to villians and vice-regal patients alike. Their personalities range from that of dominant, confident men, who were respected not only for their medical skills but for their organisational abilities, to others who seem to have been inadequate. Soon after the Fleet had put to sea, Surgeon Altree proved incapable of continuing in his surgeon's role. He had been a medical invalid "very ill for some time past ..."[16] even before the Fleet had sailed from Portsmouth. Whether physical illness was his only problem is conjectural, but it is most likely that Altree lost his self-confidence and became a psychiatric casualty. The Commandant, Phillip, was obviously worried as only the Commander of expeditions to remote parts can be when one of their medical officers loses the confidence of his fellows. Surgeon-General White discussed the problem with Phillip, and it was decided to relieve Altree of his responsibilities. White sought out Surgeon Bowes Smyth and asked him to assume Altree's responsibilities on the *Lady Penrhyn*, and to "carry the presence of Altree as best he could". Bowes Smyth subsequently described the incident:

**SURGEON – JOHN WHITE**

CAREER Entered R.N. 1778 as Third Surgeon's Mate. Saw service in the West Indies and India. Appointed Principal Surgeon 1786. Served at Sydney Cove 1788-1794. Continued Naval Service at sea, and at Sheerness and at Chatham (Kent) 1795-1820.

TIME IN AUSTRALIA

1788-1794; at Sydney, as Principal Surgeon (7 years)

EXPLORATIONS

Many collecting and scientific expeditions in the Sydney hinterland and coast.

SCIENTIFIC CONTRIBUTIONS

A keen naturalist. White's *Journal* is a major scientific record of the early Colony.

PATRONYMIC LEGACY

White's Bay, Sydney.

LAND HOLDINGS IN NEW SOUTH WALES

130 acres at Leichhardt, and at White's Bay.

NOTES As Principal Surgeon in New South Wales in 1788, White received an annual salary of 10 shillings per day, with rations and accommodation. He fought a duel with Surgeon William Balmain on August 12th, 1788. He disliked the Colony, but was an able medical administrator.

**TABLE 3.2:** *Biographic details of the First Fleet Surgeons*

## SURGEON – DENNIS CONSIDEN

CAREER — A civilian surgeon, little is known of his life before 1786. First Assistant Surgeon to White 1788-1793. He saw Army Medical Service (Europe) 1794-1800. To the Cape of Good Hope 1805-1808.

TIME IN AUSTRALIA
1788-1791; at Sydney and Norfolk Island. 1791-1793, Sydney. (6 years)

EXPLORATIONS
Numerous collecting expeditions in the Sydney region.

SCIENTIFIC CONTRIBUTIONS
Much collecting and medical experimentation with medicinal plants, all unpublished. 1804, graduated MD, University of Edinburgh with his Thesis "De Tetano".

PATRONYMIC LEGACY
*Eucalyptus considenianа* ("Peppermint", "messmate", or "white mahogany").

NOTES — An enquiring and conscientious personality – "A humane man with an innate desire to do well in his profession".[39] A "Pioneer of pharmaceutical research" in Australia.[40]

**TABLE 3.2:** *Biographic details of the First Fleet Surgeons (contd)*

**SURGEON – THOMAS ARNDELL**

CAREER

The father of 8 children, he left his wife following a family scandal, for a year's service with the East India Company. His service on the *Friendship* appears to be in part escapism from the situation at home. He was placed in charge of the hospital at Parramatta on arrival in Sydney, and enjoyed the confidence of both his medical and administrative colleagues and also the confidence and favour of all the Governors under whom he served. One of only two First Fleet surgeons known to have died in the Colony.

TIME IN AUSTRALIA

1788 – until his death in 1821 (32 years)

EXPLORATIONS

A member of Tench's expedition 1789 which discovered the Nepean River.

SCIENTIFIC CONTRIBUTIONS

Sheep-breeding was his principal concern; he introduced new Spanish strains to sheep to improve the quality of Australian wool.

MAGISTRATE OFFICES

1798 appointed Magistrate by Governor Hunter. Member of the Court which tried the mutineers of the *Barwell*. Replaced as Magistrate 1806; reappointed 1810. Numerous committees and civic duties at Parramatta, and at the Hawkesbury Settlement. He was a Trustee of Nelson Common.

LAND HOLDINGS IN NEW SOUTH WALES

In 1792, was awarded 60 acres of land at Parramatta. 100 extra acres at Dundas in 1798, making 330 in all. By 1806 owned 630 acres. He farmed at *Caddie* at Windsor, which became his family home. By 1807 he owned 750 acres.

NOTES

A man who struck Governor Macquarie for "his loyalty, honesty and exemplary manner in which he brought up his children"[20] of his convict consort (later wife). His gravestone is in St Matthew's Church, Windsor (New South Wales). Of the eleven medical men of the First Fleet, Arndell is the only one with a memorial gravestone in Australia. He served his apprenticeship as an Apothecary, in London, *c.*1767-1775. He passed – "qualified by oral examination"- an examination for Surgeon's Mate set by the Royal College of Surgeons of London, on 6th September 1781.

**TABLE 3.2:** *Biographic details of the First Fleet Surgeons (contd)*

**SURGEON – WILLIAM BALMAIN**

CAREER — Entered Royal Navy aged 18 years as Surgeon's Mate. 1786, appointed Assistant Surgeon to New South Wales. 1796, Principal Surgeon in the Colony until 1801. Died 1803, as a Naval Surgeon in London.

TIME IN AUSTRALIA

1788–1791 Sydney Cove.
1791–1795 Norfolk Island.
1796–1801 Sydney.
(14 years)

PATRONYMIC LEGACY

Suburb of Balmain in Sydney.[38]

MAGISTRATE OFFICES

Vigorous and active Magistrate, from 1791.
Served on orphans' and prisoners' committees.

LAND HOLDINGS IN NEW SOUTH WALES

1,480 acres, by 1802.

NOTES — A farmer's son from Scotland, and a career Naval Surgeon. "Able and intractable", he followed White as Principal Surgeon. A vigorous member of the Port Jackson Settlement, he clashed with the military authorities.
A strong advocate for better medical services.
An active merchant and trader, especially in spirits.
Had a female convict consort, as partner.

**TABLE 3.2**: *Biographic details of the First Fleet Surgeons (contd)*

## SURGEON – GEORGE BOUCHIER WORGAN

CAREER
Entered Royal Navy 1775.
Appointed surgeon's Second Mate 1778. Surgeon 1780.
Joined the *Sirius* in 1786.
Served Port Jackson 1788.
Cape of Good Hope 1788–1789, and at Norfolk Island 1790.
He retired in 1800.

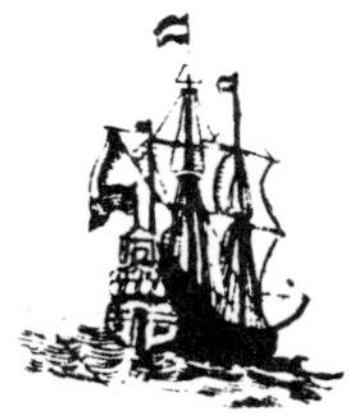

TIME IN AUSTRALIA
1788 Sydney Cove.
1790 Norfolk Island.
(2 years)

EXPLORATIONS
Exploration and survey of South Head of Port Jackson 24 May, 1788. Explored the Hawkesbury River, Broken Bay and Nepean River regions.

PATRONMYIC LEGACY
Worgan River (Upper Nepean River).

NOTES
Born in London, a musician's son. He brought the first and only piano with the First Fleet. He left the Royal Navy aged 43 years as unfit for service, and retired to farming in Cornwall. His *Journal* is a most valuable source of contemporary First Fleet observations.

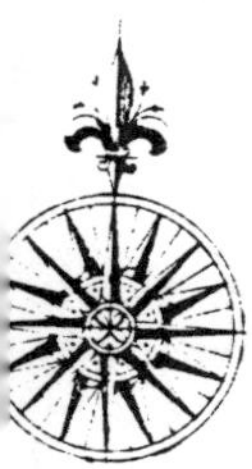

**TABLE 3.2:** *Biographic details of the First Fleet Surgeons (contd)*

**SURGEON – THOMAS JAMISON**

CAREER — University of Dublin MA, 1772. Naval Surgeon R.N. 1777. Appointed Surgeon's Mate on *Sirius* in 1786. Port Jackson 1788. Norfolk Island 1788-1799. England 1800, Sydney 1802-1809.

TIME IN AUSTRALIA
(18 years)

SCIENTIFIC CONTRIBUTIONS
Published in 1804 "General Observations on the smallpox" in the *Sydney Gazette* – the first medical publication printed in Australia.[11]

MAGISTRATE OFFICES
Appointed Magistrate 1802.

LAND HOLDINGS IN NEW SOUTH WALES
2,300 acres by 1807, at the Nepean River, and George's River.

NOTES — A strong man physically, and of resolute personality. He court-martialled two junior surgeons (Mileham and Savage) for neglect of duty in refusing to attend a woman in childbirth. He developed major commercial interests as a merchant and trader in spirits, wheat and pork, and sandalwood. He was often in conflict with authority.

**SURGEON – JAMES CALLAM**

CAREER — Naval Surgeon on the *Supply*.
Sailed for Norfolk Island in February 1788.

TIME IN AUSTRALIA
Unknown, possibly two years.

PATRONYMIC LEGACY
Callam's Bay, at Lord Howe Island.[40]

NOTES — Apparently a career Naval Surgeon. The armed tender *Supply* (12 guns) did not carry convicts, and Surgeon Callam apparently did not figure in the medical aspects of the transportation system, during the long voyage from Portsmouth. No biography of Callam has yet been attempted.

**TABLE 3.2:** *Biographic details of the First Fleet Surgeons (contd)*

**SURGEON – ARTHUR BOWES SMYTH**

CAREER — No known formal training in medicine or surgery. Known to be an experienced village midwife by 1780. On the Admiralty List of "Reserve" Surgeons by 1779. Died within a year of returning to England.

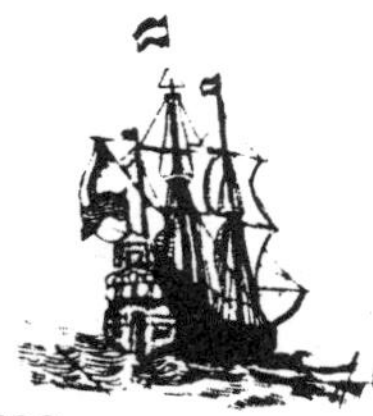

TIME IN AUSTRALIA

14 weeks

EXPLORATIONS

Explored the Botany Bay shoreline January 22, 1788.
Was a member of many local expeditions about the Camp Cove site, in the first weeks of the Colony.

SCIENTIFIC CONTRIBUTIONS

Keen naturalist, the first European to sketch and record the emu, and goanna.
First description of the carpet snake (*Python* sp).
He made some anthropological observations.

NOTES — The son of an Overseer of the Poor,[33] in the Village of Tolleshunt D'Arcy in Suffolk. Indirect evidence suggests that Arthur Bowes Smyth was well liked by the villagers to whom he was a surgeon and midwife. His writings portray him as a conservative honourable man with a sense of discipline, order and duty.

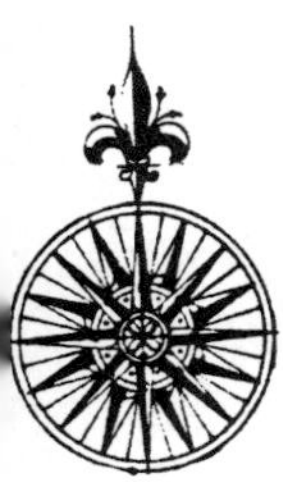

**TABLE 3.2**: *Biographic details of the First Fleet Surgeons (contd)*

## SURGEON – JOHN TURNPENNY ALTREE

CAREER

Fragmentary accounts only. He reported for duty on the *Lady Penrhyn* on 7 May 1787 but was a medical invalid even before the voyage started. He was appointed as a surgeon to convicts, but was relieved of this duty by the Surgeon General (White) 18 days after the Fleet sailed. He served as an assistant to Jamison at Norfolk Island February 1788 to February 1791, returning to England in May 1791.

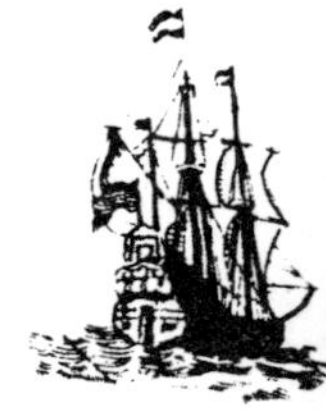

TIME IN AUSTRALIA

Served essentially at Norfolk Island.
(3 years, with several weeks only at Port Jackson)

EXPLORATIONS

Took part in an oystering "expedition" in the southern part of Botany Bay January 23, 1788.

NOTES

Knowledge about Surgeon Altree comes almost completely from Bowes Smyth's Journal.[17] The *Lady Penhryn* initially had a complement of two surgeons – Bowes Smyth "Surgeon to the Ship's Company", and Surgeon Altree "Surgeon to the Convicts". By December 1787 (in the first weeks of the voyage) Altree was unable to carry on, possibly because of illness. He narrowly escaped being washed overboard on 1 January 1788.[43]

**TABLE 3.2:** *Biographic details of the First Fleet Surgeons (contd)*

**SURGEON – JOHN IRVING**

CAREER — Surgical training unknown. Convicted at the Lincoln Assizes, for stealing a gold cup at Grantham, he escaped the death penalty and was transported for seven years. He was the first of the surgeon convicts, of whom 16 are known.[3] He served on the First Fleet voyage on the *Lady Penrhyn*. He was the first convict emancipated in Australia (1790). He served at Norfolk Island (1790-1791) and at Parramatta.

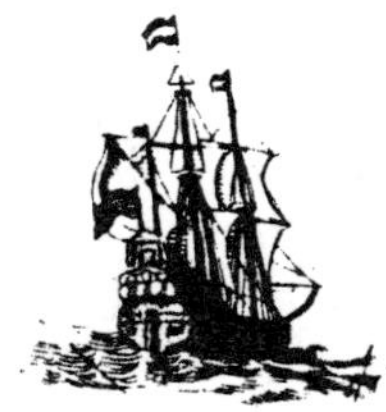

TIME IN AUSTRALIA
1788 – until his death 3 September 1795.
(7½ years)

PATRONYMIC LEGACY
Irving Street, Parramatta.
Buried in an unmarked grave at St John's Cemetery, Parramatta.

LAND HOLDINGS IN NEW SOUTH WALES
1792 – granted 30 acres at Parramatta.

NOTES — A popular surgeon in Sydney and at Norfolk Island.
Several independent reports referred to the respect with which his medical and surgical skills were regarded.

**TABLE 3.2:** *Biographic details of the First Fleet Surgeons (contd)*

**SURGEON – LOWES (JOHN)**

CAREER Details unknown. Noted first in June 1789 as "Surgeon's Mate of the *Sirius*", he may have been a Dubliner.

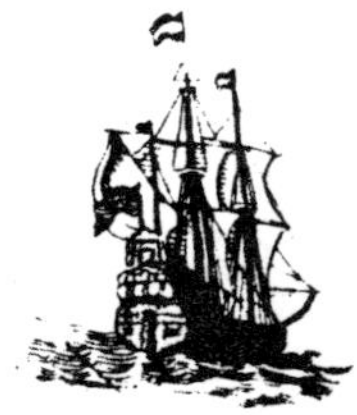

TIME IN AUSTRALIA
First records are in June 1789.[29]
(Unknown time in Colony)

EXPLORATIONS
Member of Captain Tench's six man June 1789 expedition west from Rose Hill. This expedition discovered the Nepean River. Lowes was also included in the December 1789 expedition which penetrated further west.[28]

NOTES Much biographical research remains to be undertaken about Lowes, the Surgeon's Mate of the *Sirius*. He was probably stationed at the Rose Hill outpost in June 1789, as assistant to Thomas Arndell. He appears to have been a robust person, being chosen for arduous exploration work.[31] Lowes' name does not appear on the manifest of *Sirius* in the First Fleet voyage. The first record of him is in Tench's Journal in June 1789, and it is possible that he joined the crew of *Sirius* at some time after the First Fleet voyage, possibly when the ship touched at Cape Town in February 1789, on the resupply run after the First Fleet had landed in January 1788; or was transferred to *Sirius* after October 1788 (when she left Port Jackson) from another Royal Navy ship.

**TABLE 3.2:** *Biographic details of the First Fleet Surgeons (concluded)*

> *Mr White, Surgeon to the Settlement came on board to request of me in the name of the Governor and himself to undertake the Care of the Convicts on board the Lady Penrhyn in the room of Mr Altree who he sd. shd. be provided for on his arrival at Botany Bay in some other line and in the meantime to continue on board the Lady P. and act as my Assistant. The Governor wd. reward me for my trouble in such a way as shd. prove satisfactory to me, and the Surgeon General wd. give me a Certificate ... .*[17]

When the Fleet reached Port Jackson, Surgeon Altree was further shunted off to Norfolk Island within seventeen days of arrival.

The personalities of the others ranged from the musician George Worgan (who brought the first and only piano to Australia with the First Fleet),[12] to others such as Thomas Jamison, who was a man of dominant personality. Jamison delighted in his considerable physical size, and it is known from other evidence[18,19] that he was one of the strongest men in the Colony. Two French Naval corvettes under Baudin visited Sydney Cove in 1802,[19] and one of the French Surgeon-Naturalists (Francois Péron) held a strength-testing competition using a Regnier Dynamometer, at Sydney Town. Jamison was the strongest of fourteen 'Anglois', although he was beaten by the French Botanist Michaux who was one of the seventeen 'Francois' competitors from the visiting French expedition.

It is known from indirect evidence that several of the First Fleet surgeons were very resilient men. Arndell, for example, besides being the apothecary at Parramatta, made a vigorous start in agriculture. In October 1792, a bushfire swept through his farm destroying his farmhouse, all his outbuildings, and his crops. Undaunted, he went on to establish an estate of 750 acres, which although small by the standards of the day, nevertheless showed his ability to recover after adversity. Disasters of various sorts struck the Colony in its first five years (*Figure 3.1*), and the doctors were affected directly or indirectly by all of these.

Several of the surgeons (Bowes Smyth, Altree, and Worgan) had little interest in acquiring estate in the new Colony, but others became wealthy landowners. Balmain had acquired 1,480 acres by 1802 and Jamison owned 2,300 acres by 1827 (*Table 2*). Some (such as Worgan) led uneasy financial lives and were never really materially successful. Others (such as Arndell) lived comfortably but did not leave their widows with enough independent support to care for their families after they had died.[20] In the specific case of Surgeon Arndell, it is now known that he had a total of fifteen children – eight of whom he left in England; and another seven were born in the Colony to his consort and later wife, Elizabeth Burley, alias Dalton.[21] Others (especially Jamison and Balmain) were astute businessmen, trading vigorously in spirits.

At least five (White, Balmain, Worgan, Callam and Irving) left their name on the evolving Australasian map (*Figure 3.2*). While some continued in their Naval careers after their service at Sydney (White, for example), others (e.g. Arndell) became interested in the land, and bred animals for a new style of agriculture and pastoralism that was to be the wealth of the Nation for two centuries to come.

The First Fleet Surgeons differed in their enthusiasm for biological research. Some exploited their novel opportunities in what amounted literally to a new world of natural history. Several contributed very significantly to both botany[22] and to zoology.[23] This is fortunate, as several are remembered only because of names given to creatures they discovered. The epitaph of Dennis Considen is written only in the *Eucalyptus* which now bears his name. Considen, White and Bowes Smyth described new species for a European world hungry for the wonders of an undescribed (and in many instances, unimagined) antipodean flora and fauna. Surgeon Bowes Smyth was the first white man to record (and probably to see) and draw[24] the emu, which he called "a Bird of a new genus, as large and high as an Ostrich."[25] A lizard is named after White.*

In a number of instances, historical research to date has revealed less about the clinical activities of the First Fleet doctors, than about their other contributions. The group who arrived at Sydney Cove served as clinical doctors in the Colony for an average of six years. One (Surgeon Bowes Smyth) remained in the Colony for fourteen weeks only, sailing with the *Lady Penrhyn* on the 5th May 1788. By contrast, Thomas Arndell worked as a doctor and farmed as a pastoralist in his newly adopted country for a further thirty-two years. Only two (John Irving,[14] and Arndell[1,2,21,27]) are known to have died in the Colony. Sadly, only Arndell has a memorial gravestone in this country.

*The French scientist Lacépède named the skink *Egernia whitii,* discovered by White, after the Surgeon-General.

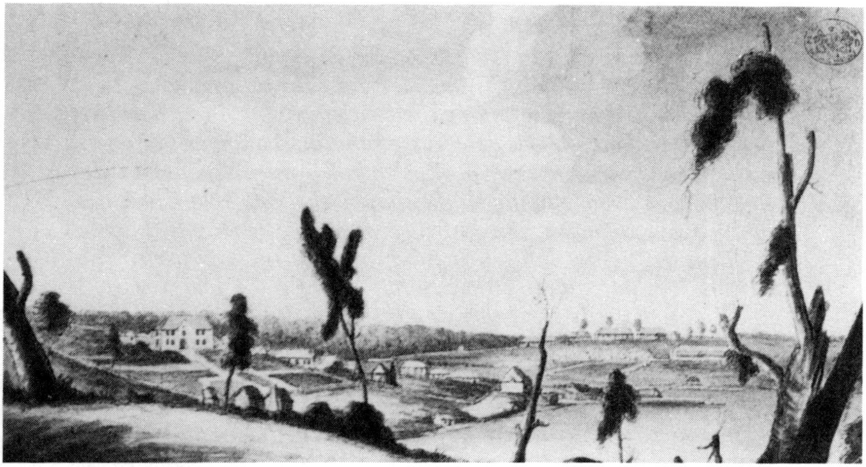

***Figure 3.2:* The evolving Australian landscape. Sydney, circa 1795. The Hospital is the building on the right. From 'A Partial View in New South Wales' by the contemporary artist Thomas Watling. By kind permission and with acknowledgements to the British Museum (Natural History)**

In the majority of cases, the clinical service which the First Fleet Surgeons gave to the new convict settlement in Australia, was in a sense a transient phase in their lives; lives which combined medicine with extra-professional interests and with high adventure.

Their origins and their professional training were as disparate as their lives in the Colony. They came from London (George Worgan), from the English Lake District (Thomas Jamison), from the village of Kingston on the Welsh border (Thomas Arndell), from Ireland (Dennis Considen, and probably John White), and from Scotland (William Balmain). Some of their early lives and their medical training exist only as shadows – Lowes[28-31] and James Callam[32] for example – and efforts to construct even fragmentary biographies of their lives have proved fruitless. An unsigned letter in the *Dublin Chronicle*, of the 13 January 1791, is now known to have been written by Lowes.[29] It, perhaps more than some formal biographies, tells so much of the privation of the first two years at Sydney Cove, but so little of the writer:

*It is now so long since we have heard from home that our clothes are worn threadbare. We begin to think the mother country has entirely forsaken us. As for shoes, my stock has been exhausted these six months, and I have been obliged since that time to beg and borrow among the gentlemen, for no such article was to be bought. In this deplorable situation famine is staring us in the face. Two ounces of pork is the allowance of animal food for four and twenty hours, and happy is the man that can kill a rat or crow to make him a dainty meal. We have raised some excellent vegetables, but such food, without the mixture of the animal, does not supply strength, but keeps us lax and weakly. I dined most heartily the other day on a fine dog, and hope I shall soon again have an invitation to a similar repast. The animals that were meant to stock the country are almost all butchered. Hunger will be appeased while any eatable remains.*

*Several of the convicts have perished by the hands of the natives, by rambling too far into the woods. I accompanied two of our gentlemen on a shooting party. We penetrated near thirty miles in two days over a delightful country, free from underwood, when we arrived at a rapid river that was not fordable.* On the other side the country seemed to be in a state of romantic and uncultivated nature. The landscape was finished by a range of hills that rise one above another, in a very grand style, to a considerable height.*

*The loss of the Sirius was the first cause of our being put to such short allowance, being obliged to supply the party a second time from the common stock. To prevent murmuring, officers and men share alike.*

*Our births have far exceeded our burials; and what is very remarkable, women who were supposed past child-bearing, and others who had not been pregnant for fifteen or sixteen years, have lately become mothers.*[29]

Letter to the *Dublin Chronicle*;
entitled 'State of the Colony 1790',
written by Surgeon's Mate Lowes.

Several of the surgeons came with very strong backgrounds of surgical experience. Some came with doubtful training in medicine and surgery, and Arndell is known to have trained as an apothecary, and was given the imprimatur of the Royal College of Surgeons of London after an oral examination on the 6th September 1781.

*The Nepean River.

Bowes Smyth came with a doubtful training in medicine and surgery but with a strong family tradition of practical philanthropy,[33] and from a strong village tradition of compassion and with personal skills in midwifery.[34]

Whilst the First Fleet was on the high seas, the various surgeons would perforce have seen only their professional colleagues on the same ship. In the case of Bowes Smyth and Altree on the *Lady Penrhyn*,[35] Bowes Smyth acted as Altree's 'minder'. Some, however, appear to have spent a deal of time also, perhaps enforced, in each other's company in the first year after disembarkation. It is known that Arndell and Lowes spent considerable time in each other's company at Parramatta, and were probably good friends. Other relationships were not so cordial. At least two fought each other, in Balmain and White's case with pistols in a public place after a Regimental Dinner hosted by the Governor.

After the Colony was established at Sydney, one of Phillip's major tasks was to explore, map and survey the new Continent. The presence of a surgeon in exploratory parties and expeditions has always been an enormous advantage, and so it proved in Sydney. It is not surprising that four of the First Fleet Surgeons (White, Considen, Arndell and Worgan) contributed significantly to geographic and anthropological knowledge as members of expeditions from the camp at Sydney Cove. Besides their clinical work, their contributions to natural history and their adventures as members of expedition parties, we know that their outdoor lives were rich and varied. Several enjoyed fishing, not simply as a hobby and sport in the early days, but as a pastime to help save the Colony from starvation itself. Some enjoyed shooting – virtually all that we know of Surgeon Altree's life at Sydney is that he "shot two curious Maccaws [probably galahs][36] on the 30th January 1788 at Sydney Cove, which he presented to his professional colleague Surgeon Bowes Smyth.

In spite of their many differences, the First Fleet Surgeons undoubtedly had a professional identity as a small brotherhood. On two recorded occasions at least, archives indicate that they regarded themselves as a 'Faculty', obviously in the connotation of the 'Faculty of Medicine'. In the context of their urgent search for new medicinal plants to treat scurvy,[22] one reads –

> *There is no doubt of this* [botanical specimen] *possessing Medicinal virtues, and it has repeatedly been made of use by the Gentlemen of the Faculty in the Settlement ... and with success.*
>
> Surgeon Arthur Bowes Smyth
> Sydney Cove, 11 February 1788.

This same feeling of identity as a Faculty brotherhood, was shown by another diary entry, at a sad incident on the anniversary four months after the initial landing at Sydney Cove –

> *I, being the Surgeon of the Sirius, and the first of the Faculty who saw the Man, whom they had so cruelly treated, was obliged to attend the Trial, to give my opinion, how far his life was endangered from his Wounds; they had nothing to say in their Defence, therefore, they were sentenced to receive 500 Lashes each.*
>
> George Bouchier Worgan
> Surgeon of the *Sirius.*
> Sydney Cove, 26 May 1788.

Some became magistrates (Jamison, Balmain and Arndell) and it is known that others aspired (unsuccessfully) to this office. Irving, for example, was not considered for this post because of his convict past. Several of the First Fleet Surgeons became active on philanthropic committees[20,37] in the new Settlement, but others (such as Considen) seemed to have shunned 'committee work', being more interested in creative pursuits.

Their personal lives also varied greatly. Some took convict wives (William Balmain[37,38] and Dennis Considen[39,40]) and the Surgeon General (John White) had a convict consort; and one, the escapee from English domestic life and subsequent widower Thomas Arndell[20,27] finally (in 1807) married his convict housekeeper who had borne him six children in the Colony by that date.[1,2,21] The fact that these men of the Settlement 'Upper Class' gave their imprimateur to marriage with convicts, by their personal example, cannot be overstated as one of the significant socialising influences operative in that society. In this respect, these four surgeons were members of that group of forebears who developed an egalitarian society from which has evolved one of the most classless populations in the Western world. Regretfully, virtually nothing of their personal writings and correspondence has survived, although three (White, Bowes Smyth and Worgan) kept diaries[5,17,41] which tell something of their work and surroundings, yet so little of their own personal lives.

Doctors exist as the servants of their patients. The profession does a disservice to the collectivity of all patients if technical standards are not of the highest order. Low technical standards amongst individual doctors lead to grave injustice to the individual patients who suffer from such inequalities. Communication skills are, in a sense, one such technical standard which is required for the practice of medicine. If variety is a virtue, it must be stated that this variety should not extend to poor technical competence or manifest inability to communicate adequately with patients. However, above these baseline requirements, a review of the lives of the First Fleet surgeons shows that advantages spring from differences. A profession which retains and fosters individuals who bring varied viewpoints, varied backgrounds and varied styles to their professional lives and to the society of patients whom they serve, can do nought but flourish.

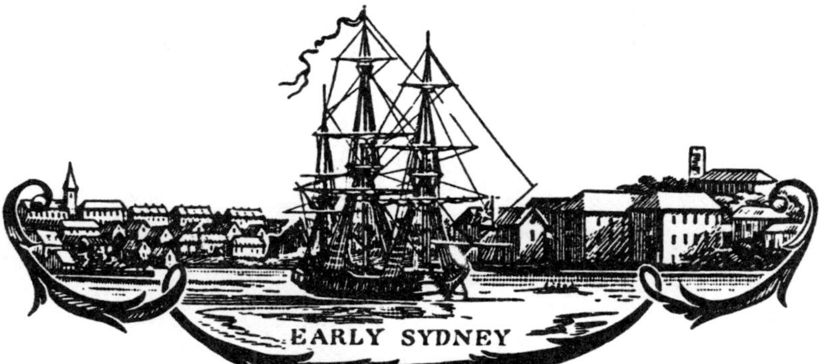

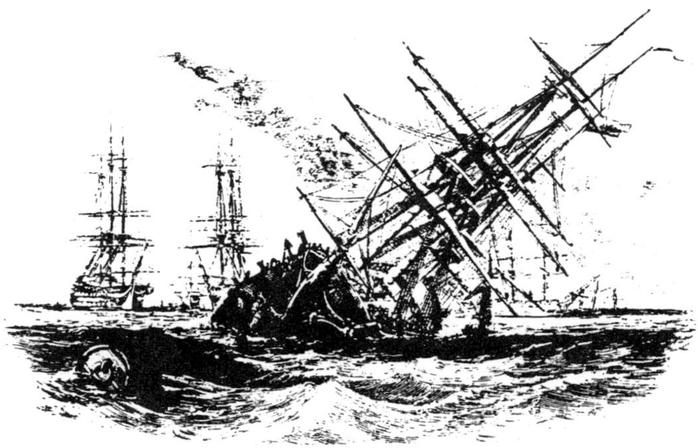

# HAMILTON OF THE PANDORA

## A Visiting Surgeon in North Queensland

**Roderick McLeod**

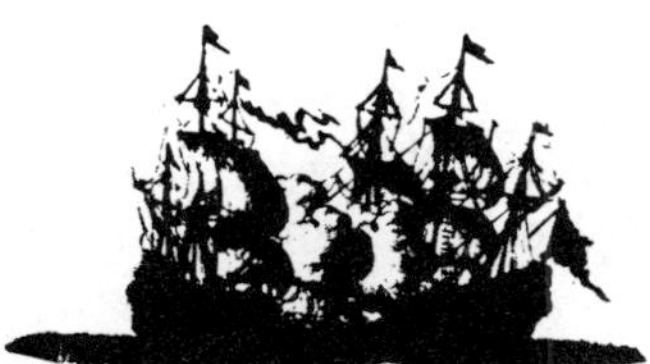

*THE* writings of several prominent navigators have informed us of the medical problems faced by ships' crews on long voyages, and the development of means to maintain health. We know little of the men whose job it was to attend to these matters – the surgeons and their assistants. The discussion of health problems usually formed part of the reports supplied by the ships' captains, and we must assume that the medical information came in part from the commander's own observations and in part from personal reports supplied to him by his medical staff.

Much of the ill-health described in these reports was caused by poor nutrition and transmissible diseases. These usually were of much greater importance than battle casualties, as far as the Royal Navy was concerned. The common diseases were vector transmitted infections or parasitic illnesses; nutritional diseases especially scurvy; venereal diseases; and the pulmonary diseases including tuberculosis. Much had been written about these problems and commanders such as James Cook RN paid particular attention to dietary matters to reduce the incidence of scurvy on long voyages.

The Admiralty appointment of William Bligh to command His Majesty's Armed Transport *Bounty* (formally *Bethia*) on an expedition to the Pacific to obtain breadfruit trees for transport to the West Indies for cultivation started a chain of events which has been the subject of reports, enquiries, courts-martial, books, films, plays and historical papers.

Bligh was a navigator who had served as an officer on the *Resolution* (Captain James Cook RN) on Cook's third and last voyage. On his homeward voyage from Tahiti, Bligh's crew mutinied, and he was set adrift with eighteen men in a 7 metre longboat, to sail 3618 nautical miles to Timor. The report of this voyage and the enquiry into its mutiny were followed by the fitting out of an expedition to search for the mutineers, recover the *Bounty*, and bring the captured home for punishment. The *Pandora*, a frigate of 24 guns, manned by 160 men, was selected and Captain Edward Edwards was appointed to the command. Among those selected for his crew was the Surgeon, George Hamilton.

Little is known of Hamilton's origins or early career. The Examination Book of the Company of Surgeons,[1] the predecessor of the Royal College of Surgeons of England, shows a George Hamilton being examined and passed, on 20 July 1758, as qualified to be 2nd Surgeon's Mate on a 3rd Rate warship (50–74 guns). At another examination on 17 May 1759 this same man failed to convince the examiners that he was qualified for high status, and remained at the same level on the Roll.

It was on 19th June, 1777 that George Hamilton was passed for 1st Surgeon's Mate of a 1st Rate ship (100 guns), and on 21st January 1779 he passed for Surgeon of a 6th Rate (a sloop, brig or small frigate). If our George Hamilton was the same man as the candidate of 1758 and 1759, he took 20 years to progress from Surgeon's Mate to Surgeon. As Hamilton of the *Pandora* seems to have been in his late 40s when appointed to the ship, it is probable that all of these dates cover the career of the one man.

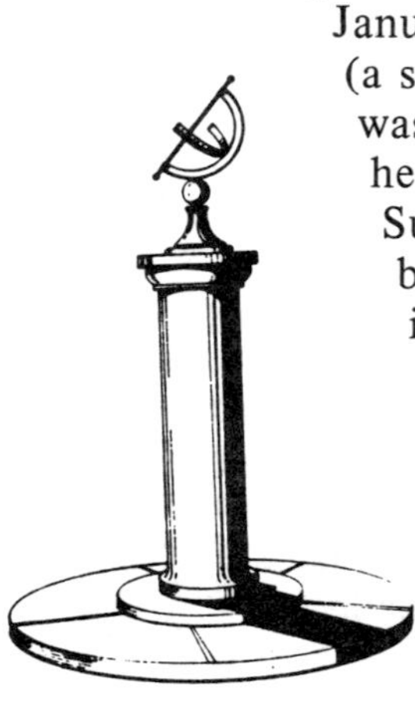

From the time of 1777 examination, George Hamilton served as Surgeon's Mate on the 6th Rate storeship *Tortoise,* of 26 guns; and on the Cutter *Ferret*, 6 guns. He then went as Surgeon to the Cutter *True Briton* (10 guns), the Sloop *Lively* (12 guns), the *Agamemnon* (3rd Rate,

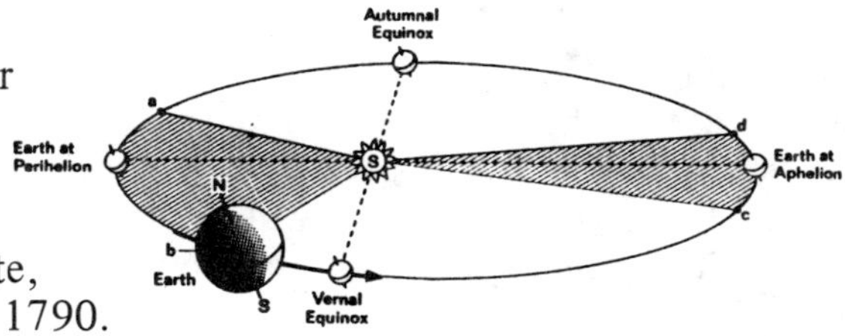


64 guns) and the Cutter *Brazen* (6 guns), a full career indeed before he was posted to the *Pandora* (6th Rate, 24 guns) on 10 August 1790.

The *Pandora's* voyage is well documented in Captain Edward's Reports, and in a short book *A Voyage Round the World* by George Hamilton – first published at Berwick in 1793.[2]

Hamilton has been criticised as "a coarse, vulgar and illiterate man" whose book cannot be relied upon, by Sir John Barrow, in his book *The Eventful History of the Mutiny and Piratical Seizure of HMS Bounty its Causes and Consequences*, which was published in 1831.[3]

The officers and petty officers of the *Pandora* were experienced people, but the major part of the crew were landsmen with no sea-going experience. All of the experienced seamen had been taken up by the ships outfitting for a major naval force which was being equipped at the same time by Lord Howe. The *Pandora* had to make do with whoever was left to recruit or press. Perhaps this led to the inclusion of men who would otherwise have been judged unfit, and men who came aboard from lodgings from which they brought their endemic insects, and the inevitable bacterial and viral parasites.

The ship was fully loaded with stores for the projected round-the-world voyage, including major stores for the refitting of the *Bounty* if recaptured. Soon after leaving Portsmouth troubles began. Fever became established and 35 men, including the only surgeon's mate, Mr Innes, were confined to bed in the crowded quarters, made even more cramped by the excess stores held in every available space.

The voyage to Santa Cruz, Tenerife, took 15 days. Here, and again at the next port, Rio de Janeiro, water, wine and fresh fruit and vegetables were taken aboard. The fever apparently continued to affect the crew until the *Pandora* rounded Cape Horn and headed north into the Pacific for Otaheite at Tahiti.

Hamilton wrote that the fever became general after the visit to Santa Cruz. Almost every man developed it in turn, many also experiencing relapses. Fortunately they were well supplied with antiscorbutics in the form of fresh fruits obtained from Santa Cruz.

In particular, Hamilton expressed his gratitude for the tea and sugar, supplied for the first time in the Service, which he believed were most beneficial for the sick. Even when the feverish men would take no food, tea and sugar were welcomed and helped sustain them. The impression gained is that the hot sweet drink helped maintain their hydration.

Another problem recorded by Hamilton was the below-decks heat in the tropics. A patent ventilator was used to provide air below decks but with little effect. Hamilton suggested modifications to Mr White's Ventilator, to render it more useful.

At the ports which the *Pandora* visited the officers were able to go ashore, but leave for the seamen was very restricted. It was too risky to let the men ashore as frequent attempts were made to abscond. The dietary normally provided for seamen was salt meat and bread or biscuits. The bread was made on board but was subject to mould and did not keep well. Sauerkraut was carried as an anti-scorbutic and made freely available to the men. Wholegrain flour mixed with sugar was used as a change to the diet, perhaps being something like a muesli food of today.

For drinks essence of malt was brewed into beer, and cocoa was used as a sweet and nourishing addition to the otherwise salted foods supplied.

From his notes, therefore, we see that Hamilton had to contend with infectious disease, dietary and nutritional problems, and poor crowded living quarters. In his medical role, he cared for the 160 men who worked and lived on this 90 foot vessel during the 136 day voyage to Tahiti, calling only at two ports to replenish fresh foods and water supplies. He does not tell us how many men died on the voyage but we must assume it was not an unusual number, or surely comment would have been made.

In Tahiti, the mutineers who could be found were captured, and the crew were able to take shore leave. While this allowed them to have free access to fresh fruits and vegetables, as well as exercise, it did produce another problem. Hamilton alluded to this where he noted that "we now began to discover that the ladies of Tahiti had left us many warm token of their affection"; venereal diseases were diagnosed amongst his crew.

The abundance of provisions on leaving Tahiti included fruit, coconuts, pigs, goats and fowls, as many as could be got

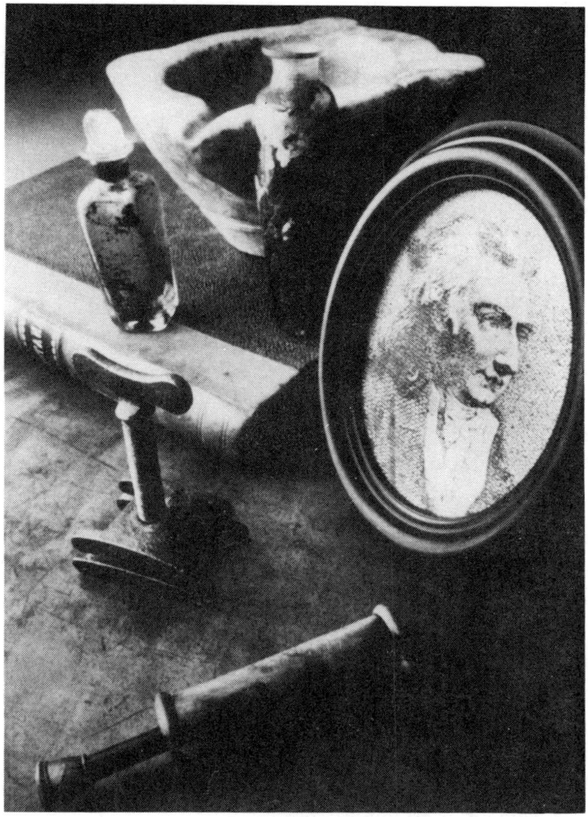

***Figure 4.1:***

***Some artefacts from the Surgeon's medical chest, from the wreck of the Pandora. Included in this tableau are two drug bottles, a stone mortar, the tightening mechanism for a tourniquet, and a syringe made of ivory. Restoration by the Division of Maritime Archaeology, The Queensland Museum, to whom acknowledgement is made for the reproduction of this photograph.***

aboard. The *Pandora* was packed with these so that the risks of scurvy and other nutritional diseases would be greatly reduced on the return voyage.

Hamilton had responsibility also for the health of the prisoners who were 14 in number. Captain Edwards had caused a low rectangular house to be built on the poop deck of the *Pandora.* It was entered through a trapdoor in the roof, and had barred ventilation openings at the side. The 'roundhouse' as it was called was so named as watchkeepers on deck could walk around it on all sides, and see across the top of it as well.

Several weeks were spent going from island to island across the Southern Pacific, seeking the remainder of the mutineers, but without success. Occasional meetings with the island inhabitants occurred, but because of the venereal disease among the crew following their sojourn in Tahiti, no association was permitted.

This discipline persisted until the *Pandora* arrived at Tonga, when it totally failed.

The voyage proceeded, with many more island visits, until the *Pandora* reached the Outer Barrier Reef on her way to Torres Strait. Here, due to attempting a night entry, with no visibility, the *Pandora* struck on a reef and was irreparably damaged.

Throughout the voyage, the order to capture the *Bounty* mutineers and bring them back to England for justice was the driving force for Captain Edwards. The 14 mutineers had been securely housed and reasonably well fed. When the shipwreck occurred, there was initial reluctance to free the prisoners from the roundhouse in case they escaped. Edwards, the Captain, failed to have them released from their irons and their prison until the last few minutes,

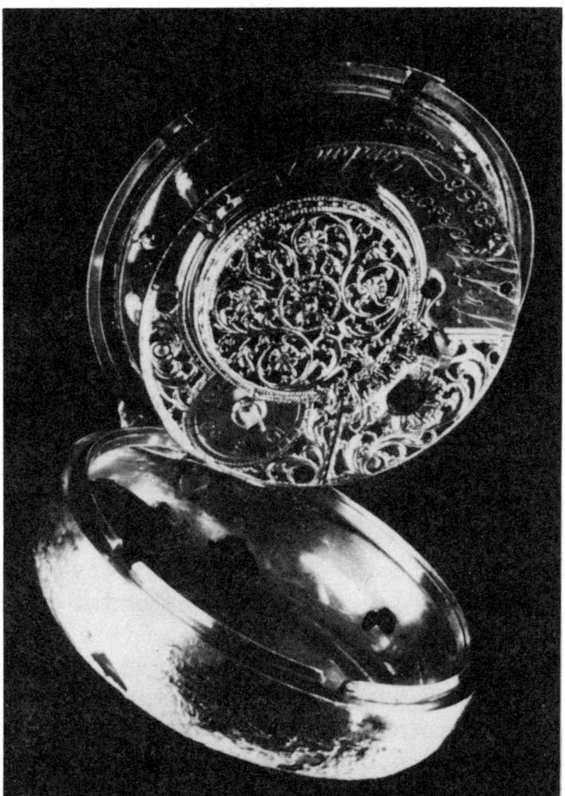

***Figure 4.2:***

***The restored silver watch from the wreck of the Pandora. Found in the sand and coral near what is believed to be the ship's medicine chest, it had a second-hand and a stop mechanism which may indicate it was the doctor's watch for taking the pulse. Photo courtesy of the Division of Maritime Archaeology, The Queensland Museum.***

and then the release was effected by a gallant crew member. Nevertheless, four of the prisoners, still in irons, drowned with the ship.

The fate of the prisoners was given little mention by Hamilton. This may have been out of deference to his Captain, who was to be accused of inhumanity to prisoners in his charge. Hamilton does give a brief story of the privations on the subsequent voyage in the four ship's boats which were saved. In a voyage almost as epic as Bligh's, these four open boats sailed overloaded, 1100 miles to Timor without loss of a man. The usual problems of water rationing, food shortage and loss of morale were overcome and a safe port was reached.

In the continuing archaeological investigation of the remains of the *Pandora*, an activity conducted by the Maritime Archaeology section of the Queensland Museum, an early discovery in a portion of the hull appears to be the contents of the surgeon's chest of George Hamilton. Items recovered include a mortar and pestle (*Figure 4.1*), an ivory syringe, a brass instrument case, drug containers, the tightening screw of a tourniquet, and a silver pocket watch (*Figure 4.2*).

These have been conserved, and in the case of the watch considerable research has produced information about it.[4] It was a watch with a second hand and a stop mechanism, which may indicate it is a doctor's or pulse watch.

The other artefacts as a group are a tantalising start to the continuing exploration of what should prove to be the surgeon's accommodation.

Hamilton's book gives some insights of the man, not always in accordance with the opinion expressed by Sir John Barrow. Hamilton lived in what could be termed a 'rumbustious' age, when the prim and proper attitudes most evident in the Victorian era had not begun to appear, where blunt discussion was usual, and possibly never more so than in a seafaring environment. Sailors have always been forthright, and the evidence suggests Hamilton was at sea for most of his adult life. To write a book without telling of good times ashore would be almost impossible for such a man. To fail to write about the consequences in his crew of such good times would be most unlikely in a surgeon describing his medical duties.

That Hamilton spoke of infections and contagious diseases, seagoing nutritional problems, and even had some quiet comments on morale would be normal for a medical man writing about his experiences on an unusual voyage. The failure on his part to talk of the men injured in the wreck may be due to their rapid death before treatment, or perhaps to a wish to avoid disturbing the emotions of the average reader. The one major omission was a detailed description of the problems of the long open boat voyage, points of interest, including the result of drinking sea water to slake thirst, and the problems of morale on such a long voyage. His failure to say much of the prisoners may have been in deference to his commanding officer, or perhaps due to the lack of interest held by most in what were in their minds guilty men waiting to be condemned, with the inevitable sequel.

Whatever the failing of his writings, Hamilton leaves an image of a man whose long experience at his profession showed in the comments he made on features of his duties.

*Acknowledgements*

The generous assistance of Dr L. Pigott and Mr Ronald Coleman, Curator of Maritime Archaeology, Queensland Museum is greatly appreciated.

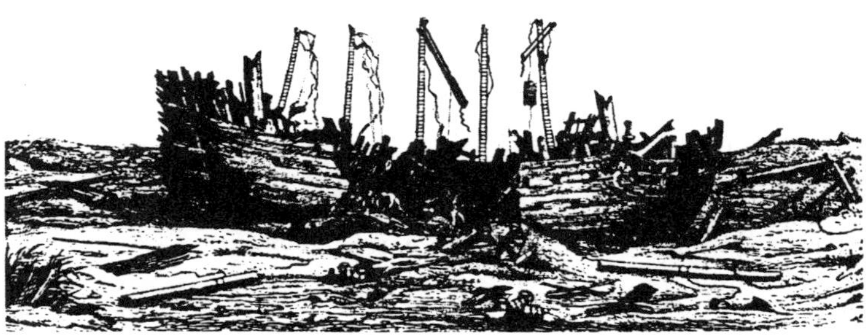

# PIONEER MEDICINE IN AUSTRALIA 5

## MEDICAL SUPERVISION ON NINETEENTH CENTURY EMIGRANT SHIPS

### The Voyage of the "Clifton", 1861–1862

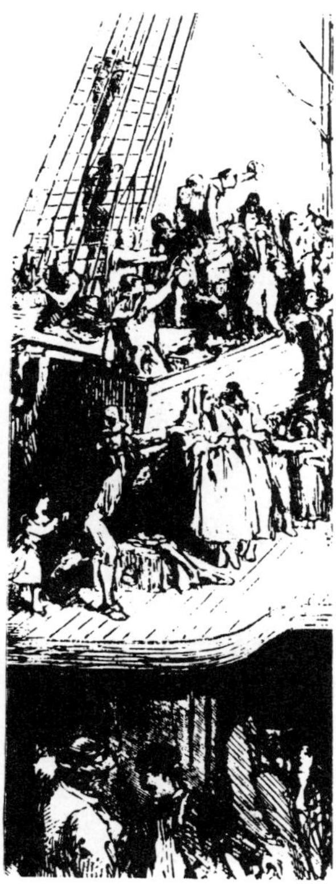

**Helen Woolcock**

*ON* a foggy November morning in 1861 the emigrant ship *Clifton* slipped from her moorings at the London docks bound for Moreton Bay. Five days later the inebriated ship's surgeon cut his throat. One of the first-cabin passengers, an unqualified practitioner, immediately accepted medical charge of the ship, and to him we are indebted for an account of the voyage.[1]

After tossing about the English Channel for another ten days, the ship finally put into Plymouth for a replacement surgeon; his unsatisfactory performance during the following four months at sea brought censure from the passengers and colonial authorities. The *Clifton's* experience, however, was not unique; reports of irregularities *en route* and other abuses raised serious questions concerning Queensland's fledgling immigration system and led to revisions in its operation. Careful passenger supervision under medical control became a key factor in the administration of a policy designed to ensure a steady stream of healthy citizens for the Colony.

The *Clifton* set sail for Queensland almost two years after separation from New South Wales. During that time an inexperienced but enthusiastic leadership, convinced of the colony's potential for progress, began grappling with the practical realities of government and the need rapidly to augment the population. Immigration was therefore high on the agenda. The existing remittance system was retained, an agent was appointed, and the Emigration Commissioners, who had been conducting migration from Britain on behalf of colonial governments for more than twenty years, were urged to forward direct to Moreton Bay as many colonists as possible.[2] In August 1860 a select committee, after investigating 'the best mode of inducing a cheap, healthy, and continuous flow of immigration' for Queensland, strongly recommended the land-order system under which anyone who paid the passage money for himself or another was entitled to a land grant in the Colony.[3] Heads nodded in approval and the proposal quickly became law. Successive extensions to the new regulations (these cancelled the remittance provisions) early in 1861, the arrival in England of Henry Jordan as the colonial emigration agent in April, and the appointment of a European agent allowed the scheme to be fully implemented.

Jordan threw himself with characteristic vigour into the task of putting Queensland on the map. He recruited young, healthy emigrants who would be willing to invest their capital or labour – or both – in the Colony. However, he soon found that, because the Commissioners' vessels operated under relatively rigid conditions and carried only steerage passengers, their arrangements simply could not cope with either the volume or class of people anxious to sail for Queensland. He finally made contact with a private shipping firm, the famous *Black Ball Line*, which had lately opened a branch office in London. Their agent entered into a rather risky undertaking. He agreed to lay on regular vessels for the Colony subject to the terms laid down in the government regulations; and to carry a proportion of selected immigrants free on each voyage in return for the equivalent in transferable land orders, provided that the remainder of the passenger complement paid the full fare. The first such vessel sailed in July 1861, followed by another in October and the *Clifton* in November. In these few months difficulties with the system soon surfaced. Exploitation and abuses meant that certain privileges had to be withdrawn, and because the age limits – forty years for men and thirty-five for women – excluded many suitable candidates, the remittance system with its higher upper level was re-established under the Commissioners' control; but private concerns could still continue sponsoring immigration to Queensland. By the time the *Clifton* departed, it was possible to reach the Colony by one of four different modes – via a private operator, with the Commissioners, or on a German or a *Black Ball* ship sailing under contract to the Queensland Government.

Although Jordan took a genuine and personal interest in prospective colonists, he was often out of London; and, submerged by the pressures of recruitment and publicity, he decided to leave the organisation of each voyage in the hands of the shipping agents. However, he was confident that the new agreement would secure the speedy and satisfactory conveyance of much needed immigrants. Almost half the 2,872 passengers who embarked in Britain and Hamburg for Queensland during 1861 sailed in *Black Ball* vessels. But all was not well; as complaints about conditions at sea began to reach Jordan, he and the colonial leaders found themselves confronting the kinds of problems that reformers of British emigration had struggled with during the previous half century – passenger rights and protection.[4] Experience had shown that sole responsibility for this could not be entrusted to either the captain, since he served the shippers' interests, or to a chaplain who might be prone to sectarian bias. The obvious choice was a medical practitioner, an impartial person, able to supervise both the physical and moral welfare of a floating population.[5]

The *British Passenger Act* (18 & 19 Vict. c.119), a distillation of decades of maritime reform, was passed in 1855 and for the next forty years regulated the lives of millions of emigrants. This statute applied to all ships carrying more than thirty steerage passengers and established minimum standards for such matters as manning and seaworthiness, embarkation and arrival procedures, dietary, water supply and medicines, space and type of accommodation for berthing and cooking, privies and hospitals.

This *Act* also stipulated that a 'duly qualified medical practitioner' (someone legally authorised to practise as a physician,

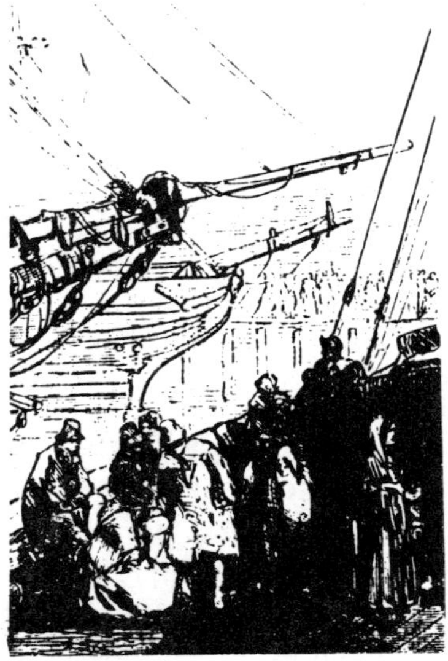

surgeon or apothecary) must accompany any vessel with more than fifty passengers and a voyage time expected to exceed eighty days under sail or forty-five with steam. Land-order immigrants for Queensland were covered by the provisions of the 1855 *Act* as well as the Government Regulations issued in January 1861:[6] These outlined eligibility criteria relating to residence, occupation and age, and required that on arrival passengers 'give proof' that they had been 'properly found' during the voyage in respect of clothing, bedding and utensils, and according to the law. In addition, the captain was obliged to comply as far as possible with instructions for the Commissioners' vessels; if there were more than five single women over fourteen years of age travelling without a parent or guardian, they had to be berthed in the stern of the ship 'behind a substantial bulkhead' and under the care of a matron; the separate male and female hospitals must remain free for use at all times; and if there were more than twenty land-order immigrants on board, a 'bona fide' doctor had to be appointed.

The doctor signed on (as a crew member) only if the emigration officer approved his credentials. The latter was a key figure: no ship could receive a clearance unless the emigration officer was satisfied that the legal requirements had been fulfilled, a procedure which included the embarkation examination of all passengers, except those in the saloon. Their personal requisites for the voyage were inspected, and the port medical officer checked for the presence of infectious disease. Once at sea it was the ship doctor's responsibility to maintain clearance standards and so ensure a healthy voyage. To this end he was expected to perform medical duties and support the master by enforcing obedience to rules 'For Preserving Order, Promoting Health and Securing Cleanliness and Ventilation' on board.[7] The Queensland regulations also required that he keep a medical log.

In early October 1861 the *Clifton*, an old wooden ship, built in 1837 and registered at 687 tons, was chartered by the *Black Ball Line* and placed on berth in London. Almost six weeks later she was ready for clearance. Captain Fillan took command, and on 17 November sailed down the Thames with 32 crew and 240 emigrants to embark 14 saloon passengers at Gravesend. Another seventeen souls, three of whom travelled first class, joined the ship at Plymouth. The total passenger complement of 271 included 203 adults (86 were married), 59 children between one and twelve years and 9 infants. Apart from 34 Scots and 15 Irish, the remainder were English, mostly recruited from the agricultural districts. Fares for the four classes accommodated on the *Clifton* ranged from £18 to £45,[8] and although at least a third of the steerage went free, all passengers had to pay travel costs to the port of embarkation and outfit themselves for the voyage and their new life in the Colony. These early immigrants did not represent the 'scum' of society. One of 'Jordan's Lambs' who sailed for Queensland in 1861 described them as 'a magnificent lot of hardy pioneers ... no wasters, no drunkards, no unemployable were to be found among them'.[9] The majority on the *Clifton* were in the prime of life, the mean age of the total complement being 21.4 years.[10] A young, hopeful and apparently robust group departed for the Colony, and if their dietary was any indication, they should have remained healthy throughout the voyage.

At the time of boarding Harry Ramsdale, the diarist, described the *Clifton* as 'the most filthy hulk'; he had never seen 'such disorder'. Foggy weather delayed departure for twenty-four hours, and once out into the Channel, contrary winds forced them to drop anchor twice in the next three days. While the passengers groaned with seasickness, the ship's surgeon, George Young, was 'raving horribly' with delirium tremens. He settled a little after Ramsdale prescribed brandy laced with opium, but at 3.20 a.m. on 22 November they found him with his throat cut and 'perfectly saturated with blood', though still alive. At first light Ramsdale took him to land and tried to contact the doctor's family. Young died two days later. His deliberate suicide suggests that he accepted appointment to the ship as a way of escape. He had, however, fulfilled the legal requirements for a ship's surgeon, being qualified as an apothecary, a surgeon and an accoucheur, and having served with the Royal Navy.[12]

Ramsdale returned to the *Clifton* drenched and exhausted,

but at the captain's request he accepted responsibility for the sick on board and attended to them without delay. His diary indicates that, although unqualified, he had medical training and experience.[13] During the next few days, as the foul weather continued, he became increasingly concerned for a fellow traveller who, in the final stages of consumption, had been shipped off alone and left to the mercy of 'the fatal November cold'. Wisely withholding medication Ramsdale gave him an invalid diet of soup and stout, but the young man's condition sank rapidly and on 26 November he died, apparently from fright when a huge wave broke over the ship. He was found by the captain who himself had begun to crack under the pressure and excitement and who needed medical attention himself. Later that day a young mother went into labour. Although Ramsdale performed the breech delivery to his satisfaction, the baby girl was still-born. Another gale sprang up and by the following day he was 'utterly fatigued', having by then been down to the steerage at least eighteen times, prescribing, dispensing and even preparing gruel. He wrote:

> *... the steerage presents a sad spectacle, one can see nothing but invalids huddled together ... hear nothing but groans and retching, smell nothing but vomitings, walk on nothing but rejected breakfasts and dinners and feel nothing but disgust.*[14]

On the 28th he attended the young consumptive's burial, a sobering event, checked between decks again and prepared lemonade which he administered with lime juice and 'a strong dose of calomel' to the third mate who was ill with 'incipient rheumatic fever'. At 5 p.m. he delivered a fine baby boy. Thankfully the weather changed for the better and from then on Ramsdale was able to record, with some satisfaction, that his patients were progressing very favourably. On 1 December the wind shifted and the next day they managed to reach Plymouth, more than two weeks after leaving Gravesend.

While in Plymouth Ramsdale saw the ship's owners about the poor accommodation on board, but they refused to listen to him or acknowledge his services. Their primary concern was to find crew replacements and obtain a speedy clearance since the ship had a clean bill of health. At midnight on 4 December the *Clifton*, with 304 souls and 500 tons of cargo, set sail for Moreton Bay and did not put into port again until she reached the Colony four months later. The 26 year-old chief mate, John D'Oyley, had taken command and John Spencer, an English doctor, sailed as the ship's surgeon. Spencer also met the legal requirements. He had served an apprenticeship, 'walked the wards' at the London Hospital, and in 1841 had qualified as a surgeon (MRCS, England). Two years later he became a Licentiate of the Apothecaries' Society, London, and then worked as a general practitioner before joining the Emigration Commissioners' Service in 1848. He appears to have remained with them until, at the age of forty-six, he signed on with the *Clifton*.[15] In every respect Spencer seemed an appropriate man for the post; the voyage was to prove otherwise.

According to Ramsdale the time at sea was exceedingly tedious; he 'never felt so wearied of anything' in all his life. The average sailing time for the seven vessels which left England for the Colony in 1861 was 107 days, compared with 124 for the *Clifton*.[16] After leaving Plymouth, she again ran into gales and stormy weather, and then spent weeks becalmed in the sultry heat of the tropics before finally picking up the trade winds and heading for the southern latitudes where, easting towards Australia, they encountered many cold, overcast and rainy days. After rounding Tasmania she hauled north to warmer climes. A 'splendid breeze' on 2 April encouraged everyone to start packing, but head winds and storms delayed them a further five days. The *Montmorency*, the *Black Ball* ship which left London six weeks after the *Clifton*, dropped anchor in Moreton Bay a few hours ahead of her. A river steamer tran-shipped the passengers to Brisbane on 9 April 1862, five months from the time they had embarked in London.

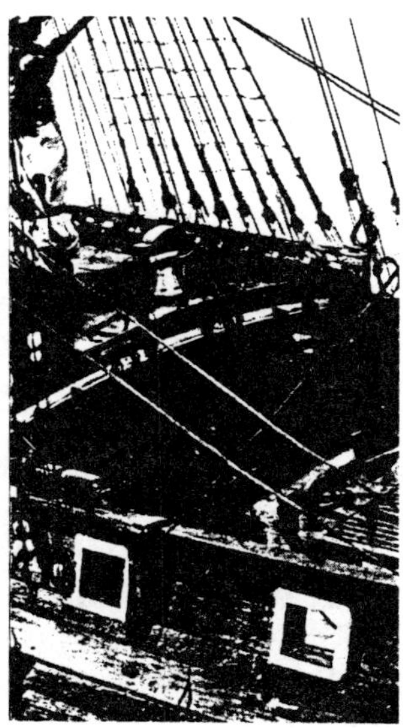

Although Ramsdale found enough to occupy his time, the constraints of shipboard life proved a sore trial to a person of such energy. It takes little to imagine how other young and healthy emigrants reacted, especially those cooped up in the steerage area. At first there seems to have been considerable flexibility regarding 'territorial rights', but friction between the different classes came to a head half way through the voyage. The captain restricted the poop to the saloon passengers and settled a dispute over bunk boundaries between decks. But we may assume that since none of the records gave any hint of 'improper conduct', segregation of the single women under the matron's care was effective. Nevertheless, maintaining law and order became a full-time job. The hot weather and many delays frayed tempers, petty thefts were common and consumption of alcohol, although forbidden by law in the steerage, was allowed in the first cabin and lay at the root of a good deal of trouble. Some of the passengers with the captain's approval formed themselves into watches to keep the several compartments under constant surveillance. Disciplinary difficulties also extended to the crew. The bosun broached the liquor supplies and was disrated, the men refused to obey his replacement, and on arrival in Moreton Bay they went on strike. And there were problems with the ship itself. The *Clifton* was an 'old tub', her decks leaked, and towards the end of the voyage the cargo shifted dangerously. Responsibility for all matters relating to the passengers' well-being, quite apart from the navigation, devolved on the captain who apparently received no support from the surgeon.

At the time of Spencer's appointment he had been assured that, in addition to the regular wage for private ship surgeons (approximately £8.10.0 a month in the 1860s), he could expect a government gratuity only for each free immigrant landed alive.[17] Not surprisingly he confined himself to medical duties between decks and took no responsibility for the sanitary state of the vessel. In view of the voyage conditions it is doubtful if the *Clifton* was ever 'sweet and clean'. Rats roamed at large, and when the pigs escaped from their pen, they trotted muck through the saloon.[18] Ramsdale's cabin was often awash with water, and he only once mentioned that it had been scraped and cleaned. Personal cleanliness would have also presented problems, since there were no baths on board. The young men took to the deck early in the morning and dowsed each other with sea water, but how did the women cope? Although passengers collected what rain water they could for washing clothes, fleas became increasingly bothersome, even in the saloon. One can understand why after reading a description of the doctor's cabin, 'a perfect jackdaw's nest'. It was cluttered with 'books & pamphlets ... phials & bottles ... trade cards ... rags & bandages, left-off clothes & chamber utensils, scissors, knives & toothpicks ... dead fleas and dirty linen'.[19]

After two months at sea everyone and everything looked the worse for wear; and as the voyage dragged on, complaints about reduced rations, putrid water and leaking casks multiplied. By mid-March the water allowance had been halved, and when the full quantity was restored some two weeks later, it was 'fearfully tarry'.[20]

Under such circumstances, if disease had gained a toe-hold, it could have ravaged the shipboard community. Yet all the reports indicate that the voyage was 'remarkably healthy', and that the medical problems were unexceptional – seasickness during rough weather, heat prostration in the tropics, and sore throats and other respiratory affections when the temperatures dropped. And there were the usual accidents – falls on deck, down the hatchway or into the hold; a lad gashed his sister's leg in a fight, and Ramsdale inadvertently hit his companion with a bucket during their morning ablutions. All such injuries apparently recovered. A threatened case of scarlet fever was immediately removed to the hospital, a second-cabin appropriated for the purpose, and despite howls of protest from adjacent cabins there were no further developments. A sufferer from heart disease fainted and a man with delirium tremens had an 'epileptic fit'. Such ailments, together with Ramsdale's own complaints (acute indigestion and severe headaches brought on by a change of dietary and too little exercise, and the return of his 'old melancholy fits'), give a general idea of the health status on board. The *Clifton* was fortunate; other vessels arrived that year reporting high morbidity and mortality rates. Only one other death occured, that of a little boy from 'teething',[21] and there were three more births, two girls and a boy.

The passengers remained healthy despite their environment and problems with medical supervision. Ramsdale withdrew his services as soon as Spencer arrived, but his previous patients implored him to continue when the doctor refused to treat them during the rough days out of Plymouth. One of the mothers, after a very difficult delivery ('her screams were terrible'), begged the captain to allow Ramsdale to care for her, but legally D'Oyley had to refuse. Nevertheless, he called on Ramsdale to attend the sick crew, including himself, and to see the matron when she 'severely injured' her hip For a sailor seized with 'violent cramp pains', Ramsdale prescribed a megadose of 'violent emetics' – enough to make 'a rhinoceros cast up' – and was surprised to find the man fit for duty the next day.[22]

Towards the end of the voyage references to the emigrants he attended became more frequent, so too did comments about the 'useless ... and lazy doctor'. When nursing mothers protested over cuts in their daily quota of porter, the captain, not Spencer, decided who needed 'strengthening'. Spencer's contribution to the passengers' welfare was seen as worthless. After two months at sea the chief mate turned on him demanding, 'What the devil use are you ... You do nothing else but lie about [the] Saloon all day & sleep, might as well have nobody as you ... you ought to be ashamed of yourself'.[23] He seems to have demonstrated no expertise, had no authority on board, and neither his age (both the captain and first mate were many years his junior) nor his experience commanded any respect. The quality of Spencer's service for the Commissioners must surely have been suspect. Moreover, he was an eccentric. His appearance was not only as curious as his disposition, but he displayed none of the gentlemanly characteristics so valued by Victorian society. Despite his qualifications Spencer's performance would have confirmed the poor public image of the medical profession in general and of ship surgeons in particular.

On arrival in Queensland the passengers were 'unanimous' in their dissatisfaction over the doctor's neglect. The immigration agent, however, would not comment on his professional competence and, being uncertain of the duties of such officers on private ships, could not determine how far he was 'culpable for the want of order and cleanliness so manifest in the vessel'.[24] Possibly Spencer received no instructions, or it may have been assumed that, given his experience, he knew what was required of him. Yet he believed he had done his duty, and wrote to the immigration agent:

> *Having been telegraph* [sic] *in London on a sudden emergency to take charge of a large body of Emigrants to this Port as Surgeon-Superintendant* [sic] *under peculiar circumstances ... I trust you will give me the usual allowance to Surgeons, having to the utmost of my ability exerted myself for the health and comfort of everyone on board.*[25]

A similar request to the Colonial Secretary received a negative reply; the evidence countervailed his claim.

Apart from medical neglect, the lack of cleanliness, poor ventilation and the shocking state of the water closets, the *Clifton's* immigrants complained of short rations, leaky decks, limited berthing and cooking space, as well as the exorbitant prices charged for shoddy bedding. Although they landed with a net increase in the shipboard population and 'spoke warmly' of the attention given by the master and his officers, the difficulties *en route* were obvious. Other private vessels arriving that year reported similar problems, but were less healthy. Conditions of travel for passengers under the land-order scheme clearly called for investigation, reform, and the careful definition of responsibility. The difference between privately organised ships and the better-managed Commissioners' vessels seemed to lie with the standard of supervision at sea. On the latter the surgeon-superintendent was expected to act as doctor, sanitary officer and moral guardian; he was invested with status and authority and remunerated accordingly.

When a report of the *Clifton's* voyage reached Jordan, he refused to blame the shippers for the alleged deficiencies since the vessel had twice been passed by an emigration officer. But the fact that one doctor had committed suicide and the other proved totally inefficient could not be ignored. Jordan had to admit that, although the men appointed to the *Black Ball* ships were professionally qualified, 'sufficient care had not always been observed in their appointment'.[27] He also conceded that the terms of the 1855 *Act* did not satisfy evolving standards for Queensland's immigration system. In a reorganisation of administrative arrangements he focused on the role of the doctor. Within a year of the *Clifton's* arrival a new contract with the *Black Ball Line* introduced regulations for the management of each vessel similar to those enforced by the Commissioners. It provided for a surgeon-superintendent, funded by and accountable to the colonial authorities for the welfare of all passengers, especially those subsidised by the Government. Jordan personally undertook the selection and appointment of the medical officers and issued them with 'letters of instruction' detailing their duties.

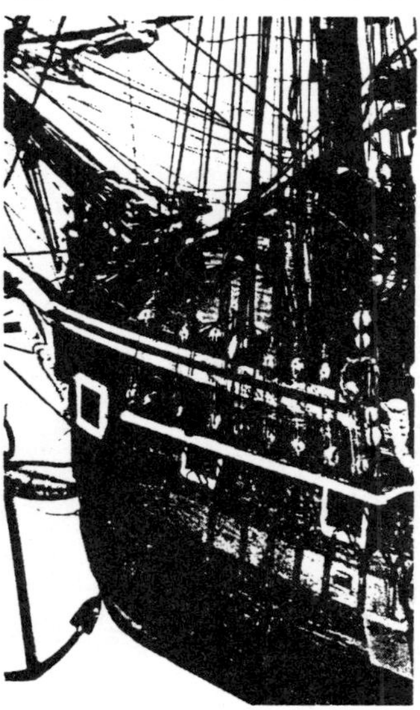

The *Clifton's* voyage not only drew attention to problems in the new immigration scheme, but demonstrated the need for improved supervision at sea in order to secure an inflow of healthy colonists. Obvious potential dangers to passenger health in the hasty or ill-considered appointment of a ship surgeon, however well qualified, gave impetus to an early reform of the system. By establishing the more comprehensive position of surgeon-superintendent on vessels carrying subsidised immigrants, and by introducing clear guidelines relating to his selection, status and responsibilities, the colonial government provided for more effective shipboard management and better control of the whole operation. Medical supervision on emigrant vessels remained a crucial factor in the execution of Queensland's immigration policy during the next thirty years.

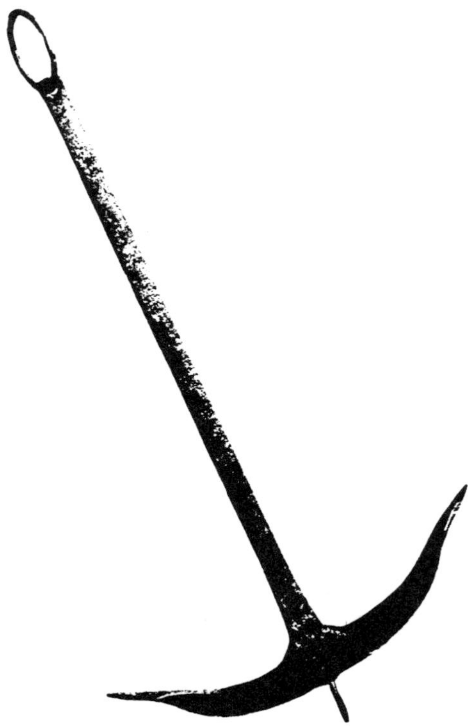

# PART II

# THE HOSTILE LAND

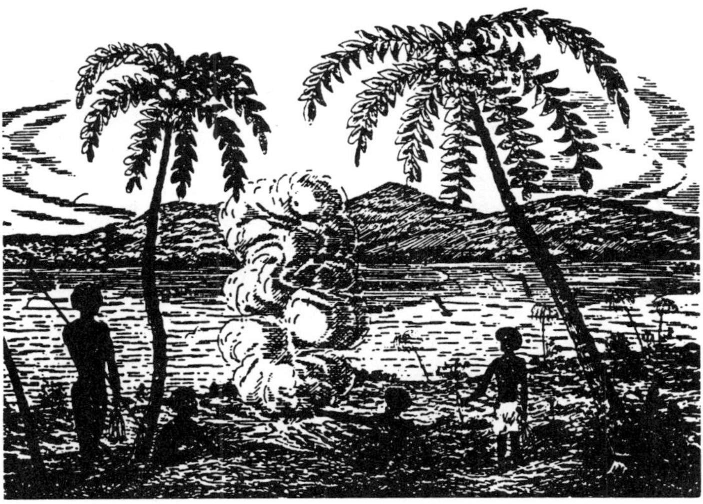

# PIONEER MEDICINE IN AUSTRALIA 6

## THE SAGA OF THE AUSTRALIAN LEECH WORM

**John Thearle**

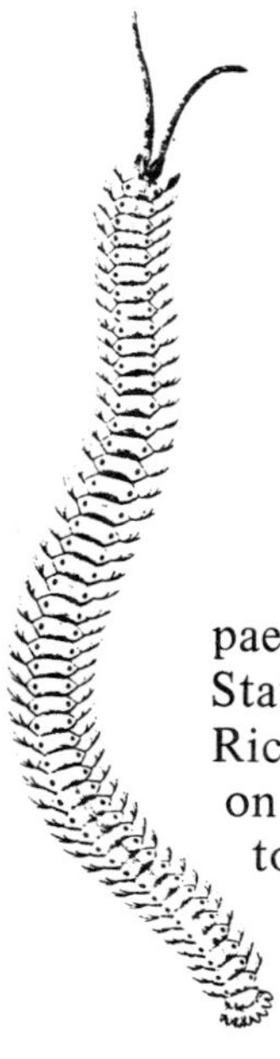

*WE hear a good deal at the present time about filling the north of Australia with a white population. How far this policy will prove a success depends mostly on the health of the second and succeeding generations of these immigrants. When our statesmen have a little time to spare for the things that really matter, I should like them to pay some attention to the reports of the United States Commission on the ravages of parasitic anaemia.*[1]

Alfred Jefferis Turner, 1909

Dr Alfred Jefferis Turner (1861–1942), a Queensland paediatrician, was referring to a report by the United States Health Commission on hookworm disease in Puerto Rico. This had shown that of one million inhabitants on the island, 800,000 were suffering from anaemia due to hookworm, six or seven thousand of whom died annually.[2] His comments were made in an address to the Queensland Branch of the British Medical Association on the prevention of anaemia due to the hookworm, *Ancylostoma duodenale*. In this paper Turner suggested that the term 'leech-worm' was appropriate to describe hookworm as the simple Anglo-Saxon language was easily understood and its meaning conveyed the blood sucking habits of the parasitic worm responsible for the disease.

Although the term did not become popular, another milestone had been reached in the saga of efforts to control hookworm infestation, shown to be present in Queensland twenty years earlier and which still had many years to run before adequate preventive public health measures became effective in Australia.

**Historical background**

Ancylostomiasis was the only helminthic parasitic disease which had been recognised for many centuries, and it had been referred to in an Egyptian papyrus as early as 1550 B.C.[3] Discovery of the worm itself had to wait until 1838 when Angelo Dubini (1813–1902), an Italian clinician and epidemiologist, identified it in the intestine of a woman dying of pneumonia in Milan in Italy. Four years later Dubini carried out a systematic examination of bodies at autopsy and found the worm in the duodenum and the beginning of the jejunum of at least 20 out of 100 cadavers dissected with the aim of finding the parasite. He reported his findings in 1843 and named the worm *Agychlostoma duodenale** because of its hooklike teeth. Dubini's reports had not attributed any particular disease to hookworm, merely describing it as an incidental finding in patients dying from other conditions.

It was not until 1846 in Egypt that a clinical association was noted between hookworm and the severe iron deficiency known as chlorosis. A few years later in 1853, also in Egypt, the zoologist T.M. Bilharz (1825–1864) postulated that hookworm was a cause of chlorosis. Bilharz's postulation was confirmed by Dr W. Griesinger (1817–1868) in the following year. The importance of these discoveries was not recognised until 1866 when O. Wucherer (1820–1873) found hookworm in the bodies of patients in Brazil who had died from tropical anaemia. A further important step was taken in

*Following discovery of the hookworm in 1843 by Dubini, it was named *Agchylostoma duodenale*, from the Greek αγχυλος (agkylos), a hook. The derivation was incorrect and should have been *Agkylostoma duodenale*. From that time many changes in naming occurred and eventually 22 variants existed. To settle the confusion, the International Commission on Zoological Nomenclature (Opinion 66 of February 1915) determined that the correct name should be *Ancylostoma* proposed by Creplin in 1845. The correct name is thus: *Ancylostoma duodenale* (Dubini, 1843) Creplin, 1845.[4]

Italy in 1878 when G. Grassi (1854–1924) and his co-workers, the Parona brothers, diagnosed hookworm disease clinically, having observed *Ancylostoma* ova in the faeces of a patient. As a result, it became accepted medical practice to examine the stools of all patients suffering from anaemia, which revealed a worldwide distribution of the hookworm parasite. At the time it was suggested that infection occurred when ova were ingested through contaminated food. That hookworm could be an occupational disease was demonstrated in 1880 when it was shown to be the cause of miners' anaemia among workmen constructing the St Gothard Tunnel through the Swiss Alps.[5]

In Australia the first recorded case of hookworm disease was described in Queensland in 1889 by Dr J.B. Hogg. Hogg, while serving as a medical officer at the Woogaroo, later Goodna, Lunatic Asylum, reported that the parasitic worm was present at autopsy in the duodenum and jejunum of a patient originally from Denmark who, when admitted to the mental institution, had been suffering from chronic anaemia.[6] Three years later, in 1892, two sisters, aged two and four years, with chronic anaemia were sent for investigation from Cairns to the Hospital for Sick Children in Brisbane. Their faeces were examined by Dr A.J. Turner, the Resident Medical Officer at the Children's Hospital, and the ova found reported to be those of hookworm. These cases were reported to the Medical Society of Queensland in April 1892 by Dr John Lockhart Gibson, a visiting Honorary Medical Officer to the Brisbane Hospital for Sick Children.[7]

Later in 1892 Gibson and Turner presented a detailed scientific paper entitled "Notes on the occurrence of *Anchylostomum duodenale* in Queensland" in which they emphasised their belief that hookworm was a frequent cause of anaemia in North Queensland.[8] They showed that its presence could be demonstrated easily by microscopic examination of the faeces for ova, and they provided clear illustrations of the appearance of the ova as seen through a microscope, making diagnosis easy. The clear diagram of the hookworm eggs was annotated in Turner's handwriting with the microscope setting appended, as shown in *Figure 6.1*. At the same time Turner and Gibson discussed the difficulties associated with treating the condition. Successful treatment was only achieved by administering combinations of some of the known anti-helminthic

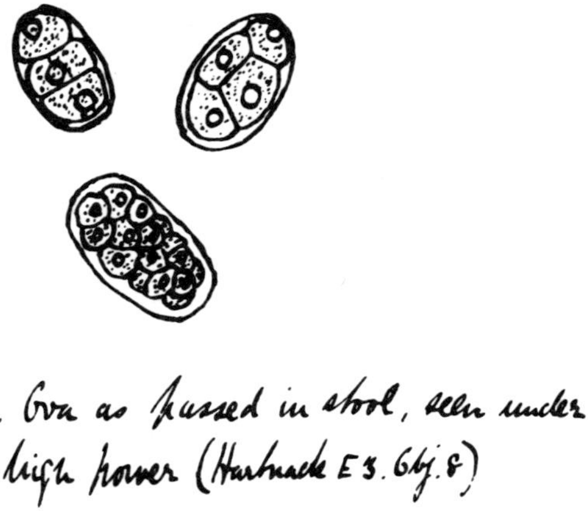


***Figure 6.1:* Alfred Jefferis Turner's sketch of hookworm eggs, together with the settings for his microscope.**

preparations such as an extract of the male fern (*Felix mas*), spigelia, santonin and a purgative calomel (mercurous chloride). Large doses of arsenic had been administered to lower the parasite's vitality and protochloride of iron was given for the associated anaemia which was caused by the ingestion of blood from the duodenum through the hooklike teeth of the parasite. Turner's and Gibson's paper notified the medical profession of Queensland (and Australia) for the first time that hookworm infestation in children existed in Australia.

Within the next few years many cases of hookworm were reported in children and adults in Queensland from Cairns to Brisbane.[9] In 1895 Dr Turner delivered a lecture to the Royal Society of Queensland in which he expressed his belief that, in the interests of preventive medicine, the general public should be acquainted with a serious but easily preventable parasitic disease, hookworm, and described current knowledge and opinions world-wide about *Ancylostoma.*[10] Further cases of hookworm infestation were reported from the Brisbane Children's Hospital.[11] In 1898, at the Annual General Meeting of the Queensland Branch of the British Medical Association (B.M.A.), the President stated that it was vital for people to be aware of diseases peculiar to their own country;

he cited ancylostomiasis as the most important recent example and praised the valuable work on the disease which had been done by Dr Turner and others.[12]

Four years later, in 1902, as the result of his research in Brisbane, Dr T.L. Bancroft published a significant paper on hookworm infection in humans. He produced epidemiological evidence which supported the epoch-making observation of Arthur Looss (1861-1923), a German helminthologist working in Egypt, that hookworm larvae could infect man by penetrating the skin. Bancroft was possibly the first person to emphasize the danger inherent in children going barefoot, recognising the high probability of the young *Ancylostomum duodenale* entering its subject through the feet.[13] Looss had made his original observation in Cairo in 1898 when he accidentally infected himself with a hookworm culture, but his discovery had gained acceptance very slowly.[14] It was not until 1911, when he published a monograph on the anatomy and life history of *Ancylostoma duodenale*, that his discovery was more widely accepted.[15]

Hookworm disease became the subject of public debate in Queensland. In May 1903 Dr T.F. McDonald, a medical practitioner in northern Queensland, wrote to the *Brisbane Courier* imploring the Commonwealth and State Health Departments to intervene to combat the troublesome disease.[16] The Hon. A.H. Barlow, M.L.C., replied that as early as November 1900 he had asked questions in Queensland's Legislative Council on the subject of the 'earth eating disease' (hookworm) and had received a lengthy reply to the effect that there was no cause for public anxiety.[17] However, he felt it was time the matter was investigated as the disease was a most serious one.[18] Turner supported McDonald and Barlow and also wrote to the Editor of the *Brisbane Courier*, praising Dr McDonald for the service he had rendered by once again directing general attention to the 'earth eating disease', so called because of the unusual habit of its victims of eating soil (pica).[19] He reminded the public of the lecture he had given to the Royal Society of Queensland in 1895 on the subject of hookworm and gave details regarding the number of cases admitted to the Brisbane Children's Hospital over the previous 11 years. There had been 59 admissions, although some had undoubtedly been readmissions, with the majority coming from the coastal belt of Queensland between Brisbane and Gympie there had been no cases from Brisbane. Turner described the symptoms of lethargy from anaemia, the stunting of growth and the predisposition of these children to intercurrent disease. He also believed that a considerable number did not attain adulthood and reiterated his earlier advice on ways to prevent the disease, adding the most recently discovered need to avoid allowing the infective hookworm larvae to penetrate the skin of the feet. In conclusion Turner remarked that during the present time of retrenchment there was not much hope of preventive work being done by the State. However, he thought that the disease was one which should receive attention from the Federal Government which was trying to encourage the growth of the Queensland sugar industry by using European (white) labour. Turner described the hookworm scourge as one of the most serious hindrances to acclimatisation of the white race in the tropical sugar growing districts.

In January 1901 Dr Burnett Ham was appointed the first Commissioner of Public Health in Queensland. He had many public health problems to deal with, including hookworm, although at the turn of the century there was no real idea of how widespread infestation was in Queensland because accurate mortality rates from the disease were not available. As Dr Ham's annual reports were published, the extent of ancylostomiasis was revealed; one particularly able and comprehensive account was that of R.A. O'Brien, a health officer in the Department of Public Health, in 1904.[20] He described the disease chiefly in the Cairns-Townsville district, at scattered places in the coastal district between Brisbane and Maryborough, and also some isolated cases in the extreme south eastern part of the State. It was O'Brien's opinion that, although incidence of the disease was not increasing rapidly, the spread was insidious and new areas were being infected. He believed the problem could be solved by proclaiming ancylostomiasis an infectious disease in certain areas and using the appropriate regulations to isolate cases. In 1906 five more cases of ancylostomiasis were reported from Gympie.[21] The following year the Commissioner for Public Health reported that no reliable estimate of the mortality from ancylostomiasis was available but that many deaths which were attributed to dropsy, debility and anaemia were due to the disease, and reiterated O'Brien's opinion that compulsory notification of the disease would serve a useful purpose.[22]

Dr T.F. McDonald's unabated concern about hookworm disease in Australia led to his being invited in 1907 to address the Society of Tropical Medicine and Hygiene in London, under the chairmanship of the noted authority on tropical medicine, Sir Patrick Manson (1844-1922).[23] McDonald outlined the seriousness of the problem in North Queensland in the Johnstone River district between Townsville and Cairns where he practised. He deplored the reluctance of the Queensland and Federal Governments to give assistance to combat the disease. His experience showed that 90% of school children were affected and he mentioned their craving to eat dirt. As well as emphasising the physical features of the anaemic children, McDonald expressed concern for the mental aberrations noted in them ranging from disobedience, cunning, through to lying and stealing, and gave several amusing but rather sad illustrations.

> *A young girl of highly imaginative character, under the influence of the disease, forged letters to her mother, a widow, setting forth proposals of marriage from supposed admirers, coupled with the information that she must be kind and lenient, even indulgent, to her charming little daughter. This charming daughter went so far with her forging propensities, that it was necessary to take steps to stop her. I recommended thymol as a first 'punishment', which resulted in the expulsion of quantities of ankylostomes and, later on, regeneration of character slowly ensued.*
>
> *Another little maid of nine summers developed a faculty for finding half sovereigns. One of these happened to be a coin which I had marked, and missed. Nothing was said to the child, but thymol having been exhibited, with the usual result, careful watch was kept for developments. In order to study her case, it was arranged that the girl should stay with my servants for some months, and from being quite the 'naughtiest' girl at school, she grew into a really bright and lovable child.*[24]

Dr A.J. Turner's unflagging interest in the battle against hookworm was once again voiced publicly in July 1909 when he read his paper entitled "The prevention of parasitic anaemia" to the Queensland Branch of the B.M.A.[25] In the same month Dr A.G. Salter, an Honorary Physician at the Brisbane Children's Hospital, published a paper summarising the hospital's experiences with hookworm over the previous ten years. He pointed out that the number of admissions for the disease was increasing and that the world picture generally was depressing because known preventive measures were not being practised.[26] Dr Turner and Dr Salter were requested by the Queensland Branch of the B.M.A.[27] to compile a leaflet on the subject called "Instructions to Parents" which was distributed throughout the State by the Public Health Department.[28] Finally, in September 1909, ancylostomiasis was listed as a notifiable disease in Queensland and accurate assessment of its extent became possible.[29]

The establishment of the Australian Institute of Tropical Medicine in Townsville, North Queensland, in 1910 gave the fight against ancylostomiasis further scientific support. The Austrian doctor, Anton Breinl, who had gained experience in the field of tropical medicine as Director of the Liverpool School of Tropical Medicine in England from 1907 to 1909, was the first Director of the Institute.[30] As the result of field trips and research at the Institute, the prevalence of ancylostomiasis in Townsville and surrounding areas was established. It was found to be particularly severe among children in Cairns, from where Turner's and Gibson's first cases had come in 1892. In 1911 the Institute reported a wide distribution of *Ancylostoma duodenale* and that speciments of *Necator americanus* (American hookworm) had also been found.*[31] In the same year Dr Breinl presented a paper to the Australian Medical Congress on the practical and economic impact of hookworm in Queensland,[34] and he addressed a special meeting of the Queensland Branch of the B.M.A. regarding important diseases which he felt required immediate attention. In his list he included ancylostomiasis, filariasis and mosquito-borne diseases.[35]

*In 1902 Dr G.W. Stiles (1867-1941), an American zoologist, described *Necator americanus*, subsequently called the New World Hookworm as it was thought to have been introduced into the western world by the slave trade. Prior to this *Ancylostoma duodenale* (the Old World Hookworm) was thought to be the only genus of hookworm. The differences between them can be distinguished morphologically on microscopic examination, in particular on mouth parts. *Ancylostoma* has prominent buccal hooks whilst *Necator* has semilunar plates rather than hooks. Their life cycles are similar with *Ancylostoma* showing a predilection for dry environments; *Necator* prefers moist conditions.[32] In Australia both types of hookworm were found to exist. *Ancylostoma duodenale*, the predominant species, are believed to have originated from Chinese and southern European sources whilst *Necator americanus* is thought to have been brought in by Kanakas who came from Melanesia to work on Queensland's sugar plantations.[33]

In 1909 the philanthropist, John D. Rockefeller, Sr, with a gift of US$1,000,000 had established the Rockefeller Sanitary Commission (later the International Health Board of the Rockefeller Foundation) in the United States.[36] In 1916 the Commonwealth of Australia requested the Rockefeller Foundation to undertake a hookworm survey of Papua. Hookworm had been reported there in 1911 and during 1916 its existence had been confirmed by the Australian Institute of Tropical Medicine in Townsville. The survey was made in 1917 under the supervision of Dr J.H. Waite. The help of the International Health Board was then enlisted for an attack on the disease in Queensland, a sum of £1552 having been contributed by the Queensland Government over a 12 month period. This was known as the Queensland Hookworm Campaign within the Department of Public Health, working in close affiliation with the Australian Institute of Tropical Medicine, Townsville.[37] The results of the first survey of the wet coastal belt between Cooktown and Townsville are shown in *Table 6.1.* Then for two years the Commonwealth Government subsidised the State's work to eradicate hookworm. With the cooperation of the International Health Board, the Australian Hookworm Campaign was inaugurated on 1 October 1919. The object was to determine the prevalence of hookworm infection and advise on treatment and control. A secondary objective was to promote interest in public health. The results of the Campaign's survey of States and Territories are shown in *Table 6.2.*

**TABLE 6.2: Queensland Hookworm Campaign**
*(First Survey:* 17 April 1916–20 September 1919)

| | Number in census | Number of persons examined | Number infected with hookworm | Percentage infected with hookworm |
|---|---|---|---|---|
| Population | 17864 | 15654 | 3479 | 22.2 |
| Aborigines included in above population | 1479 | 992 | 803 | 80.9 |

*Source:* Final Report of the Australian Hookworm Campaign, Part I, 1 October 1919 to 30 September 1924. p.17.

**TABLE 6.2: Hookworm infection in Australia and its Dependencies Australian Hookworm Campaign, 1919-1924**

| State or Territory | Number of persons examined | Number infected with hookworm | Percentage infected with hookworm |
|---|---|---|---|
| Victoria | 2497 | 0 | 0 |
| South Australia | 3281 | 0 | 0 |
| Tasmania | 2209 | 2 | 0.1 |
| Western Australia | 2846 | 306 | 10.8 |
| Northern Territory | 886 | 148 | 16.7 |
| New South Wales | 23573 | 774 | 3.3 |
| Queensland | 167290 | 15472 | 9.2 |
| Papua | 17905 | 10601 | 59.2 |
| New Guinea | 28234 | 20951 | 74.2 |
| **Totals** | 248721 | 482256 | 19.4 |

*Source:* Final Report of the Australian Hookworm Campaign, Part I, 1 October 1919-30 September 1924. p.17.

**Results of the Australian Hookworm Campaign**

1. It was shown that overall there was a 19.4% infection rate. Detailed analysis revealed that in Victoria, Tasmania and South Australia hookworm was not endemic.

2. A small endemic area around Beagle Bay, near Broome in Western Australia; of the 306 infected cases in Western Australia, 303 came from Beagle Bay and 300 of these were Aborigines.

3. Hookworm was endemic in the northern part of the Northern Territory and in the islands off the coast, and the majority of infected cases were found among Aborigines.

4. The general endemic area in Queensland stretched from Cape York Peninsula (Cooktown) down a Pacific coastal strip with an average width of about 60 miles as far south as Coolangatta. An area around Rockhampton and another around Brisbane could be excluded, but the Ipswich coal mines and an area around Nambour had to be included.

5. The endemic area in New South Wales was along a coastal strip from the Queensland border to the Myall Lakes north of Newcastle.

6. Hookworm was endemic in the whole of Papua and New Guinea.

As part of the survey, further important statistics revealed the existence of other intestinal parasites, including: *Trichuris trichiura* (whip worm) – 4%; *Oxyuris vermicularis* (pin worm) – 1.4%; *Ascaris lumbricoides* (round worm) – 2.3%; all others – less than 1%.[38]

**The effects of hookworm infection in Australia**

The Australian Hookworm Campaign's survey revealed the following effects:

1. Anaemia: in infected cases the average haemoglobin was 72.9%, but some were as low as 20%. In 892 school children, 60% had a haemoglobin of 70% or less.

2. Prolonged anaemia resulted in arrested physical growth and sexual development.

3. Among infected children, mental development could be retarded by as much as two years.

The survey concluded that these effects were visible in only a small percentage of the affected white population, and most of these were children.[39]

**Treatment**

As part of the survey, treatment was carried out and assessed. The conclusion was that one dose of carbon tetrachloride, given in water with a dose of purging salts, was cheaper and more effective than oil of chenopodium which necessitated two doses taken as capsules.[40]

**Malaria and Filariasis**

As a result of a resolution passed by the Australasian Medical Congress held in Brisbane in 1920, the Australian Hookworm Campaign was extended in 1922 to include the investigation of filaria and malaria.[41] This enabled valuable work to be done in eradicating these serious tropical diseases. The results of this campaign which ended in 1924 are shown in *Table 6.3.*

**TABLE 6.3: Results of examinations for malaria and filaria**

| **States** | **No. of persons examined for:** | | **No. of persons infected with:** | | **Percentage infected with:** | |
|---|---|---|---|---|---|---|
| | **malaria** | **filaria** | **malaria** | **filaria** | **malaria** | **filaria** |
| Western Australia | 111 | 111 | 0 | 0 | 0 | 0 |
| Northern Territory | 273 | 273 | 4 | 0 | 1.5 | 0 |
| Northern Rivers District of New South Wales | 145 | 203 | 0 | 6 | 0 | 2.9 |
| Queensland | 8493 | 14362 | 40 | 373 | 0.5 | 2.6 |
| **Grand total** | 9022 | 14949 | 44 | 379 | 0.5 | 2.5 |

*Source:* Final Report of the Australian Hookworm Campaign, Part II, 1 October 1919-30 September 1924. p.17.

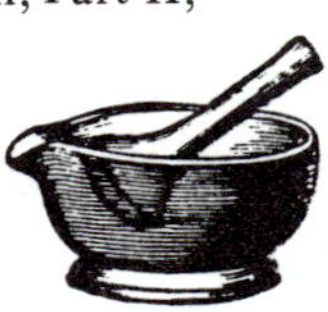

**Conclusions and outcome of the Australian Hookworm Campaign**

The campaign cost £100,000 over five years, 20% of which was contributed by the International Health Board, 40% by the States and 40% by the Commonwealth Government. In the final report it was recommended that vigilance continue for control of the disease, especially in tropical areas. This should include regular annual examinations for hookworm ova in the faeces of school children aged from six to eighteen years, education programmes, improved sanitation and adequate treatment.

When the agreement between the Commonwealth, the States and the International Health Board terminated on 30 September 1924, hookworm control in Queensland and New South Wales continued to receive Federal support and produced a marked reduction in the incidence of hookworm, although as recently as 1955 the disease remained a problem amongst Queensland's Aborigines.[42] Even today it occurs sporadically in a few Aboriginal communities, particularly in north western Queensland.[43]

The Australian Hookworm Campaign eventually achieved its aim, in spite of the delays in its inception; Dr Alfred Jefferis Turner summed it up well when, in 1938, he recalled the days of the battle against hookworm:

> *Our statesmen did nothing, until 1917* [sic] *the Rockefeller Foundation sent out a team to teach us how to do the job. By that time I had learnt something about the obstacles in the way of preventive medicine.*[44]

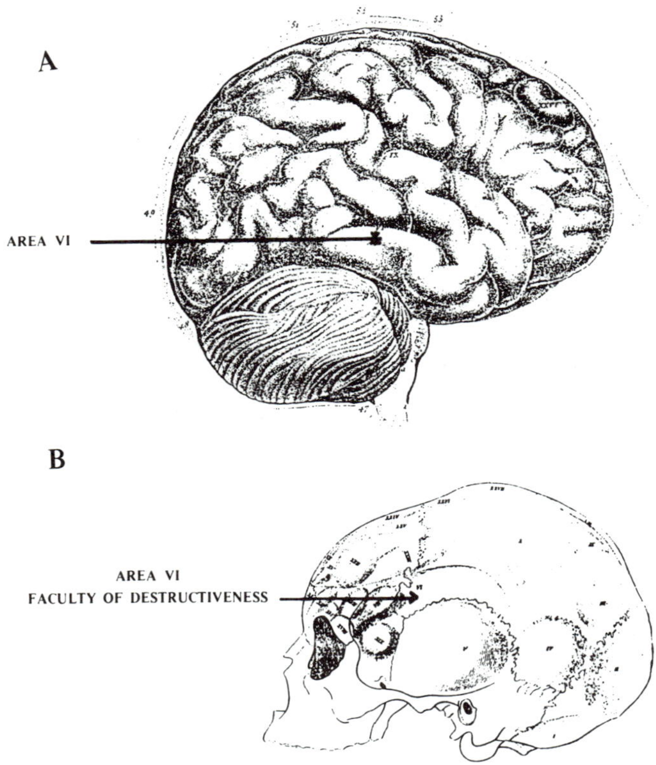


*Figure 7.1: Illustrations from "Anatomie et Physiologie du Systeme Nerveaux en General, et du Cerveau en Particulier". Gall FJ et Spurzheim G Paris Chas. F. Schoell 1810*

*A. Plate XXVII identifying some of the "faculties in the brain".*

*B. Plate SCIX showing the surface representations of these "faculties on the skull".*

# PIONEER MEDICINE IN AUSTRALIA 7

## MURDERERS' SKULLS

**Neville Parker**

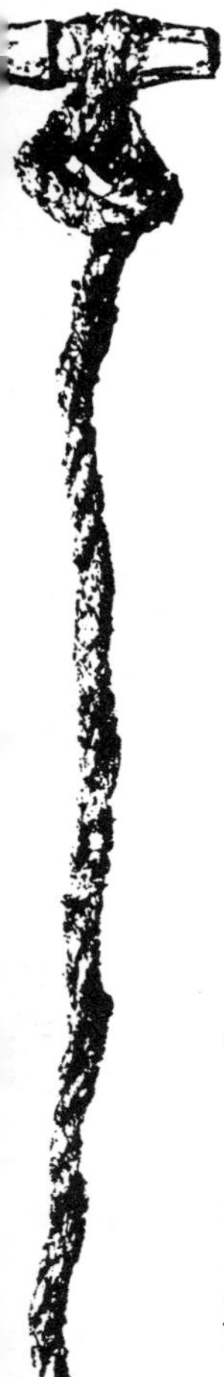

*ON* the 29th September, 1826 the ship *England* berthed at Sydney Cove bringing 148 transported convicts without loss of life. Some of them were prisoners within this prison population for there had been an uprising and attempted mutiny on the voyage.[1] That it had not led to bloodshed was attributed to the efforts of Mr De Ville, a phrenologist who had examined every convict on board before sailing. He identified a number of 'desperadoes' whom he warned should be kept under close scrutiny; one Welshman in particular was singled out as a most dangerous character.

Perhaps it was a coincidence, but all but one of the mutineers were the convicts De Ville had called 'desperadoes' and the Welshman was their leader. The exception was a former sailor who had been persuaded to join them so he could steer the ship to South America. Dr G. Thompson the ship's surgeon, who admitted that he had been sceptical about these phrenological examinations, wrote a grateful letter to the London doctor who had made this innovative suggestion, adding "All the authorities here have become Phrenologists and I cannot get my journals out of their offices until they have perused and re-perused De Ville's report."[2]

Phrenology had arrived in Australia but for various reasons did not flourish here as was the case in Great Britain and in America. Our forebears were concerned with practical problems, and when it came to murderers our administrators and intellectuals were preoccupied with their disposal rather than speculating about the causes of their crimes. Phrenology was seen as a ludicrous passing fad supported by an occasional clergyman and doctor. It was seen to be in the main promoted by a number of self-styled 'Professors' who travelled the country giving public lectures and reading the bumps on people's heads. A central belief of the phrenologists was that the skull could be shaped by the growing brain; after all, they argued, a tender blade of grass can thrust itself through thick soil and a growing tree can displace a solid wall – soft structures can mould the hard.

The founder of phrenology, Dr Franz Joseph Gall (1757–1828) had identified twenty-six areas of the brain, each with a special function and represented on the cranial surface. The strength of these 'faculties', Gall concluded, could be determined by observing the skull for its exterior contours corresponded with the conformation of the brain (*Figure 7.1*).These areas or faculties were increased to thirty-five by his first follower Dr Johan Gasper Spurzheim (1776–1832) an anatomist from Treves. Casts of the head with the skull covered in numbers mapping the 'Cerebral Atlas' were widely used by phrenologists and have now become collector's pieces (*Figure 7.2*).

However it was an Edinburgh lawyer and educationalist George Combe who spread the gospel of phrenology. His book *The Constitution of Man* (1828) became a best seller and found its place alongside The Bible and *Pilgrims Progress* in workers' homes to be studied by the upwardly mobile artisans of the day. Phrenology was the new religion purporting to be objective and neutral, divested of all social and ideological interests. Combe travelled in the United States from 1838 to 1840 lecturing extensively and studying the heads of American prisoners; with emotional fervour he won over converts to phrenology wherever he went. While there he became a close friend of Dr Samuel Morton (1799–1851) Professor of Anatomy at the Pennsylvanian Medical College at the time when Philadelphia was a major centre of medicine in the western hemisphere.[3]

Morton had his reservations about phrenology; however, he felt that Combe's contribution to the mental and moral aspects of human behaviour, based on a study of the skull, complemented his own studies on the ranking order of different races as determined by cranial capacity. When he wrote his monumental work *Crania Americana* he invited Combe to provide an appendix.[4] It was published in 1839, fifteen years after Alexander Pearce, a celebrated Australian convict was hanged for murder. It transpired that Morton was to examine Pearce's skull, following the wide impression that this book made throughout the English speaking world. If the leading authority on the skull was to be found to study Pearce's skull then Morton had no rival and it was sent to him in Philadelphia.

**ALEXANDER PEARCE**

Pearce's head was kept by Dr Henry Crockett, an assistant surgeon in Hobart after he had completed the assignment of 'anatomising' the body. It was not routine to conduct an autopsy on executed murderers at the time (1824), but the Judge had given an additional punishment to Pearce – "Your body is to be delivered over to the surgeons for dissection". The records put it more bluntly – "Sentence of Death pronounced on the Prisoner and that his body when dead be disjointed".[5] Crockett was not the only doctor in Australia to steal a murderer's head; a Rockhampton general practitioner, Dr Callaghan had dug up a grave with help from his brother-in-law, (a Bank manager) and a local businessman to obtain Griffin's skull, which he displayed on his consulting room desk for the rest of his professional life.[6] However, Crockett was motivated by scientific curiosity; he wished to learn why Pearce had resorted to cannibalism and believed that he must have been insane; a study of the skull and its bumps could perhaps provide the answer.

Alexander Pearce was an Irishman from County Monaghan convicted for stealing seven pairs of shoes and transported to Van Diemen's Land for seven years. After absconding from service in Hobart a magistrate decided that Pearce was incorrigible and he was sent to a maximum security prison on a small island in Macquarie Harbour on the West Coast. Escape across the closely wooded and mountainous country, so inhospitable that birds and animals were difficult to find, was considered impossible; but escape Pearcc did,

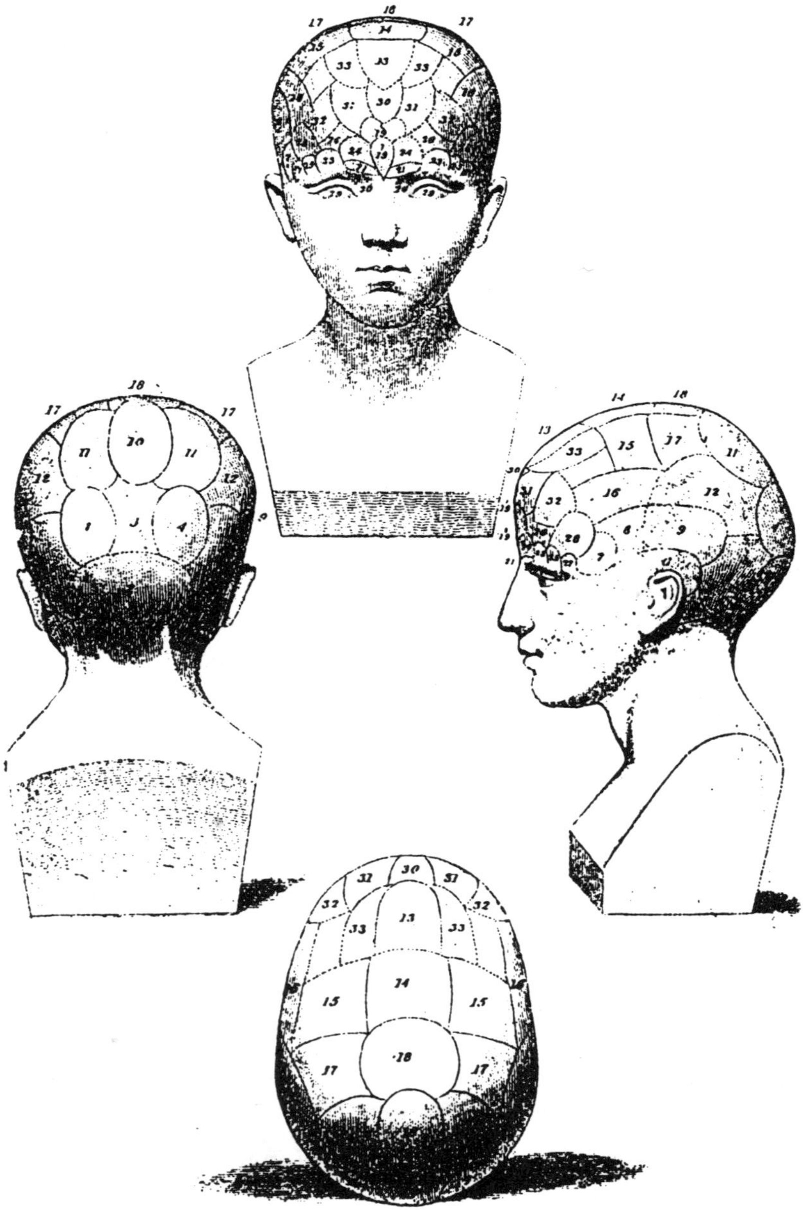

*Figure 7.2: Relative positions of the Phrenological Organs*
*(Reproduced from the Transactions of the Phrenological Society 1824)*

with a small party of convicts. Some reached the settled areas on the eastern side. During the journey with virtually no provisions, one by one they killed and ate each other; Pearce was the sole survivor but nobody believed his story and he was sent back to Macquarie Harbour. He escaped again nine months later, this time with only one other convict, but gave himself up after five days. In his pocket was a piece of human flesh and this time they did believe him for he took his captors to a clearing in the bush where the mangled remains of his fellow escapee were there to see.

Why had Pearce committed these atrocious crimes? Could Dr Morton in Philadelphia provide the answers? Pearce's skull (*Figure 7.3*) was one of the earliest to be examined by Dr Morton and

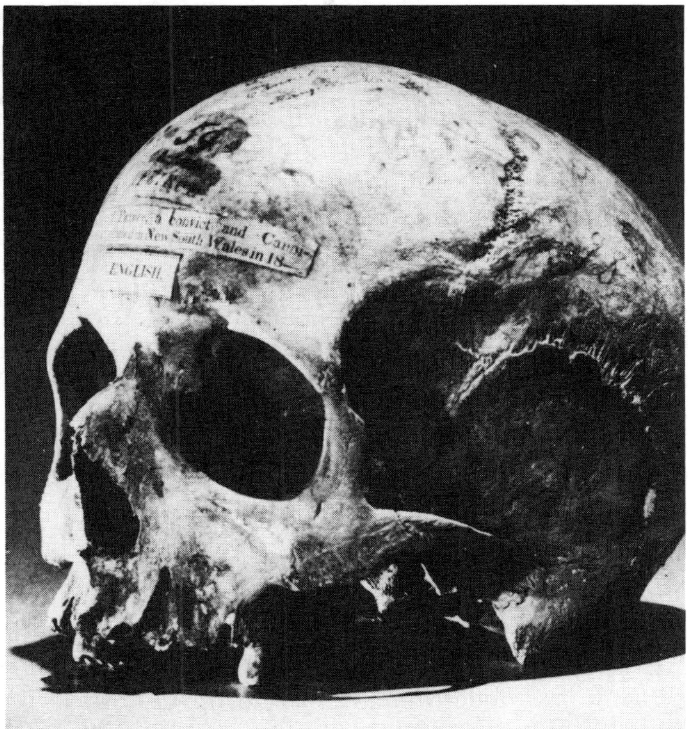


***Figure 7.3:** The skull of Alexander Pearce, No 59 in Samuel Morton's Collection held in the Museum of the University of Pennsylvania, Philadelphia.*

at that stage he was measuring cranial capacity with sifted white mustard seed and the volume recorded in cubic inches. It did not pack well and had other disadvantages, so the seed was later replaced with BB lead shot. Morton was able to classify the races of man in this way and by 1849 (when he presented his final analysis of 623 skulls) he claimed to have identified a pecking order of racial groups headed by the Teutonic Family – Germans, English and Anglo-Americans (with a mean cranial capacity of 92 cubic inches) down to the Negro Group with the Australian aboriginals at the bottom of the list level with the Hottentots (mean cranial capacity of 75 cubic inches).[7]

In these days with apparently faked research results emerging, it is an interesting aside that Stephen Jay Gould, a contemporary paleontologist with strong anti-racist views re-analysed Morton's data and concluded "To put it bluntly, Morton's summaries are a patchwork of fudging and finagling in the clear interest of controlling *a priori* convictions".[8] So much for the objectivity of measurements. For the record Alexander Pearce's cranial capacity was 99 cubic inches placing him in the upper range of the Teutonic Family. Another measurement recorded in Morton's Catalogue of Skulls against Pearce's name, (No. 59) and sandwiched between the entry of a German lunatic and the embalmed head of an Egyptian lady from the Catacombs near Thebes,[9] is the phrenometrical angle of 85 degrees, a high figure in keeping with those for murderers and violent criminals. Had George Combe or some other phrenologist examined Pearce's skull their attention would have been directed to the size of Area VI (*see Figure 7.1*). It was that area that purported to represent the 'faculty of destructiveness' and it is of interest to learn how this area was singled out.

## Dr F. J. GALL

Dr Gall, the founder of phrenology, was an outstanding naturalist whose observations of animal behaviour are reminiscent of the studies of his modern counterpart Konrad Lorenz; both made deductions about human aggression using analogies from their studies of animals. Gall noticed a striking difference between the skulls of carnivorous birds and animals when compared with herbivora (*Figure 7.4*). The former had much larger skull development behind

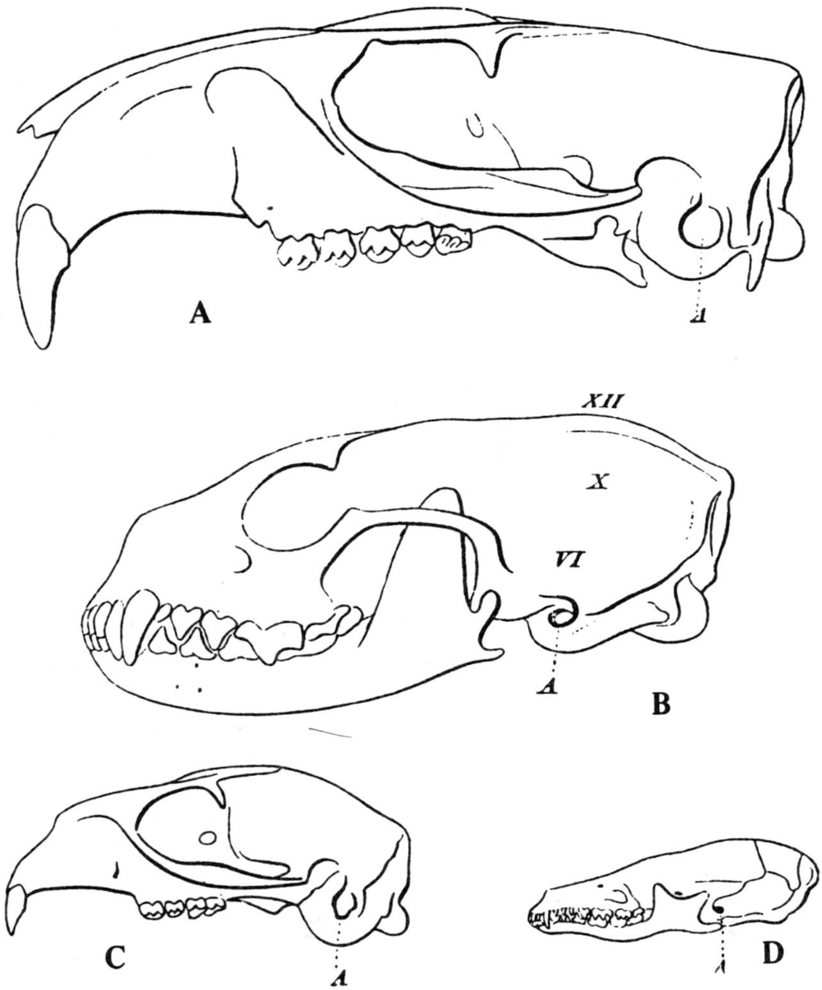


*Figure 7.4: Plate LXIV from Gall and Spurzheim's Folio demonstrating examples of the difference in skull shape between herbivorous animals (Marmot and Squirrel) and carnivorous animals (Marten and Mole).*

*A, Marmot; B, Marten; C, Squirrel; D, Mole.*

a perpendicular line drawn through the external auditory meatus, and there was a prominent bulging above the ear, unrelated to muscle development. At the time he made these findings he was given two murderers' skulls and both had well developed protuberances in the petrous temporal bone.

"Can it be" Gall wrote "that there is any connection between this part of the brain and the propensity to kill?"[10] He had been launched into an investigation of the causes of murder. Gall had a dread of theorising and making generalisations. Like Charles Darwin, he spent years collecting his facts before publishing the findings. Preconceptions, metaphysical theories, codes of morality or theological dogma did not appeal to him and, also like Darwin, when his results were published he was attacked by the Church.

Gall, dedicated scientist as he was, examined all the murderers' skulls he could lay his hands on. There were many available for it was the custom in Europe at that time to give criminal bodies to medical schools and to keep the skulls. He also visited prisons and studied the heads of murderers; they all had the same overdeveloped protuberance above the ears, and the area of brain immediately underneath (designated number VI) he concluded was the seat of murderous impulses. He named it 'instinct carnasier, penchant au merture' and this French word 'merture' was incorrectly translated into English as 'murder'. It should have been called 'the act of killing', phrenologists commented, for big game hunters also had this faculty well developed. To avoid such a judgmental translation Spurzheim renamed it the 'Faculty of Destructiveness'.

Unlike his detractors and many of his followers Gall was prepared to modify his hypotheses. By 1823, towards the end of his career, Gall was able to write –

> *Birth, social position, education, laws usages, and religion exert the greatest influence on the occupations, on the mode of actions of the organs and upon the normal character of man. It would be rash to conclude that the actions of the individual respond simply to the predominant features of the cerebral organisation.*[11]

Innate behaviour could be modified by the environment and this became the thrust in the teaching of the phrenologists about the causes and prevention of murder. Indeed the faculties which the phrenologists described were little different from the driving forces or 'mental mechanisms' used today by psychoanalysts to explain human behaviour.

**FREDERICK DEEMING**

Another murderer's skull, that of Frederick Deeming (*Figure 7.5*) will now be mentioned to illustrate a different approach to an understanding of the murderer which emphasised the importance of an examination of the skull. When Deeming murdered his wife in Melbourne in 1892 it attracted world-wide publicity. After he had bludgeoned his wife he cut her throat and buried her in cement under the hearthstone in a house they were renting near the Prahran market. In that part of the city solid rock is but a few feet from the surface and Mrs Deeming's decomposing body cracked the thin layer of cement leading to such an unpleasant smell that the cause had to be found.

A crumpled dinner invitation found in the backyard of the Prahran house led an enterprising journalist to visit Rainhill (a village in the English midlands) to interview the deceased woman's mother. Further enquiries resulted in another digging under the kitchen floor in a house nearby and this unearthed Deeming's first wife and four children embedded in cement. When Deeming was arrested he was living in a shanty at Southern Cross diggings, a remote mining outpost in Western Australia. He was expecting a visit from a young woman who had agreed to marry him and shortly beforehand he had paid for a consignment of cement.

His trial was perhaps one of the most important cases where the defence of insanity was used in the Australian colonies. Deeming was defended (unsuccessfully) by Alfred Deakin, three times elected Prime Minister of Australia, and he ended his final speech at the trial with a plea that it was impossible to say that Deeming was human in anything more than form, and could not therefore be held responsible for his actions.

Permission was not given for an examination of his brain after the execution. By a happy chance in 1930, however, while excavating to make alterations to the Old Melbourne Gaol, Deeming's skull and left femur were dug up. They were sent to Sir Colin Mackenzie (1877–1938) the first Director and Professor of Comparative Anatomy at the Institute of Anatomy in Canberra. Mackenzie used these bones in a lecture to the Anthropological Society of New South Wales in February 1934.[12] He assembled the casts of a number of skulls – white Australians, Aboriginals, a male gorilla,

A

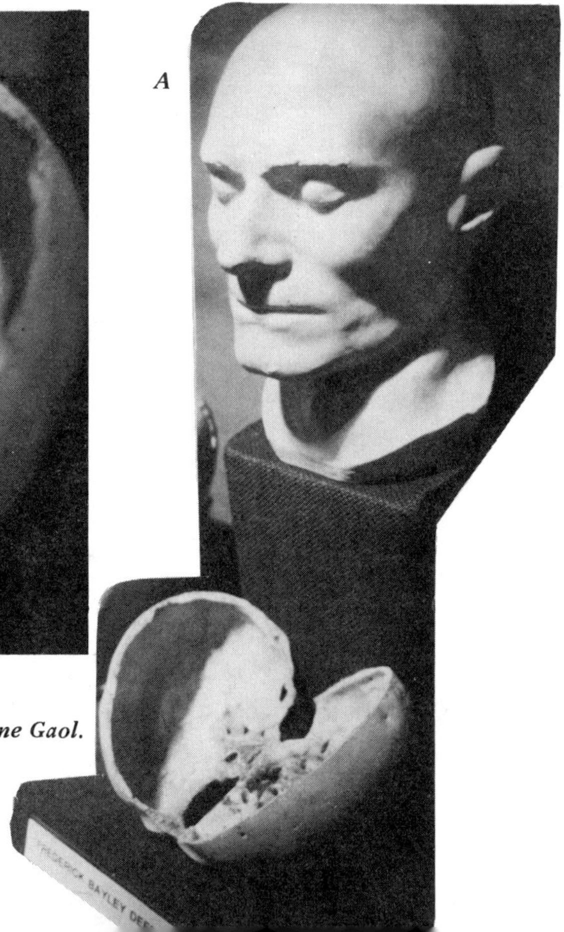

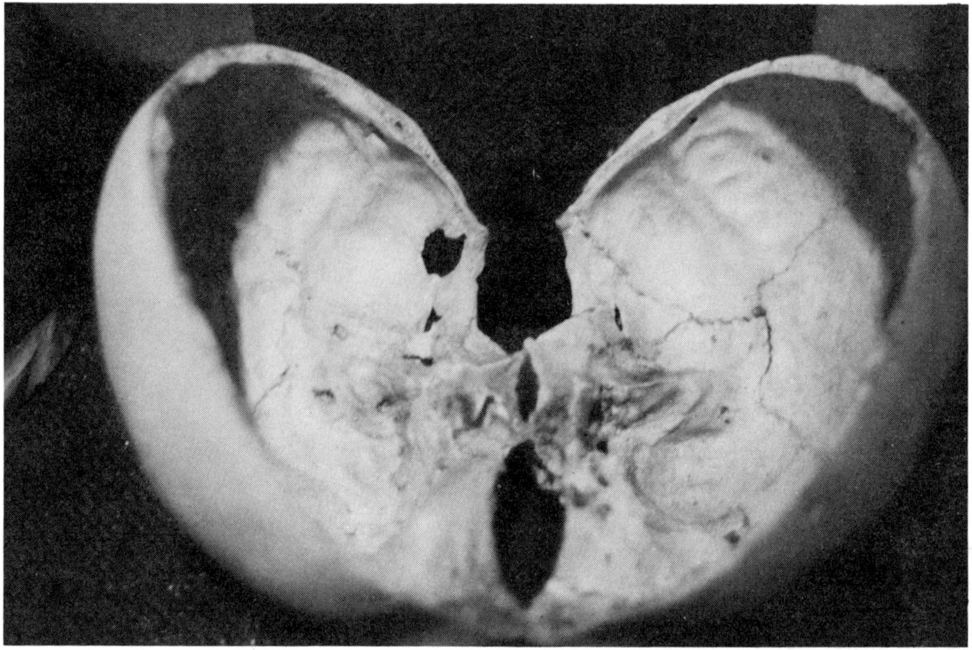

B

*Figure 7.5: Frederick Bayley Deeming's skull — Displayed at the Old Melbourne Gaol.*

*A. Death Mask & Skull. B. Skull*

a prehistoric skull which he had found in the Jervois ranges in Central Australia (which at that time was the most primitive human skull to be found), and for good measure a brachycephalic German soldier's skull a 'souvenir' from the First World War. These were compared with Deeming's skull and Mackenzie concluded –

> *The explanation of his conduct seems to lie in the fact that he was a case of delayed development. It would be an insult to primitive man to say he resembled Deeming, but Deeming can best be described as a primitive man living in the present.*[13]

**CESARE LOMBROSO**

Criminal anthropology in Australia had not progressed for more than half a century when Cesare Lombroso (1835–1909) was lecturing about 'born criminals' who were throw backs to primitive man determined by the size and shape of their skulls and identified by their flattened noses, scanty beards, tattoos, lopsided skulls and other 'stigmata'. As he explained –

> *Suddenly one morning on a gloomy day in December, I found in the skull of a brigand a long series of atavistic abnormalities ... analogous to those that are found in inferior vertebrates ... the problem of the nature and generation of criminals was resolved for me.*

He had identified –

> *... an atavistic being who reproduces in his person the ferocious instincts of primitive humanity and the inferior criminals.*[14]

Lombroso, like Gall, had moved away from abstract reasoning about guilt and responsibility when considering murderers. Stimulated by the discovery of fossil skulls and a study of primitive tribes he measured the skulls of criminals concluding that the 'born criminal' had a primitive brain structure bearing many resemblances to the features in fossil skulls and contemporary Stone Age people; a primitive type of humanity. His followers using ill-defined measurements, unwarranted deductions, and inadequate control groups gave support from their research to Lombroso's theory. It was not until an Englishman, Dr Charles Goring, under the direction of Karl Pearson studied and tabulated material from 3,000 criminals and controls that Lombroso's conclusions were effectively challenged –

twenty years before Sir Colin Mackenzie was talking nonsense about Deeming's skull to a scientific gathering in Sydney.

Goring measured the skulls of 802 prisoners and compared them with 108 Officers and men of the Royal Engineers. He concluded "From those comparisons no evidence has emerged confirming the existence of a physical criminal type such as Lombroso and his disciples have described".[15] Apparently Mackenzie had not heard of that study. Goring however, was too anxious to disprove Lombroso's theories and like Morton in Philadelphia had done some 'fudging and finangling in the clear interest of controlling *a priori* convictions'. Like Gould who re-analysed Morton's findings, another Harvard anthropologist, E. A. Hooton, checked Goring's hypothesis with an even more impressive sample of 14,000 prisoners and over 3,000 non-criminal controls, reaching the opposite conclusion. His statistics showed that criminals are 'organically inferior',[16] but then Hooton's critics found fault with his methodology and demonstrated that there were greater differences in measurement between prison populations than between criminals and non-criminals; Hooton had also been 'fudging and finangling'. Numbers are not as objective as we would like them to be.

**CONCLUSION**

The skulls of Alexander Pearce and Frederick Deeming are a symbolic reminder of the mistakes of the past in our understanding of the murderer. In their time Gall's and Lombroso's scientific studies were models to emulate; many present-day research projects do not measure up by comparison. These two pioneers of criminology relied on careful observations unprejudiced by prevailing dogmas. They used the inductive method coupled with good intuitive judgement and intellectual honesty, and yet their original hypotheses slavishly adhered to by their followers proved to be absolute nonsense.

There were two reasons for this: serious deficiencies in their methodology and an inability to study the brain adequately. Today our measurements are more accurate and control groups carefully selected. However, it cannot be concluded that statistical methods have achieved perfection and it is doubtful whether they will ever provide the answers to questions posed by the social sciences. Just as Morton's, Goring's and Hooton's measurements of the skull were distorted by their personal prejudices so today the collected data turned into numbers may be influenced by the same factor.

The phrenologists were limited to an examination of the skull to make inferences about the underlying brain. Today we have the advantages of directly investigating the cerebral cortex and in the future the mysteries of deeper structures will be open to scrutiny. Meanwhile we must accept the limitations of our current theories; there is too much smug acceptance that we have arrived at the ultimate truth, defending our position with an uncritical belief in the infallibility of the scientific method. If a paper on murder is delivered at the Australian Tri-Centennial Medical Congress our current beliefs may well appear as ridiculous as the conclusions of the phrenologists and cultural anthropologists of the nineteenth century.

**ACKNOWLEDGEMENTS**

Miss Brenda Heagney, Librarian of the Royal Australasian College of Physicians was most helpful in obtaining references and the Mitchell Library Sydney provided access to early records. Mr Dan Sprod, Hobart, author of *Alexander Pearce of Macquarie Harbour* gave me relevant information from his collection of references and correspondence and an Edinburgh friend, Dr William Boyd arranged visits in his city to obtain access to the literature on phrenology and see the Henderson Trust Phrenology Collection at the University Medical School. My understanding of phrenology was considerably influenced by two books: *A Vindication of Phrenology* by W. Mattieu Williams published in 1894 and an excellent recent contribution *The Cultural Meaning of Popular Science* by Roger Cooter (Cambridge History of Medicine 1984).

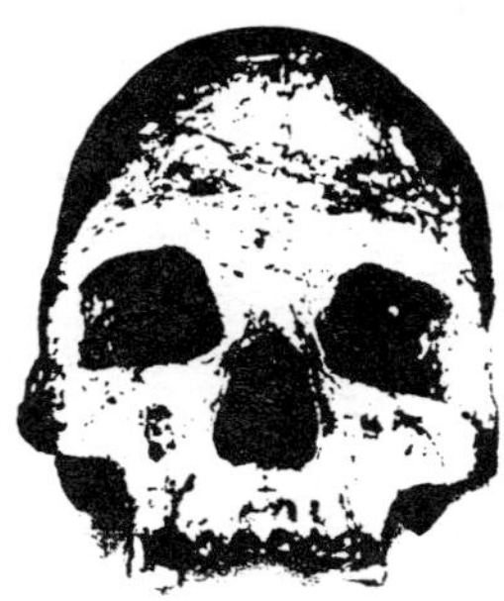

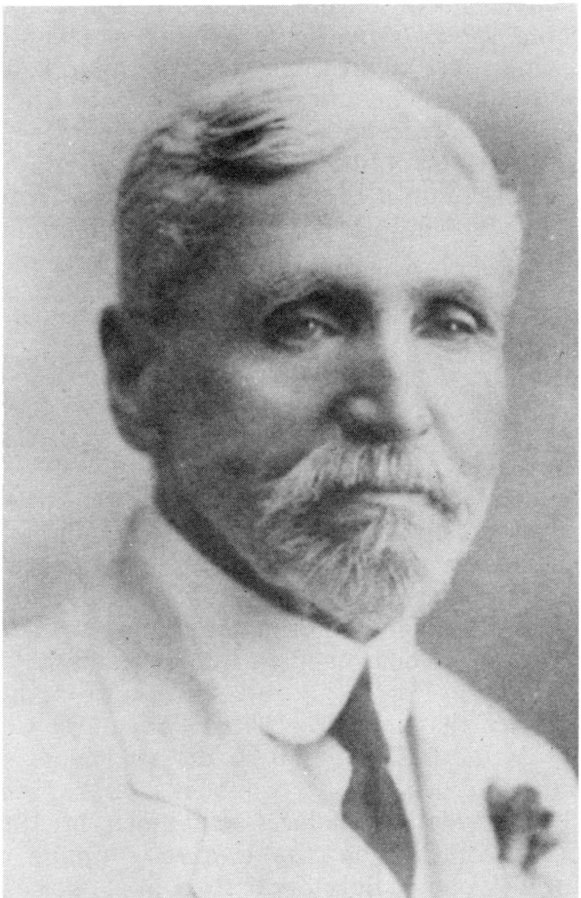

***Figure 8.1: The Honourable Doctor W.F. Taylor MD, MRCSE, DPH, LSA, first President of the British Medical Association (Queensland Branch) (from 1894);***
***President of the Queensland Medical Society 1891, and first Consultant Ophthalmologist to the Brisbane Hospital.***

# PIONEER MEDICINE IN AUSTRALIA 8

## THROUGH THE EYES OF AUSTRALIAN COLONISTS
### TRACHOMA - A Public Health Problem in Northern Australia

**Ronald Wood**

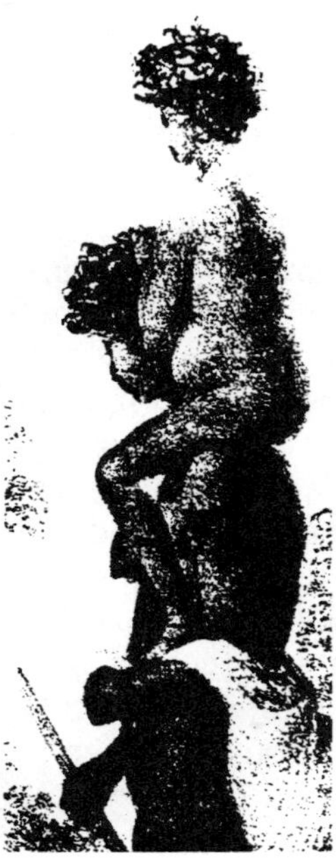

*QUEENSLAND* occupies the north eastern one sixth of the continent of Australia and was originally part of the British Colony of New South Wales whose Bicentennial we celebrated in 1988. It became the British Colony of Queensland in 1859 and the State of Queensland in 1901 when the six Australian Colonies federated.

The Great Dividing Range, the eastern highlands of Australia extends from Cape York Peninsula in the north to the southern part of the continent and separates the short coastal rivers from the longer sluggish streams west of the range which mainly feed into the Murray Darling River system.

In present day practice, the ophthalmologist spends much of his time dealing with cataracts, glaucoma and macular degeneration.

The operation to remove a cataract and insert an intraocular lens may well be the commonest operation performed in western countries today. These three ocular conditions are age-related, occurring mostly in the seventh and eighth decades of life. In 1986 the expectation of life for the Australian male was 73 years and for the female 79 years. In 1901 it was 55 years for the male and 58 years for the female. Because fewer people lived long enough in the early 1900s these three ocular conditions were not common.

What then were the commonest eye conditions treated by the pioneer doctors in pre-Federation Australia? Apart from trauma they were the eye infections of which trachoma was the most troublesome.[1] Trachoma is a specific communicable infection of the anterior aspect of the eye caused by an organism, *Chlamydia trachomatis*, which was not isolated until 1957. If untreated, it causes a follicular conjunctivitis with vascularisation of the upper part of the cornea (pannus), corneal scarring and distortion of the eyelids. It is a potential cause of blindness.

Trachoma[2] was first described in China in the 27th Century B.C. and became well established in Arabia from where it was carried by the followers of Mohammed to other parts of the world. In 1798–9 Napoleon invaded Egypt at the height of the season of severe eye infections. Almost all his 32,000 men fell victim to them. Many in the British Army that followed were similarly affected. Many British soldiers were sent home blind, were discharged from the Army and carried the infection throughout the general populations of Great Britain and Ireland. Ida Mann[3] the great British and later Australian ophthalmologist found no evidence that the Aborigines had trachoma before the coming of white men. The Europeans were responsible for its introduction into this country.

In 1867, Aubrey Brown,[4] co-founder of the Royal Victorian Eye and Ear Hospital in Melbourne described an epidemic of ophthalmia at the Industrial School in Melbourne and recognised two forms of infection, the epidemic and the endemic. The epidemic type was the more severe, lasted a short period of time and was probably caused by organisms such as the Koch-Weeks bacillus. The endemic form of ophthalmia ('sandy blight') was well recognised as being not as severe and yet was a disastrously common cause of total blindness. That 'sandy blight' was contagious was certainly known by Bowen but others did not properly understand this.

In 1941, Sir James Barrett,[5] a distinguished Melbourne ophthalmologist wrote "When I commenced practice in about 1888, trachoma was easily the most common disease met with and occupied most of the time and anxiety of the oculist."

The late Dr E.G. McGuinness told me that when he started in practice in Brisbane in 1923 more than half the eye operations performed at the Brisbane Hospital were to deal with the complications of trachoma which was widespread throughout Australia.

There exist many accounts of eye infection in nineteenth century Australia. The names used to describe these included ophthalmia, blight and sandy blight. One such account was written by W.H. Corfield[6] of an incident near Hughenden in 1862.

> *I was suffering from a severe attack of sandy blight in both eyes, so had to ride a horse which was tied to the bullock dray. I was hors-de-combat for over a week. Not having any eye-water, the only relief I could get was cold tea leaves at night. Fortunately we met the McKinlay expedition returning from an unsuccessful search after Leichhardt. The doctor gave me a bottle of his eye water which he informed me contained some nitrate of silver. This he instructed me how to use, and I soon regained my eyesight, but the eyes continued very weak.*

In 1906 the 'blight' was concerning teachers,particularly those teaching under the trying conditions of western Queensland. The education authorities asked the Queensland Health Department if it were possible to prepare an efficacious lotion which might be obtained at small cost and applied by teachers or parents to the eyes of affected children.[7] The Health Department recommended Citrine Ointment, two eye washes containing zinc sulphate and bi-sulphate of quinine and 'the installation of gauze doors in the schools'. The 1907 report of the Commissioner of Public Health commented on the serious and increasing damage arising from blight among the children in western Queensland. A deputation from the west met the Home Secretary and asked that children with eye infections who could not be treated locally be brought to the coast for treatment. Many parents could not afford to pay for this. Dr Reginald Row from Thargomindah recommended that the best way to eradicate the evil was to have children examined at school by a doctor and for the parents to be compelled to look after their children at home.

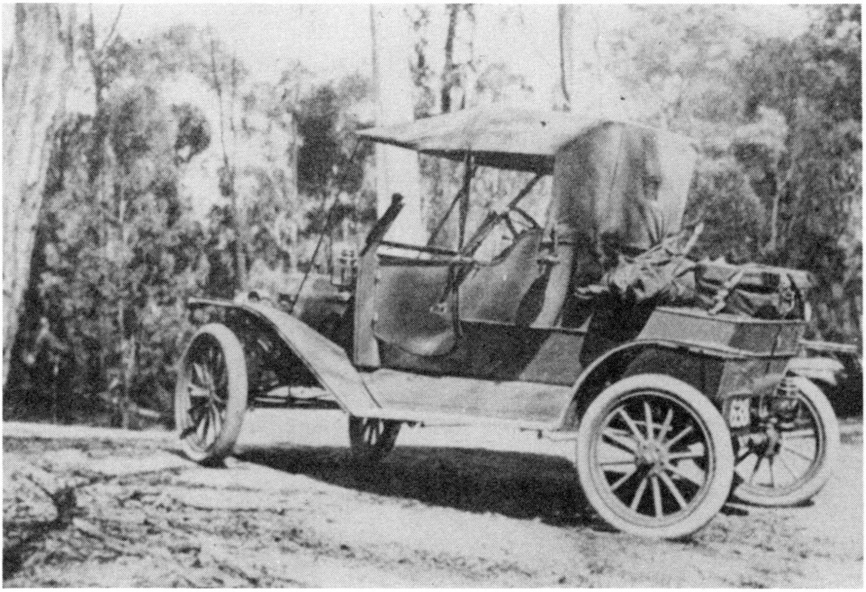

*Figure 8.2: The campaign against trachoma. In this car Dr Douglas Rodger travelled throughout Outback Australia, on his School Health Clinic runs 1913–1915. A contemporary photograph (circa 1914) of his medical and personal kit on a trachoma survey.*

*Photo, courtesy Works Department, Queensland.*

The response of the Queensland Government was fairly prompt. It appointed Hon. W.F. Taylor M.D., (*Figure 8.1*) a member of the Legislative Council to make a survey of the affected areas.[8] Taylor was an ophthalmologist who held a Diploma of Public Health and was a Fellow of the Royal Sanitary Institution. His visit to eleven towns in October and November 1907 took eight weeks to complete. Although he found no sign of acute ophthalmia, 90% of the 1932 children examined had unhealthy eyelids, the result of previous eye disease, 20% had permanent impairment of sight from corneal opacities and 10% were free from the effects of eye disease.

Amongst the twelve recommendations were[9] –

1. Notification of acute contagious ophthalmia be made compulsory.
2. Provision be made for the treatment of all such cases on the spot.
3. Chronic cases be treated locally as are likely to be benefited by treatment.
4. All cases certified by the resident doctor be moved to the coast for treatment.
5. The resident doctor be paid a salary for attending all cases of ophthalmia.
6. A sanatorium be erected on Moreton Bay near Brisbane for treatment of chronic eye cases unable to pay for private treatment.
7. The verandahs and windows of schools be enclosed with wire gauze.

What was the Government response to these recommendations? Like most governments they accepted some. Many schools were screened with wire gauze. Local doctors were appointed part-time ophthalmic officers by the Education authorities at a salary of thirty pounds a year to carry out treatment on school children with eye infections. Routine medical inspection of school children began in 1911 with the appointment of Dr Eleanor Bourne as medical officer. A dental officer and nurse were appointed at the same time. There were 100,000 children in 600,000 square miles to be examined. Bourne[10] later wrote –

> *The reason for establishing the scheme which appealed with most effect to a somewhat sceptical Cabinet was the large amount of eye disease ... on the vast inland plains ... It was ... sufficient to justify the appointment of an ophthalmic surgeon to supervise controls.*

Dr Douglas Rodger,[11] an ophthalmologist trained in England, was appointed. On his first tour of Western Queensland (*Figure 8.2*) 20% of the 1477 children examined had trachoma while 4% had

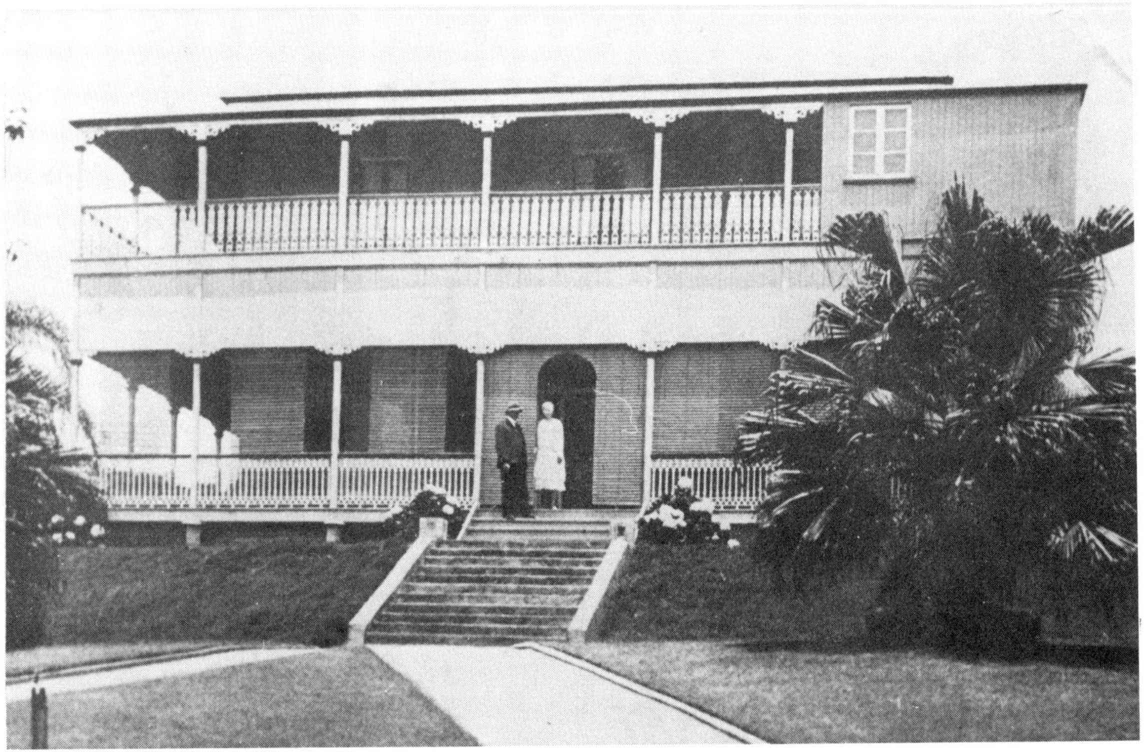

*Figure 8.3: The Wilson Ophthalmic Hostel, Wilston, Brisbane.*
*Named in 1927 after a former Minister of Public Instruction, Queensland State Government.*
*Photo, c. 1928.*

suspected trachoma. Many more had conjunctivitis. In 1915 Rodger reported that the incidence of trachoma had dropped to 9.46%.

Rodger enlisted in the Army in 1915 and was killed in the fighting in France in the following year. Bourne enlisted in 1916 and did not return to the position. She resigned in 1920 leaving the Directorship vacant until Dr Leslie St Vincent Welch was appointed in 1926. On a tour Welch found that eye infections were prevalent and that there was no uniformity of treatment. He recommended the establishment of an Ophthalmic School Hostel in Brisbane and the appointment of an ophthalmic surgeon. Both recommendations were accepted, the Wilson Hostel being established at Wilston twenty one years after Taylor's report (*Figures 8.3 and 8.4*); Dr R.F. Johnson from England was appointed ophthalmic surgeon.

On the Central railway line Johnson[12] found no trachoma before Jericho and Alpha. The incidence around Blackall was 9.1%, Barcaldine 15%, Longreach 27.3%, and at Ilfracombe and Winton an incredible 26%. In the South Western area 32% of children were affected. The incidence at Charleville was 5%, and at Cunnamulla 27.5%. Most children in this area suffered from conjunctival infection.

Johnson proposed specific treatment – painting the lids with 2% silver nitrate using protargol drops, irrigations and Golden Eye ointment along the eyelids. Johnson was killed in a motor accident on the Toll Bar Road near Toowoomba in 1930 and no one was appointed to replace him.

In 1932 Dr Edward Oswald Marks (*Figure 8.5*), a Brisbane ophthalmologist, made a six weeks survey of the South Western area of the State while Dr Charles Victor Watson Brown of Longreach was appointed part-time Ophthalmic Inspector of Schools in the Central West. Watson Brown treated up to one hundred children a day in his surgery for eye infections. Blue Stone (Copper Sulphate) was the treatment recommended for the chronic eye infections! Watson Brown and Ted Marks later came to question the efficacy of this. In the South West, Marks[13] found –

*Active Trachoma in South West Queensland*
*0% Talwood, Morven*
*0–10% St George, Bollon, Wyandra, Mitchell, Charleville*
*10–20% Cunnamulla, Eulo, Quilpie, Windorah, Jundah, Thallon, Dirranbandi, Adavale*
*Over 20% Thargomindah, Eromanga, Nindigully.*

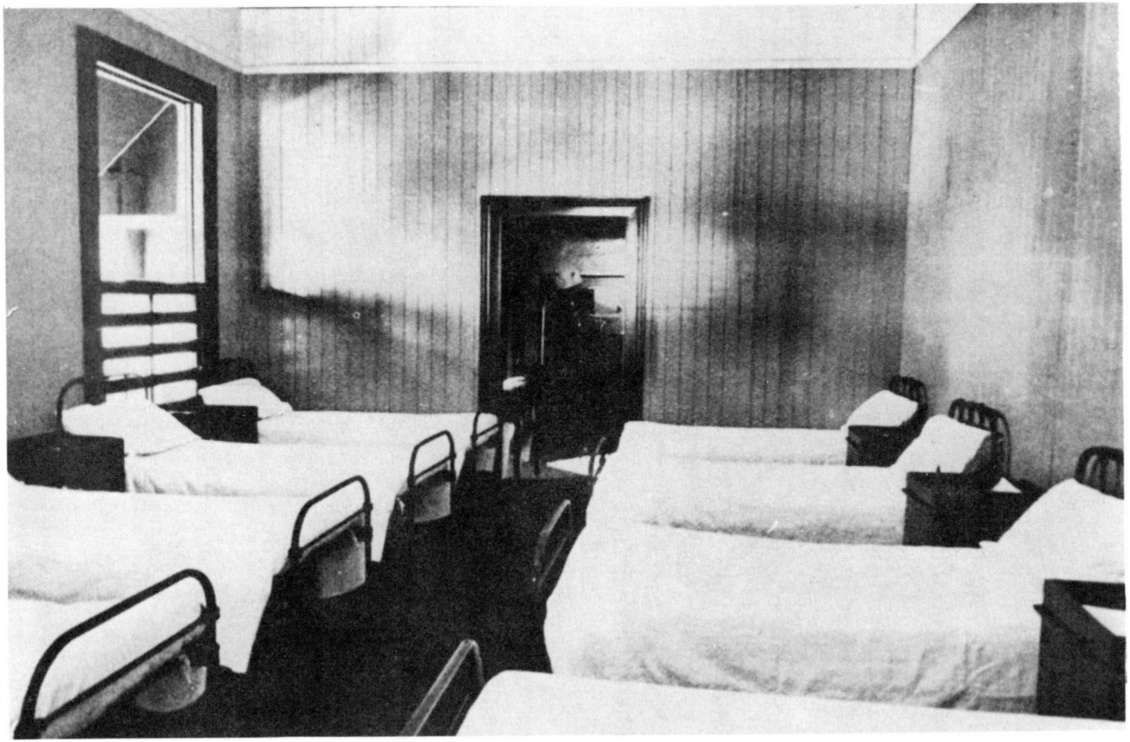

*Figure 8.4: Dormitory for child inpatients at the Wilson Ophthalmic Hostel, Wilston, Brisbane, circa 1928. This stark dormitory bedroom was the home of hundreds of country children, sufferers from trachoma, who were referred to Brisbane for treatment and schooling.*

At St George, 11 cases were found in 150 children but 8 came from one family.

During his 1932 tour Marks examined 1716 children of whom 124 had trachoma (7%); another 56 (3%) were suspicious but doubtful cases.

In his report Marks stated that while not entirely restricted to the poorer classes, very few cases occurred among the well-to-do and well cared for children. In the homes of trachomatous families the conditions were often found to be very bad. There was insufficient accommodation for large families, with a general lack of cleanliness and hygiene. It was not a matter of poverty alone but the lack of care and lack of desire for anything better. Other contributing factors were the dryness and the dust which irritated the conjunctival surfaces, the myriads of flies which were effective carriers of contagion, and the prevalence of acute conjunctivitis. Some centres were comparatively free of trachoma showing that the condition could be eliminated if a vigorous preventive health campaign could be mounted. Marks reported that school children were not the only ones affected by the disease and recommended that this was a matter for the Public Health Authorities rather than the schools alone.

In the nineteen thirties, treatment for trachoma was carried out by the local doctor, hospital matron, bush nurse or head teacher of a school. Severe cases were sent to the Wilson Hostel for treatment by Marks. In 1937 the School Medical Service was transferred to the Health Department.

World War II began in 1939 and the work of the Service was hampered. In 1942, after the Japanese spectacular military successes and arrival in New Guinea, many schools in North Queensland were closed and the children at the Wilson Hostel returned home. When World War II ended in 1945, the incidence of trachoma in Western Queensland was unknown. There had been no survey since 1932 and many towns had been without a doctor during the War.

Marks undertook four tours of the schools in Western Queensland in the eight years following the War.[14] In 1946, 151 of 4,413 children examined (3.4%) had trachoma. The infection was less severe, not one child having corneal involvement. In 1948, 201 of 5,430 children examined had trachoma with further diminution of severity. After each tour, Marks recommended the admission of some children to the Wilson Hostel. After the 1950 tour the parents of one third of the children recommended would not let their children go to Brisbane because of the mildness of the infection.

In 1953 Marks then aged 73 years made his last tour. He diagnosed 143 cases of trachoma from 7264 children examined and only two needed special treatment. The Central Western area was virtually free of trachoma (0.3%) while the South West had 1.7% and the North West 3.9%. The Wilson Ophthalmic School Hostel was closed in 1952.

Although trachoma is the greatest cause of preventable blindness in the world, it produced little blindness in Queensland and was milder than similar infections in Europe and Egypt. In Australia it produced defective vision in affected people,preventing them from engaging in the more lucrative skilled trades. Bacterial transmission was largely from person to person by the use of the same washing water, towels and handkerchiefs. There was little trachoma near the coast where the average rainfall was about 40 inches. The rainfall in Western Queensland was only about 15 inches,occurring mostly in two months of the year. The water collected in tanks was in short supply for most of the year. The importance of bodily cleanliness only became appreciated towards the end of the nineteenth century and was not known by many people. Eye infections were a major health problem and needed the attention of the Queensland health authorities for almost fifty years. Trachoma was finally overcome by the recognition of the problem, and by improved economic conditions resulting in a reticulated water supply in many communities and better hygiene in the towns and in the homes. Although it was not then generally realised that the sulphonamides cured trachoma, the widespread use of these drugs for general infection helped to eradicate it from the late 1930s.

Education of the people 'at risk' from the problem was important in the eradication of trachoma. This was carried out by teachers in schools, by doctors and nurses and by the health authorities. While there are still small pockets of trachoma present in Australia, it is no longer a major health problem.

**ACKNOWLEDGEMENT**

This account could not have been written without the generous support of Dr Elizabeth N. Marks of Camp Mountain who lent me precious original reports of her late father, Dr E.O. Marks.

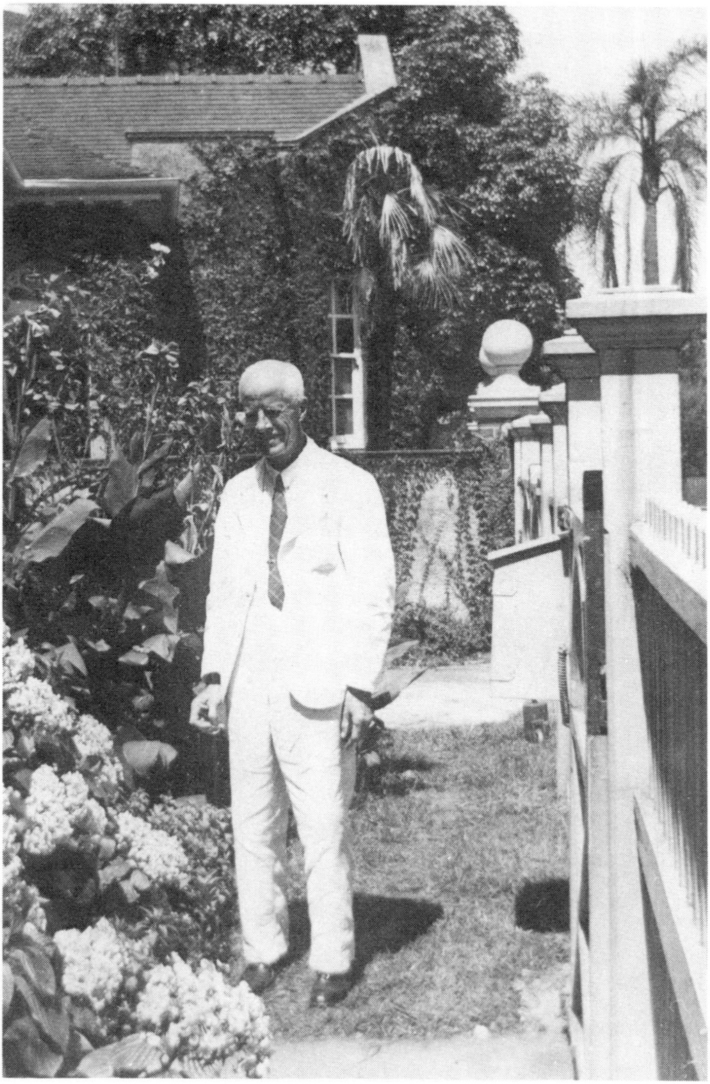

***Figure 8.5:*** ***Dr Edward Oswald Marks, esteemed Australian ophthalmologist and geologist, in his garden on Wickham Terrace, Brisbane. Photo, circa 1965.***
***He led the campaign against trachoma in northern Australia.***
***Photo, courtesy of Dr Elizabeth Marks.***

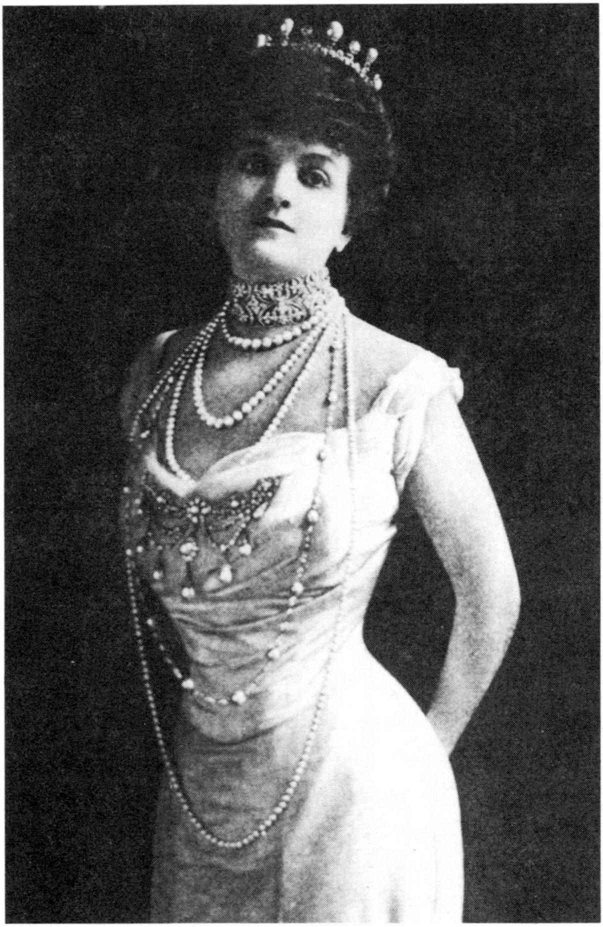

*Figure 9.1: Pearls were formally 'a girl's best friend'.*

*From "The Book of Pearl" (1908) with acknowledgements.*

# FULL FATHOM FIVE

## A Medical History of Australia's Pearling Industry

**Mervyn Cobcroft**

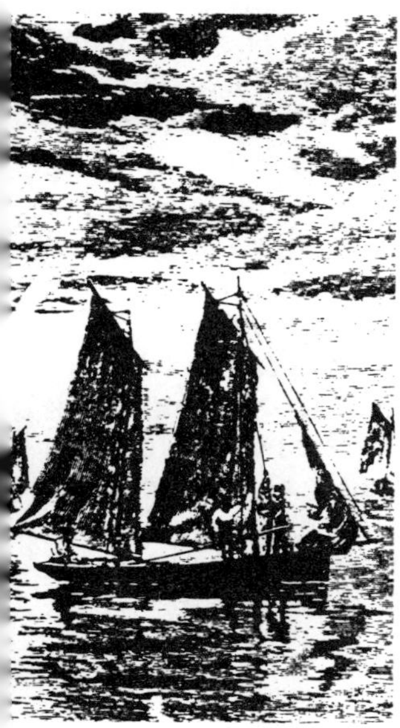

*Full fathom five thy father lies:*
*Of his bones are coral made;*
*Those are pearls that were his eyes ...*

Shakespeare: *The Tempest.*

*MAN'S* infatuation with the pearl, itself a pathological product, occurred prior to recorded time. By the Classical Era, the pearl was, in the opinion of Pliny the Elder, 'the first rank and the very highest position among all valuables'; Cleopatra amazed Mark Antony by dissolving a large pearl in wine and drinking it in a demonstration of the world's most expensive dinner.[1] (I dare say today this cheeky little wine would be said to have a 'strong acid finish' – acetic!). Christ himself employed it as a parable on valuing holiness: "neither cast ye your pearls before swine lest they trample them under their feet".[2]

Only comparatively recently have diamonds surpassed pearls as a 'girl's best friend' (*Figure 9.1*). Today the natural pearl is accorded gem status and despite the enormous quantity of imitation and cultured pearls, a prime example of the natural type is 'sufficiently uncommon to tax the deepest purse'.[3]

This mystique, in part, derives from the great dangers inherent in recovering these rarities from tropic seas half a world away. While jewellers might weigh pearls in carats (or pearl-grains; 4 equalling one carat), it could as well be in drops of blood. It is this equation we will consider (so to speak) 'in depth':

> *The lugger* [returns, the diver dead] *or he's brought back paralyzed for life. He'd have been better dead, though.*
> *"That's one reason why pearls are not cheap," I commented.*
> *"They're never half paid for," he said contemptuously, "whatever the price".*[4]

**The Development of Australian Pearling**

Precisely by whom and when the first pearl-oysters were taken in Australian waters is unknown. Aboriginals or Malay fishermen walking along sandbanks at low tide picked them up for food.[5] The beautiful mother-of-pearl shells attracted them while any pearl was a tooth-crunching annoyance to be vigorously spat out. The Aborigines developed an extensive network to trade pearl shells over an area now including the whole of Australia save the eastern States.[6] The shells had decorative and ritualistic properties. Later white men, on seeing these shells, went to exploit their source from the 1860s on.

It is little known that White Australia had an interest in pearling from the start of colonisation. Entrepreneurs like John Macarthur and Simeon Lord needed commodities for sale in China in return for goods bought for the Sydney market. The penal settlement could and would not (East India Company monopoly) supply this trade. Traders turned to the newly discovered Pacific Islands for such things as sandalwood, bêche-de-mer, and pearl shell; all highly prized in China.[7] For example, Arnold Fisk in the *Favorite* was cutting sandalwood and pearling in the central Pacific before 1810.[8] Fanning even then noted the effects of barotrauma among the native divers despite wildly over-estimating their staying powers:

> *... the length of time they are able, by being accustomed to it, to remain under water, is truely astonishing, varying from twenty to thirty minutes* [!]*; they also take great pride in striving to outdo each other in these duties ... it certainly must injure their constitutions, for on attaining the deck, their eyes appear to have started from their sockets while blood ofttimes oozes from the mouth, nose, and ears.*[9]

Modern pearling began in Western Australia in the 1860s predominantly for shell used in buttons and decorative inlays (*Figure 9.2*). Gem quality pearls, while highly desirable, were purely a bonus. Closely allied were trochus shelling for the same purpose and the harvesting of bêche-de-mer, the Chinese delicacy. The industry exploited tropical seas and reefs around Australia but came to be centered on Broome, Torres Strait, and (to a lesser extent) Darwin.[10]

At first shell was taken from easily accessible areas by either low-tide wading (stonefish and stingrays, notwithstanding), dredging, or unaided diving – 'swim diving'.[5] Some regions soon became depleted necessitating other collection methods which touched the limits of the shell's natural habitat (down to 90 metres) throughout its geographic distribution. This required long periods at sea and 'apparatus diving' based on the diving helmet and airpipe from the surface. (SCUBA – Self-Contained Underwater Breathing Apparatus – is a post-war innovation and never had any currency.) Swim diving, however, continued the whole time in the shallows of the Great Barrier Reef.

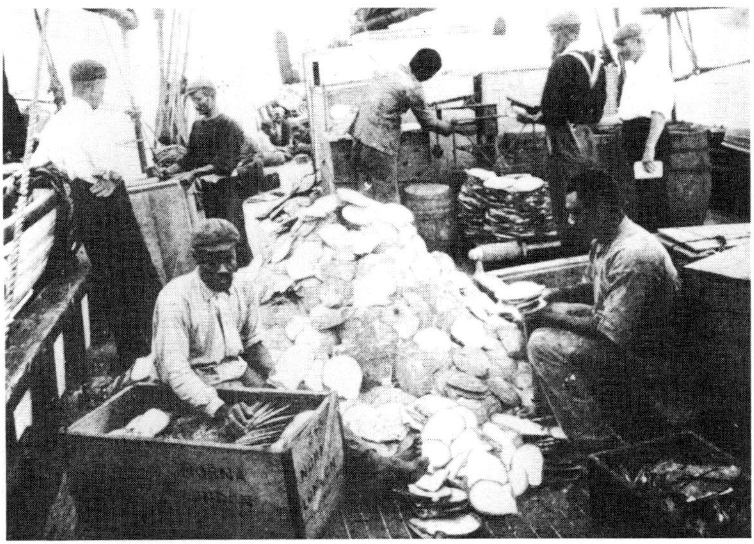

***Figure 9.2:* *Grading and packing pearl-shell, for eventual use in buttons and decorative inlays.***

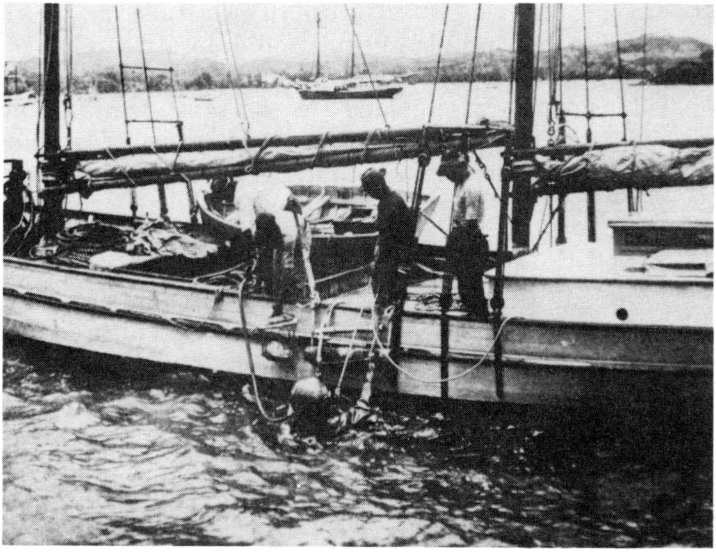

***Figure 9.3: A pearling lugger off north-western Australia, with the diver surfacing.***

Pearling was dominated by Asiatic and Islander divers. As Coombs wrote in 1946 –

> *Although British and Australians are physically able to undertake the work, they have been neither temperamentally nor economically successful and were replaced by Asiatic divers. Gradually the crews of pearling luggers came to be composed wholly of coloured workers.*[10]

In other words, such men cost less and were expendable. For example, in 1947 a diver earned just £5 ($10) a month plus a bonus of £25 per ton (tonne) of shell, well under the whites' basic wage. As for racial origin, those involved at the time of the West Australian peak of 1907 were: Chinese 100, Japanese 1000, Filippino 400, Malay 700, Aboriginal 50, and European (British) 250. And in Queensland in 1933: European 14, Aboriginal 105. Torres Strait Islanders 742, Japanese 352, Malay 24, Filippino 2, Papuan 199.[10]

All these aspects had a profound influence on the risks inherent in the industry.

## Hazards on the surface

### *The pearling fleet*

To work the vast remoteness of the pearling beds required a fleet, typically of several luggers (*Figure 9.3*) or collecting vessels and a mother-ship, usually a schooner:

> *Schooners go out with the lugger fleet and act as floating stations for the deposit of the shells and storehouses for the supply of food-stuffs. In many cases these larger vessels seek the shelter of some mangrove-fringed creek within easy access to the working craft ... The average lugger from which all diving operations are carried on is a two-masted craft about 35 feet* [10m] *long and 12 feet across: its chief pecularity lies in a very small free board rendering its life on a moderately rough sea extremely dangerous. Yet this risky design is found necessary to allow the heavily-weighted diver to descend over the gunwale with freedom and to permit his being dragged on board without the use of blocks and tackle. It occasionally happens that these boats become swamped when a distance from shore and then the entire crew take refuge in the dinghy.*[11]

Normally the fleet would lay-up over the summer cyclone period but sometimes unseasonal cyclones would descend. These ungainly vessels were no match for the fury of such storms. The greatest single disaster to befall any Australian pearling fleet occurred on the night of the 4th–5th March, 1899 when it is believed two cyclones met head-on at midnight over Cape Melville, Princess Charlotte Bay on Cape York Peninsula. By storm's end, sixty-six luggers and seven tenders were destroyed with the loss of 307 men of whom only 12 were white. Those who initially struggled ashore were then swept out to sea by a huge tidal surge.[12,13]

### *Poor facilities, worse food*

With a crew of six and the large amount of diving apparatus, the small luggers offered little space to each individual:

> *Living quarters were cramped and uncomfortable, the life utterly monotonous ... It was taken for granted that lugger crews usually spent part of their lives as physical wrecks ... This probably explains why almost 100% Asiatic labour composed the crews of pearling fleets ...* [10]

Coombs, who wrote this report in 1946 [!], recommended providing such crews with 'wireless sets' to alleviate their sufferings (assuming, of course, they all understood Radio-Australian English!). If they were lucky, the men might sleep each night at a base camp on some lonely northern beach or river bank certainly with mosquitoes, perhaps even crocodiles.

Life afloat guaranteed no freedom from pests. Centipedes, scorpions, black ants, and cockroaches went to sea in droves upon these wooden luggers, causing no comment unless they bit or got into the tea. One diver complained sourly about the cockroaches chewing the skin from his toes giving him agonising pain like 'stubbing my toes against a ring-bolt' each time he entered the salt water. His solution was to pull on washed flour-bags for bedsocks.[14]

These annoyances echoed the lot of common sailors a century previously in that equally dangerous colonial enterprise, the sperm whale fishery.[15] Surprisingly, another mutual, disease-producing factor had not fallen to the thrust of 100 years' progress: food of the poorest quality. In the 1930s, food could be refrigerated, canned, and roaded, railed, or even air-freighted with some freshness. But still men of the northern pearling fleets perished from beri-beri and scurvy. Why? Two forces were at work: (a) the cost of freighting fresh supplies to remote locations meant owners would not cut profits to benefit what some regarded as expendable foreigners and (b) failure to appreciate the subtleties of the exotic and totally different diets of the divers from such diverse ethnic origins. Orientals seemed to eat a diet exclusively of rice so owners were satisfied to supply bags of the vitaminless, polished variety:

> *Food on these pearling boats was mainly fish, in all forms, with rice instead of bread. Beri-beri was one of our big worries on the pearling luggers.*[16]

Coombs recorded the typical provisions supplied in 1935: 'rice, flour, sugar, meat, dripping, jam, condensed milk, tinned fish, vinegar, tea, coffee, pickles, curry, mustard, salt, potatoes, and onions'.[10] (A bit like a shopping list for a fast-food franchise and about as nutritious!)

### *And no doctor*

Unlike their whaling predecessors who occasionally took surgeons to sea,[15] pearlers had little or no access to trained medical staff. In the remote expanse of ocean, they relied solely on the skill or otherwise of the lugger captain or schooner master and the contents of his medicine chest.

Idriess[17] catalogues the everyday complaints which masters dealt with as a matter of course: headaches, stomach pains, tropical ulcers, poisoned limbs from sea stingers, knife cuts, tomahawk lacerations, gunshot wounds, and spear barbs buried deep in the flesh. A friendly lot, those pearlers.

A knowledgeable master was a priceless asset to a pearling fleet. He could and did work miracles. Captain Gregory saved a Japanese diver with severe decompression sickness who had been given up for dead by his crew. Gregory's treatment, in the days long before decompression chambers, was to order the a-reflexic diver re-submersed to the depth he came up from. After careful re-staging, the diver made a complete and totally ungrateful recovery (so we are told). Lou Marshall did the same, keeping the diver down 34 hours, again with complete (but this time, grateful) success. In 1922, Captain Goldie drained a life-threatening quinsy with sail-needle and pocket-knife, the anaesthetic being a knock-out blow to the head. The patient, McBryde, was able to 'walk half-way to the hospital' when they reached Broome.[17]

Not that pearlers got much sympathy when doctors were at hand. As one bitterly commented:

> *The doctor's a white man and probably a friend of the boss, and he knows that a pearling lugger laid up for want of a diver is not earning her keep. He passes the Jap as fit* [even after the 'bends'] *and everybody's happy.*[4]

## Hazards under the sea

### *Apparatus diving*

This consisted of three major elements.[17,18] On the surface, the lugger crew operated an air compressor either manually or motorised. The crew, under the diver's command, guided the vessel as it passed across the pearl beds, either with the help of sail and anchor or later with in-board motors.

The diver wore an all-encasing suit (*Figure 9.4*) over layers of underclothing and woollen garments to combat heat loss in the cold depths. The diver often sweated profusely leading to obvious problems with skin maceration and, I should imagine, salt and water imbalance. Coupled with the inability to drink at depth, this latter

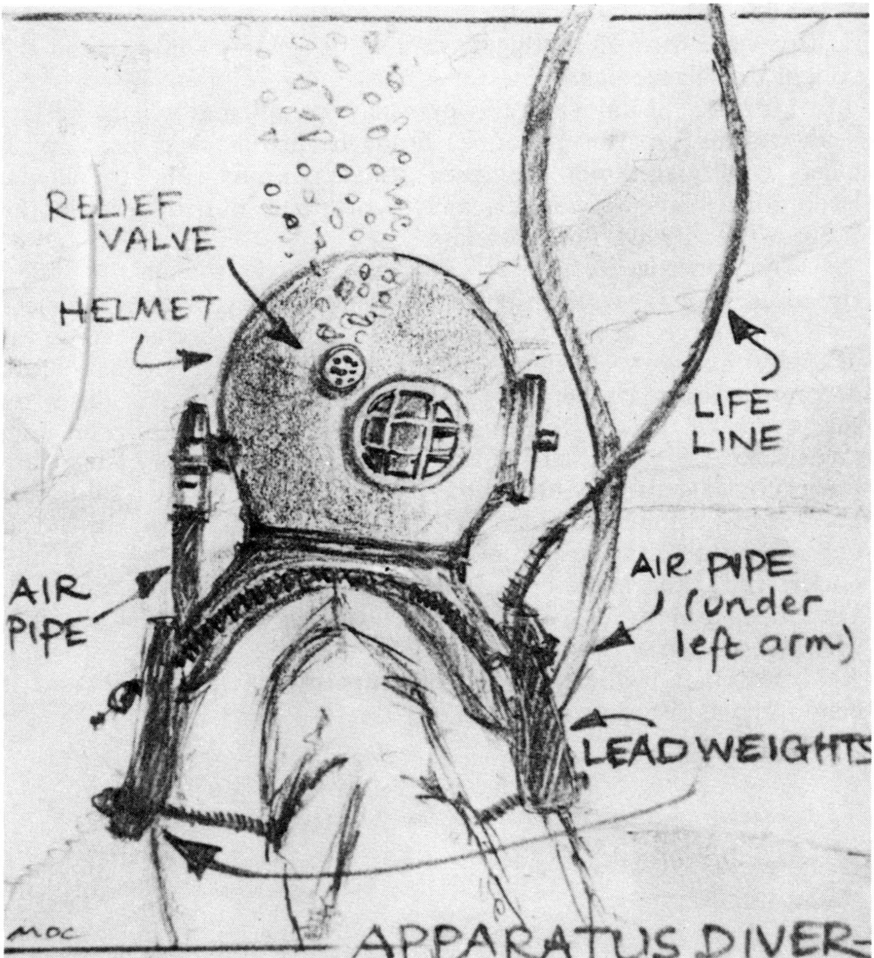


***Figure 9.4:*** ***The apparatus diver on the bottom, in the pearling beds of northern Australia. Pencil sketch by the author, M.D. Cobcroft.***

would not have helped renal function although I have never heard of a case of kidney stones or infection. The heavy helmet which enclosed the head was bolted to a corselet over the shoulders. Vision was through thick glass plates. A diver's 'sinkability' was further enhanced with leaded boots and chest weights.

The most important component was the diver's link with the surface. His life-line was used to haul him up and for communication via a complex language of jerks and tugs (throat microphones belong to the Space Age). The air-line was of rubber and ran from compressor to the diver's helmet. A controllable relief valve let spent air escape; if closed, the suit inflated allowing the diver to clear obstacles or to float to the surface. This pocket of air was sometimes used as an emergency supply should the diver be in dire trouble.

Such a complex system required great skill. There were no diving schools where a team went to acquire proficiency. It was all 'on-the-job training'. Inexperience obviously courted disaster; equipment malfunctions were a significant contribution to man loss, none more so than problems with air-pipes. Air-pipes were made from rubber, not from today's high-pressure, kink-resistant synthetics. Pipes would sometimes rupture or become hopelessly entangled on coral outcrops.

Foul play was not unknown. Benham[14] tells how he murdered an innocent Japanese diver by kicking his face glass in with leaded boots, such was the intensity of rivalry between crews. More than once, rumour had it, a crew eliminated a troublesome diver by 'accidentally' allowing engine exhaust to be sucked into the air intake.

*Diving physiology*

It has been a long road (?swim) to an understanding of man's adaptability to a sub-aquatic existence. It is a journey which quickened with the advent of SCUBA equipment but one which has not yet finished. This is an enormous subject,[19] the details beyond this historical review. Little wonder pearling divers, with either non-existent or limited knowledge, succumbed with a resignation born of ignorance.

All the first-hand accounts mention two feared medical complications of pearling. The first, *barotrauma* (worst just under the surface by virtue of the Boyle's Law), is dismissed as an inconsequential annoyance be it in swim divers who learned to burst ear drums or apparatus men who noticed blood from nose or ear inside their helmets.[20]

None makes light of the second, the result of too deep diving or too rapid ascent – what we now call *decompression sickness.*

Swim divers (*Figure 9.5*) worked to four or five fathoms (7 to 9 m) for just over a minute. Apparatus divers were wary of depths over 20 fathoms (36 m) with only the most experienced venturing beyond 30 (54 m) – the pressure increases by a factor of one atmosphere with every 10 m descent.[18-21]

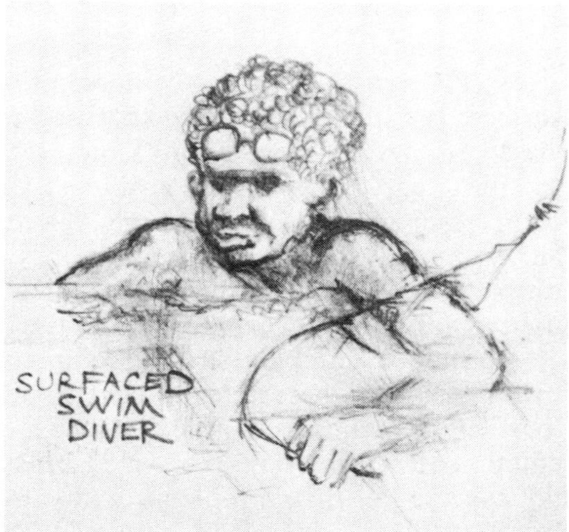


***Figure 9.5:* *The swim diver surfacing after the quest for pearls. Pencil sketch, by the author, adapted from Bartlett's 'The Pearl Seekers'.*[18]**

Too deep descent was sometimes accidental: a life-line might part, perhaps cut by a boat propeller; a diver might plummet into an unexpected crevasse on the sea floor; or a large tidal rise such as the 15 metre increase caused by the topography of King Sound ('The Graveyard') north of Derby might catch a diver out. At other times it was a deliberate, calculated risk taken for those elusive large shells, left to grow to that size by more cautious men. The infamous 'Darnley Deeps' of Torres Strait lured many a diver to his death. The result was a body horribly twisted and crushed up into the unyielding brass diving helmet. It had to be unceremoniously hacked out or buried as retrieved, suit and all. (*Figure 9.6*)

Decompression sickness was caused by too rapid an ascent, nitrogen bubbles forming in body tissues like the fizz of champagne when the cork is popped. The symptoms depend on which organs are involved, and are complexly related to dive time, depth and rate of ascent. Most cases in the pearling industry either affected the muscles and joints (the painful and crippling 'screws' or 'bends') or the spinal cord (paralysis) although other types did occur. Clark's description of the fatal pulmonary 'chokes'[20] makes frightening reading for divers and doctors of today.

Little was known of this phenomenon prior to the First World War; for instance, there was a 10% mortality per year amongst divers at Broome.[18] With the advent of 'staging' (resting a diver at various levels on his ascent to allow dissipation of dissolved gas), the situation improved dramatically. However this did not meet with universal approval as many divers saw it as an unproductive waste of time. These men cut corners, and were prepared to endure the aches and pains of the mild 'bends' which they eased with massage and embrocations. Inexorably, their bodies withered provided they did not kill themselves in the process. Policeman Hall recalls the shock of seeing a long-time Japanese diver remove his suit to reveal the lower portion of his body as a wasted, contorted skeleton.[13]

As we have seen, serious decompression problems could only be treated by re-submerging the diver. Mortality remained high despite this.

*Creatures of the deep*

While shark attack[22] looms large in the public imagination, research shows that most pearling injuries or deaths were due to air-line or pressure–decompression accidents.[18] Sharks generally avoided helmeted divers. It was generally believed that they were scared off by the constant stream of air bubbles or they found the vibrations set up by the pulsating air-pipes unpleasant. In the few recorded attacks (less than five), the diving suit may have been inadvertently smeared with fish slime or the remains of a boiled beef breakfast.[18] For the swim divers of the Barrier Reef the situation was marginally worse: 45 attacks, 12 fatal, in nearly seventy years.[13] Some escapes were almost miraculous, the most celebrated being those of two Torres Strait Islanders, Treacle and Iona Asai. In both attacks, the shark had the diver by the head but let go when the victim gouged the shark's eyes.[23] (*Figure 9.7*)

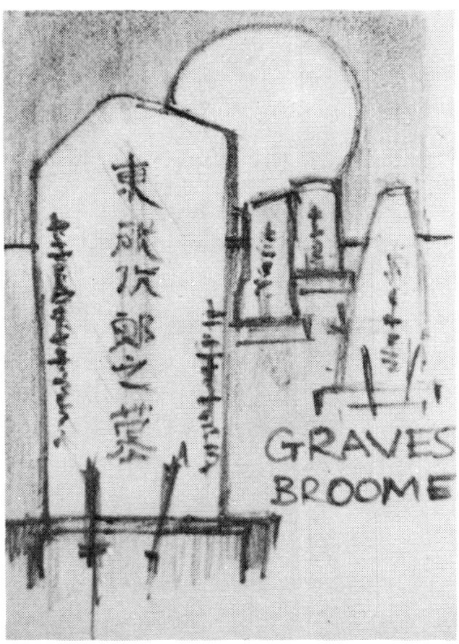


***Figure 9.6:* Many of the best pearl divers in Northern Australian waters have been Japanese. Their graves are to be found in pearling towns throughout the North.**

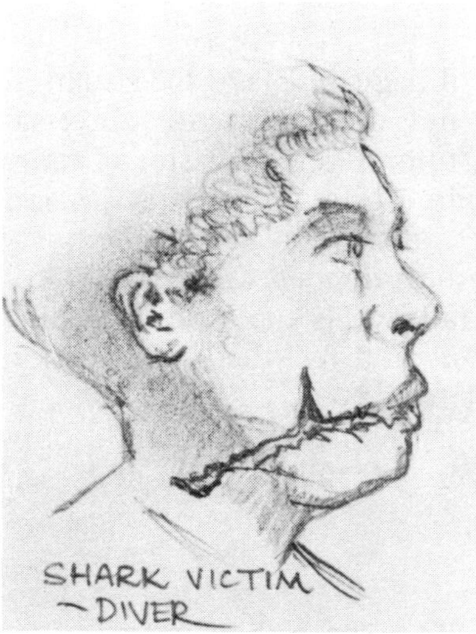


***Figure 9.7:* Healed keloid scar on the face of a Torres Straits pearl diver following a shark attack. Pencil sketch from a photograph in Bartlett's 'The Pearl Seekers'.**[18]

There were isolated reports of other sea creatures blundering into divers and their lines – a whale,[17] manta ray,[18] and octopus.[24] These harmless encounters did more to quicken the pulse of the book-buyer than harm the diver. The first edition of Idriess' *Forty Fathoms Deep* (1937) came with a dust-jacket illustration* of a struggling diver wrapped in the wings of a Devil Ray like some apocalyptic horseman's cape (and a fish with luminous tentacles from the abyssal depths!); the 1984 edition has but three sharks!

The tropic seas are full of stinging organisms[25] but these barely rate a mention in contemporary accounts.

## Hazards on the land

The home bases of pearling fleets were rough-and-ready towns spaced along the northern coastline, places like Broome, Darwin, and Thursday Island (the 'sink of the Pacific' as one aptly called it).[18] It was here that shell and pearl were traded, provisions bought and boats restocked; here it was that dying or dead divers were unshipped and new crews taken on, luggers and equipment stripped and repaired, and here fleets laid-up while summer storms whipped up seas and muddied bottoms.

> *Broome is the great centre for all pearlers. It is a blistering little settlement, situated on the edge of Roebuck Inlet – a mangrove-lined salt-water creek, which harbours a most powerful species of mosquito – and a population made up of fifty whites and five hundred of mixed ... race.*
>
> *Such a population, as may be imagined, is a somewhat dangerous one, and it appears all the more so when it is known that the pearlers' 'hotels' are but villainous drinking-saloons, run, alas!, by one or two unscrupulous white men.*

*Oh that the cover of this book of Australian medical history would sell as many copies. [Ed.]

> *Details of life in this out-of-the-way township may well be spared the reader. It is one of the hottest corners on the face of the earth, which statement is true in the double sense, thanks to the miserable influence of the renegades mentioned...*[11]

The numerous ethnic groups ('seventeen over the known human races') congregated in shanties or squatter camps, the Japanese 'Yokohama' of Thursday Island being a typical example. Boredom, especially during the lay-up, was as stifling as the dust of the dry season and the humidity of the wet. Men found diversion in gambling, opium or alcohol, and women. Among the divers there was, quite rightly, a 'live today, die tomorrow' fatalism.[13,17,18]

It was a recipe for disaster.

Broome witnessed one such calamity. For three blazingly hot December days in 1920, a war raged between hundreds of rampaging Japanese and defending East-India Koepangers. The Japanese accused the Koepangers of the deaths of some of their number (which was probably true). Boredom, alcohol, and the heat intensified the acrimony. Police Inspector Thomas and a band of hastily-sworn special constables stood between the two. It is to their credit that they managed to keep the killing to a few on each side although there were many battered and bleeding casualties. Ironically, Thomas was the only European to die; he suffered a massive heart attack as peace was being restored.[17]

Murder was by no means uncommon. The usual motive was either disputes over women or underhand dealings in stolen pearls.[17] Sometimes an Asiatic (mostly Malay) would run 'amok' for no apparent reason; a hospital doctor narrowly missed having his throat cut in one such incident in which three others died.[4,18] Provided the victim was not white, very little notice was taken but, if he were, justice was swift and deadly.[13,18] In the early days, there were occasional attacks by tribal Aborigines; retribution was likewise fast, furious, and excessive.[18]

Venereal disease was the greatest, single, 'land-based' malady preventing divers putting to sea. The main reservoir was the group of professional prostitutes who serviced the larger settlements.[13,14,18] The loss of working time was so bad at Thursday Island at the beginning of this Century that the 1868 *Contagious Diseases Act* which required obligatory medical examinations and imprisonment of positive cases was invoked. This created so much protest and cost so much that it had to be rescinded in favour of voluntary checks.[13]

Alcohol was always troublesome. Binges on return to port were thought of as normal behaviour and led inevitably to problems, both acute and chronic.[14,18]

*Dived in the depths of the Darnleys, down twenty fathom and five;*
*Down where by law and by reason, men are forbidden to dive;*
*Down in a pressure so awful that only the strongest survive:*

*Sweated four men at the air pumps, fast as the handles could go,*
*Forcing the air down that reached him heated, and tainted, and slow –*
*Kanzo Makame the diver stayed seven minutes below;*

*Came up on deck like a dead man, paralysed body and brain;*
*Suffered, while blood was returning, infinite tortures of pain:*
*Sailed once again to the Darnleys – laughed and descended again!*

*Down in the ooze and the coral, down where earth's wonders are spread,*
*Helmeted, ghastly, and swollen, Kanzo Makame lies dead:*
*Joe Nagasaki, his 'tender', is owner and diver instead.*

*Wearer of pearls in your necklace, comfort yourself if you can,*
*These are the risks of the pearling – these are the ways of Japan,*
*'Plenty more Japanee diver, plenty more little brown man!'*

A. 'Banjo' Paterson; *The Pearl Diver*; 1902.

★

*Acknowledgements*

The author wishes to thank the following for their assistance in researching this paper: A.J. Cobcroft; CPO P. Lane RAN; Professor John Pearn; also the Staff of the John Oxley Library, Brisbane, and Lansdowne Press, copyright holder of Paterson's poem *The Pearl Diver*.

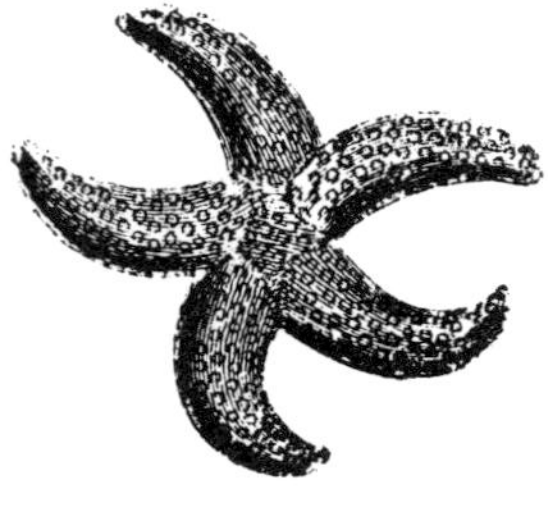

# PART III

# PUBLIC HEALTH AND TROPICAL MEDICINE

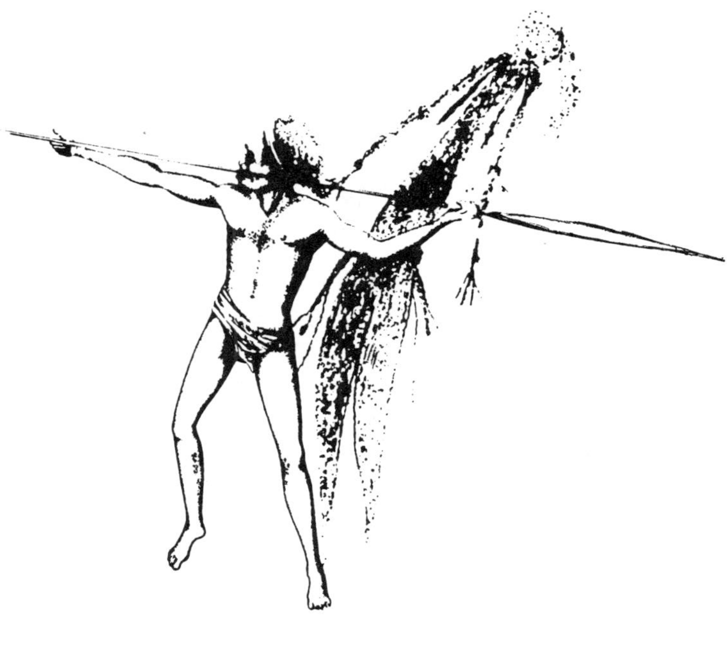

# PIONEER MEDICINE IN AUSTRALIA 10

## *ONE DAY IN THE MEDICAL LIFE OF QUEENSLAND*

### *The Opening of the Australian Institute of Tropical Medicine*

**Robert Douglas**

*ON* the 28th June, 1913, were gathered together a group of individuals, in the grounds of the Townsville Hospital. Their presence and contiguity has been preserved, from that instant in time (*Figure 10.1*) when they attended the official opening of the new building specifically erected to house the Australian Institute of Tropical Medicine.

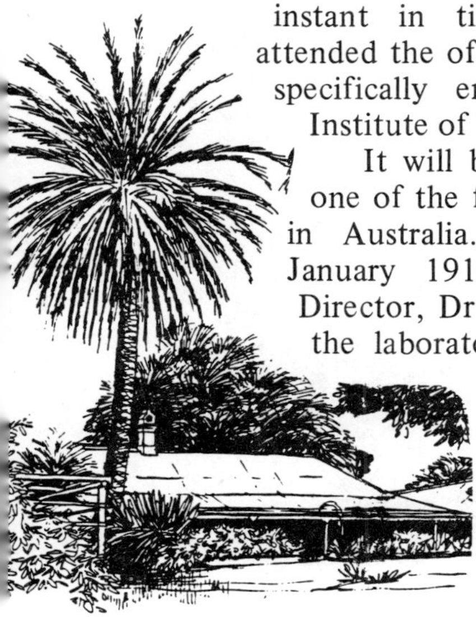

It will be recalled that the A.I.T.M. was one of the first institutes of medical research in Australia. It commenced operations in January 1910 with the arrival of its first Director, Dr Anton Breinl, and his only help, the laboratory assistant John Fielding. As a result of a 1911 recommendation by Professor W.A. Osborne, Professor of Physiology at the University of Melbourne, it was decided to widen the scope of the Institute. There was thus the need for the new building to

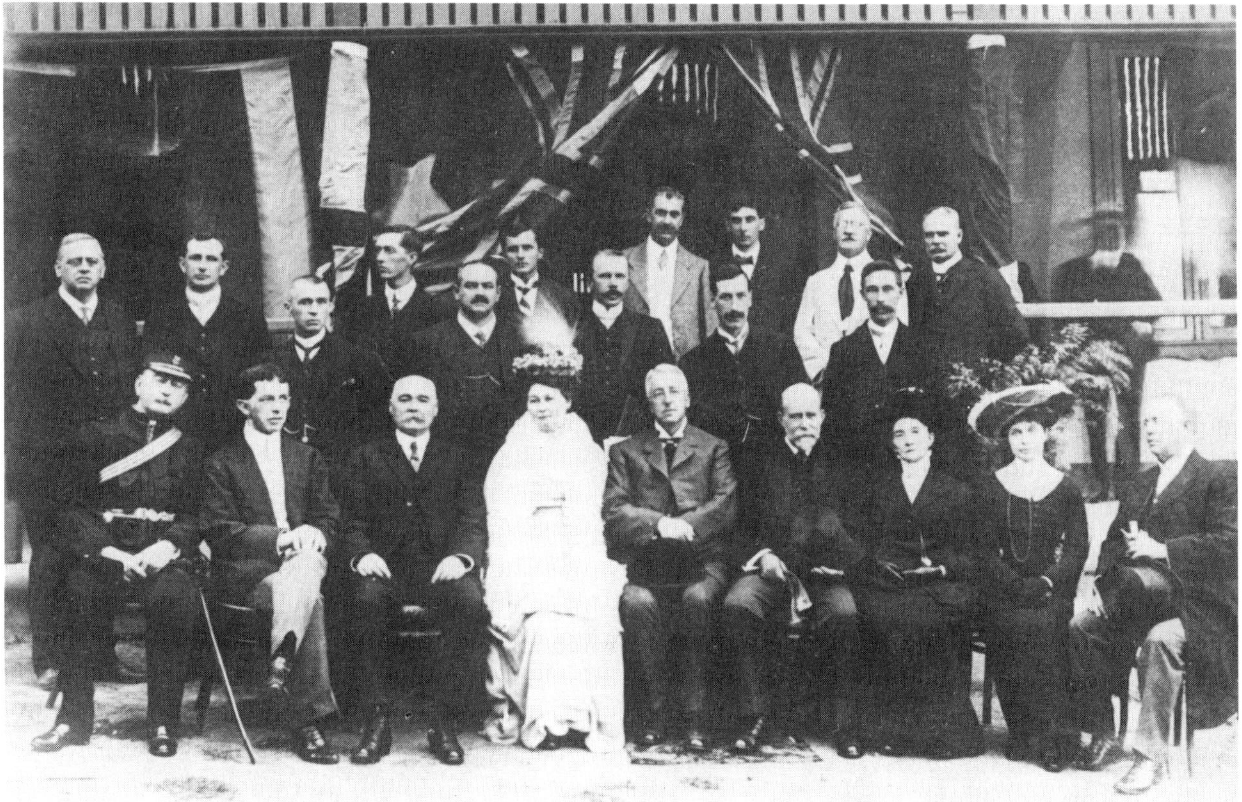

*Figure 10.1: Photograph of Opening of the Australian Institute of Tropical Medicine, Townsville, 28th June 1913.*

*BACK ROW (left to right)*

*Mr F.H. Taylor, FRES, Entomologist to A.I.T.M. 1911–1918 and 1925–1945.*
*Mr J.W. Fielding, FRMS, Laboratory Technician, A.I.T.M. 1910–1954.*
*Dr C.H. Cormac, Bowen.*
*Dr W.J. Young, Biochemist to A.I.T.M., 1910–1919.*
*Dr R.B. Huxtable, Charters Towers.*
*Dr E. Humphrey, Townsville.*

*MIDDLE ROW (left to right)*

*Dr C.J. Parkinson, Townsville.*
*Dr T.G. Ross, Townsville. (Superintendent of the Townsville General Hospital).*
*Mr Jacob Leu, Townsville (Solicitor), President of the Townsville Hospital Board.*
*Mr H.C. Johnson, Town Clerk of Townsville.*
*Captain Foxton, (ADC to Sir William MacGregor).*
*Dr W. Nicoll, Parasitologist to A.I.T.M., 1912–1915.*
*Dr H. Priestley, Bacteriologist to the A.I.T.M., 1912–1917.*

*FRONT ROW (left to right)*

*Dr J. Ahearne, Townsville.*
*Dr A. Breinl, Director, A.I.T.M. 1910–1920.*
*Mr R.W. McCelland, Mayor of Townsville.*
*Lady MacGregor, Wife of the Governor of Queensland.*
*Professor T.P. Anderson Stuart, Professor of Physiology at the University of Sydney, Founder of the Medical School at that University and one of the founders of the A.I.T.M.*
*Sir William MacGregor, MD, Governor of Queensland, 1909–1914.*
*Mrs McCelland, wife of the Mayor of Townsville.*
*Mrs Anderson–Stuart, wife of Professor T.P. Anderson–Stuart.*
*Dr Wilton Love, Brisbane.*

house the additional staff who had been recruited in England in 1912 by Professor T.P. Anderson Stuart and Professor H.B. Allen. The new members of staff, who all appear in the photograph (*Figure 10.1*) were Dr W. Nicoll, Dr W.J. Young and Dr H. Priestley.[1,2].

On an overall inspection of this photograph the exact instant in time cannot be identified, but I would think from the light at the western end of the building, it was probably late afternoon at an exposure time of 1/40th second, because of the blurred figure in the background. Above Breinl there hangs what was for long thought to be a piece of bunting, but is of course the flag of his native Austria.

Although the whole idea of having an institute of research was first suggested to Bishop Frodsham by Dr R.A. O'Brien of Cairns, no one in the Official Party was from Cairns. In 1910 Townsville had a population of 10,000 people and the population of Cairns would have been less than half that number. Representatives are present in the photograph from Charters Towers, Bowen and Ayr. It is not known why Cairns was not represented.

Dr Anton Breinl was the first Director.[1-3] His greatest achievement in medicine occurred before he came to Australia and was the successful use of the pentavalent arsenical drug Atoxyl against trypanosomiasis. This work was undertaken in conjunction with Dr H. Wolferstan Thomas at Liverpool in 1905. Paul Ehrlich came from Germany to learn about this work at first hand as he was interested in trypanosomiasis. On his return to Germany he resolved to try Trivalent Arsenic in syphilis. From this work he developed Salvarsan which was the first really effective therapy for this disorder. Hence Thomas, Breinl and Ehrlich were the pioneers of the immensely important subject of chemotherapy.[4] Breinl was cured of an accidental laboratory infection with sleeping sickness by the use of his own Atoxyl. I remember him well, as a patient when I was a teenager. He gave me a course of tin injections for acne; painful though they were, I bore him no resentment, doubtless because of his charming manner. I am told by my sister that as a child I had some type of severe fever and Breinl stayed up all night with me; such a happening was consistent with his intense concern for patients. There are many legends about him. He was a most adventurous, courageous and humble man.

Next to Breinl in the official photograph of that 'instant in time' is a man who eventually turned out to be an enemy. He is

Dr Joseph Ahearne who had practised in Townsville since 1881, having arrived in Queensland in 1876. He was involved in the North Queensland Separation Movement and was Principal Medical Officer of the Northern Military District as a Lieutenant Colonel. He was to retire from his military duties in the year of the photograph. In 1915 he went to Greece and Serbia with the Red Cross. One can almost imagine him rattling his sabre. Certainly he seems to be dozing off and got caught by a blink of the eyelid when the camera clicked. Mrs Breinl told me that he was under the influence of alcohol at the time of the ceremony. During and after the war of 1914-18 he was to show a lot of xenophobic hostility to Breinl, as did some other members of the medical profession in Townsville.

Dr E. Humphrey was a product of St Bartholomew's Hospital in London and surgically inclined. He was present at my birth and operated on my leg at the age of five, though neither episode do I remember. He was our family doctor and had a magnificent reputation. He was one of those old general practitioners who could do most things. He is said to have carried out the first successful cataract operation at the Townsville General Hospital in 1914.[5] Humphrey was a great friend of Breinl, and Breinl being single until 1919 used to have dinner every Sunday with the Humphrey family. During the war and after, Humphrey was most supportive of Breinl.

Mr John Fielding was one of the most important men in the photograph. He was then aged twenty-three, and was probably the lowest paid of all at £100 a year. He was the laboratory assistant Breinl had brought with him from the Runcorn Laboratory at Liverpool. Medical historians should be eternally grateful to him as he remained with the Institute when it was transferred to Sydney in 1930 and produced a hand-written manuscript of one hundred and twenty-three pages dealing with the history of the Institute from its inception to the time of its transfer to Sydney.[6] The manuscript was probably written in 1953 following his first heart attack. He was to die the following year from a further heart attack. His manuscript is a mine of information. Fielding himself became a self-taught biological scientist and published important findings in his own right. He worked out that the vector for the eye worm in poultry (an important disease in northern Australia) was the Surinam cockroach. He wrote Health Department Service Publication (Tropical Division) No. 9 on Australasian ticks. In the 1940s Fielding published his findings on the transmission of rat leprosy on which he had worked for many years. Fielding was a remarkable man and no doubt his reminiscences will be admired for years to come.

Dr R.B. Huxtable was a visitor from Charters Towers. Earlier he had been medical officer to the Kennedy Regiment but later transferred to infantry and commanded the Regiment. When on the 5th August, 1914, war against Germany was declared, the Kennedy Regiment, under its commanding officer, commandeered the steamer *Kanowna* and set off on the 8th August, 1914 for its battle station at Thursday Island. The accounts of this episode contain, in retrospect, many hilarious features. The Colonel transferred back to the Medical Corps in 1915 and was sent to Gallipoli and later France where he had a very distinguished career as ADMS 1st Division A.I.F. He was awarded the CMG, DSO, VD and the Croix de Guerre. Some years ago when rummaging through an old storage room at the restored Stock Exchange Building in Charters Towers, I came across a large unnamed photograph which I recognised as being that of Huxtable. The local people had never heard of him. *Sic transit gloria mundi.*

Another soldier was Dr T. Gordon Ross. He was the Medical Superintendent of the Townsville Hospital from 1907 to 1923 with a five year gap for the War. He was one of the earliest movers in the Bishop's project to establish an institute of medical research. Two years after the photograph (*Figure 10.1*) he was at Gallipoli serving with the 5th Field Ambulance together with Dr William Crowther. Crowther stated that Huxtable and Ross were most interested in Breinl and often spoke of him while at Gallipoli.

Breinl had been appointed to hold Ross's former job as Hospital Superintendent in an entirely honorary capacity during the war, in addition to being Director of the Institute.[8] Ross finished the war as a Lieutenant-Colonel in command of the 12th Field Ambulance and was awarded the DSO. After the war he returned to Townsville entering private practice in 1923. He opened a private hospital in North Ward but later transferred it as the Lister Hospital to West End, where in the fullness of time it was to become the present Townsville Mater Hospital. Ross moved to Sydney in about 1928. He was a Foundation Fellow of the Royal Australasian College of Surgeons.

Dr W. Nicoll was the parasitologist and was academically the best qualified of all the staff. He was a Master of Arts, a Doctor of

Science and a Doctor of Medicine. Unfortunately the glass bottle was his downfall and he was dismissed in 1915. He went to Brisbane to enlist in the forces and was inducted but discharged after two days as he was in a constant state of inebriation over this period of time. At the commencement of the war it is thought that he would have wished to oust Breinl and become Director himself. Later he was to write a most vitriolic condemnation of the Institute and the Australian tropics in general.[2,9]

Dr W.J. Young was, with Dr H. Priestley, recruited from the Lister Institute in London in 1912. Dr Young was a biochemist and a MSc of Manchester University and a DSc of London University. He left the A.I.T.M. to be Associate Professor of Physiology to teach biochemistry in Melbourne in 1919. Professor W.A. Osborne, Professor of Physiology in Melbourne, had met him when he visited and worked at the Institute in 1918. I remember him well as he was my professor of biochemistry and was affectionately known to the students as 'Youngie'. Perhaps he was recruited by Osborne not only because of his expertise in biochemistry but also because of their mutual interest in literature, particularly Shakespeare. Both were active members of the Shakespearean Society of Melbourne. His major scientific work in Australia after his Townsville work was devoted to the carriage and ripening of bananas, the refrigeration of meat and the carriage of citrus fruit.[10] He became full Professor of Biochemistry in 1938.

As an example of the high academic standards of the staff of the A.I.T.M. we may cite Dr H. Priestley,[11] who was the only Australian graduate on the staff. He graduated in medicine from Sydney University in 1909 at the top of his year and with first class honours and the University Medal. He had come top of each year in the course with high distinction. Prior to studying medicine he graduated in science with first class honours and with University Medals in chemistry and geology. Nominally he was appointed as a bacteriologist to the A.I.T.M. but really was engaged in much general investigative work. Professor Anderson Stuart, Professor of Physiology at the University of Sydney must have been well aware of his capabilities, and in 1917 persuaded him to join him in Sydney as lecturer. In 1921, Priestley was appointed Associate Professor. From 1930 under Professor H.W. Davies he was in charge of the Department of Biochemistry and was appointed McCaughey Professor of Biochemistry in 1938.

Nineteen thirty eight was the year when biochemistry became a separate department at both Sydney and Melbourne Universities; both Foundation Professors had commenced their Australian careers at the A.I.T.M. As Professor E.C. Slater pointed out,[12] Townsville was the home of Australian biochemistry. Both professors were described as being practical men and both became expert wood workers, Priestley certainly learning his craft during his time in Townsville.

In the middle of the photographic group (it would seem occupying the position of honour – perhaps to the chagrin of the Governor of Queensland, as one might judge from his expression) is Professor T.P. Anderson Stuart. Certainly Anderson Stuart was a very important man indeed, important enough to have a six page obituary in the *Medical Journal of Australia* when he died in 1920.[13] I believe that this constitutes a record. He was knighted in June of 1914. Anderson Stuart was the founder of the Sydney Medical School and its first Professor, a post encompassing both anatomy and physiology,when the School commenced in 1883. In fact many regarded him as 'the School' from the time of his appointment until the time of his death. He was a man of outstanding influence and organisational attainment, besides being a teacher of distinction. Anderson Stuart was always of the opinion that the A.I.T.M. should have been in Sydney and not in Townsville. However when the decision was made to site it in Townsville he gave the project his wholehearted support. He was a member of the original committee formed in 1908 and was its foundation Chairman.

Dr Wilton W. Love was the Queensland Government medical representative on the Committee of Management of the A.I.T.M. as there was no University of Queensland at the time. From 1910–1916, he served as a foundation member of the Senate of the University of Queensland. He was a surgeon to the Brisbane Children's Hospital, the Lady Lamington Hospital for Women and the Lady Bowen Maternity Hospital. He was a pioneer in the use of x-rays and a Foundation Fellow of the Royal Australasian College of Surgeons.[14]

Last but not least is Sir William MacGregor, himself a medical man, and Governor of Queensland. He was the son of a Scottish crofter and owed his eminence entirely to his own efforts. He played a prominent part in the establishment of the University of

Queensland, and in 1911 became its first Chancellor. One matter that interests me is that exactly one hundred years ago this year he took over from my grandfather, John Douglas, as the Administrator of British New Guinea.

Professor Anderson-Stuart was eventually proved right, as in most things, and the A.I.T.M. was moved to Sydney University in 1930. It was incorporated into the School of Public Health and Tropical Medicine of the University of Sydney. With the dismemberment of that School a portion of it has returned to Townsville under the aegis of the James Cook University of North Queensland and is entitled the Centre for Australian Tropical Studies. The building forming the background of that 1913 photograph has been named 'The Anton Breinl Centre for Tropical Health and Medicine' and recommenced operation in 1988 in the role of a research building. Prior to this time it had functioned as part of the Commonwealth Health Laboratory attached to the Townsville General Hospital. A few years ago it narrowly escaped demolition to form a parking lot for the great god 'car', but was saved by being classified by the National Trust of Queensland.

*Acknowledgement*

Thanks are due to Professor R.K. Macpherson, formerly Head of the School of Public Health and Tropical Medicine of the University of Sydney who in 1974 supplied me with the group photograph illustrated.

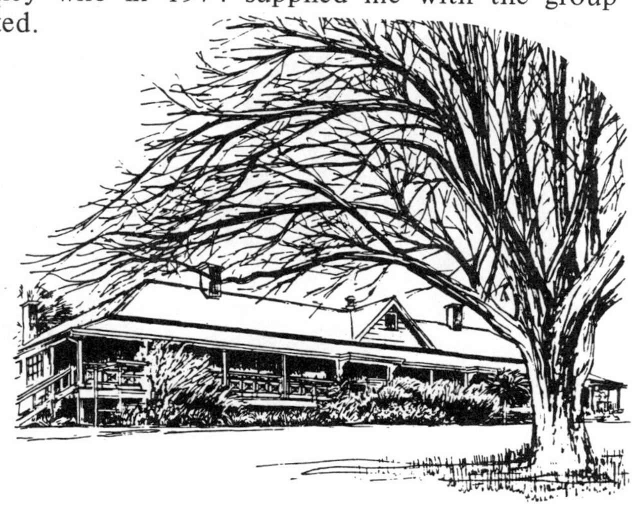

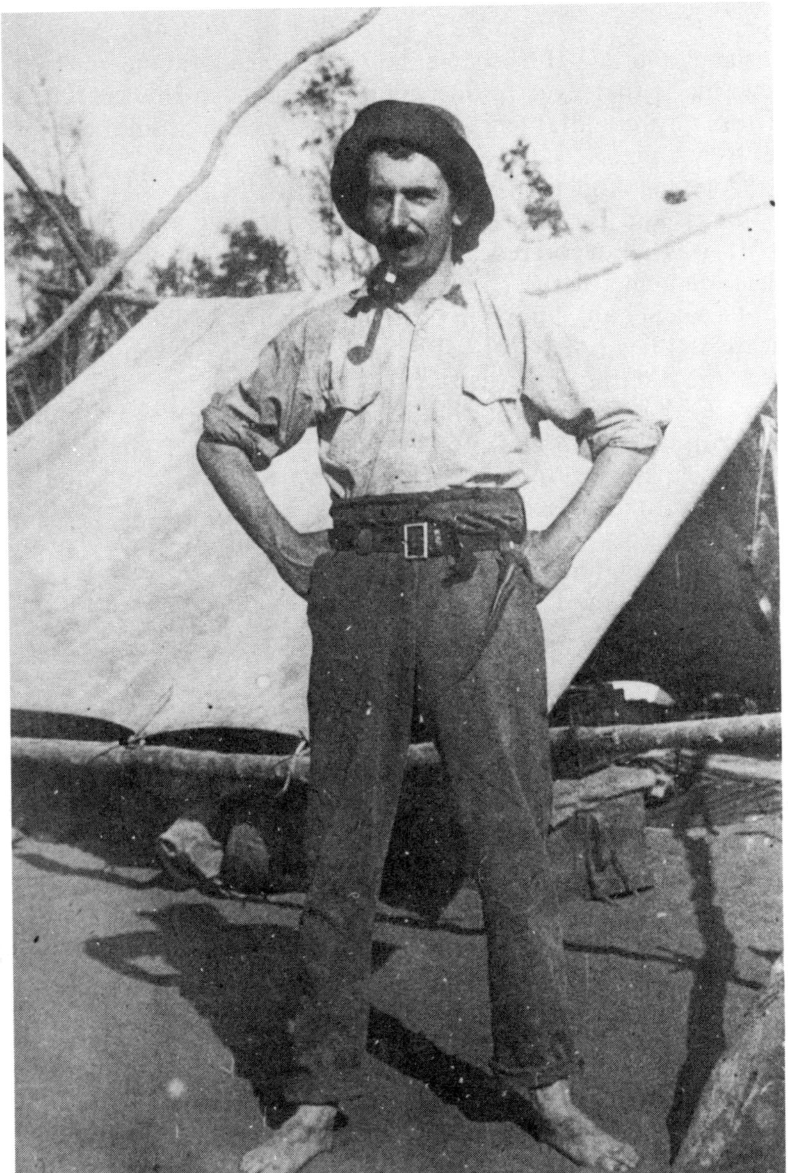

*Figure 11.3: Dr Anton Breinl 'On Safari', Papua, circa 1913. Photograph from a glass plate negative, in the Breinl Collection. (Courtesy of his son, Dr John Breinl)*

# FROM NORTH TO SOUTH
## The Translocation of the Australian Institute of Tropical Medicine

**Lori Harloe**

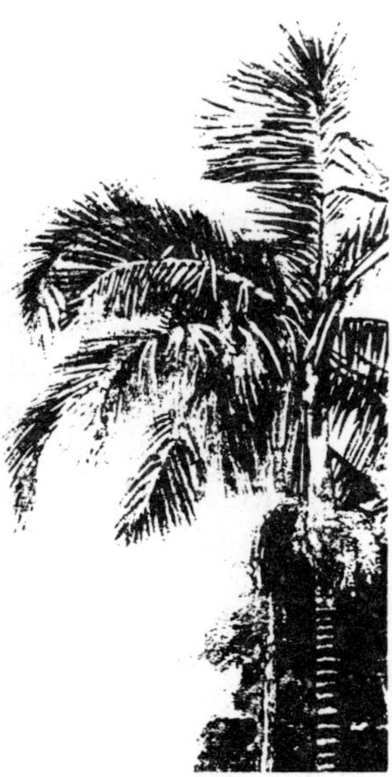

*IN* recent years historians have begun to adopt a strategy for dealing with the integration of science, culture, and statecraft.[1,2] The application of their techniques brings into focus the interplay between imperial cultural perceptions, the quest for local autonomy, and the development of nationalism. In the Australian context, medicine has been largely underestimated in the study of the development of our national consciousness. That the broader aspects of cultural history have, until recently, ignored the history of medicine is to the detriment of Australian history. This has tainted our historiography, as has the 'writing out'[3] of women and the cultural ignorance displayed towards the original Australians.[4]

North Queenslanders believed they were disadvantaged by the removal of the Australian Institute of Tropical Medicine from Townsville to Sydney in 1930, yet little has been written about this phenomenon. Lack of comment stems possibly from the perspective that tropical medicine was a failure and that 'the north' was irrelevant to most historians.[5] It could be argued that 'translocation' is a misnomer: the Institute ceased to exist once it was subsumed into the School of Public Health and Tropical Medicine. Nevertheless, the term does convey the sentiment of the Townsville community nearly sixty years ago. In those days the symbolism attached to the Institute was such that the idea of its relocation was preferable to the notion of no facility at all. Moreover, most northern Australians were oblivious to the fact that the Institute had itself become moribund by 1920. By that time, Anton Breinl, the inaugural Director, had provided evidence which resolved affirmatedly the major research question – 'could a white race live and work in tropical Australia?'[6] Indeed, once this had been determined, the Institute had served its original political purpose. Translocation to Sydney justified other political aims.

The choice of Townsville as the location of the Institute (*Figure 11.1*) may be interpreted as a gesture by politicians to placate a Bishop and a small band of supporters. However, two factors are relevant: the prominence Australian nationalism attached to Anglo-Saxondom, and the prejudice against the tropics as optimum for white habitation. In time, the latter concept became obsolete and was converted into a rationale for south-centred Australian health care.

**Problems of Location**

The successful impetus for the establishment of an Institute to study tropical diseases in Australia came from the Anglican Bishop of North Queensland, Rev Dr George Frodsham. By 1907 he had the support of northern community groups, business men, and almost all of the local medical practitioners.[7] It was his intention that investigations be made of –

> ... *infectious diseases different to those prevalent in colder regions* ... [because ... immigrants] *are more susceptible to their malefic influence than the natives who are more or less racially immune.*[8]

To increase the comfort and health of the white race, who had made their homes north of the Tropic of Capricorn, Frodsham proposed that 'clinical observations of the diseases of the Australian Tropics'

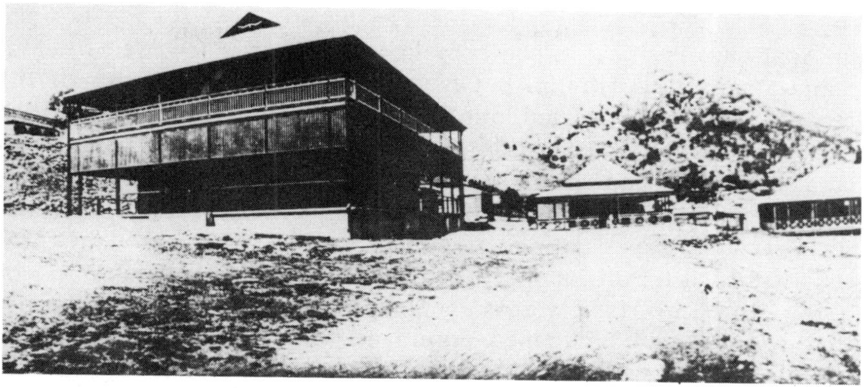

*Figure 11.1: The Australian Institute of Tropical Medicine, Townsville. Photographed in 1912, by Frank Taylor Esq., Entomologist at the Institute. The Institute was situated in the grounds of the Townsville Hospital, two out-buildings of which are at the right. Castle Hill is in the distance, right. (Courtesy of Dr Robert Douglas AM)*

be undertaken at Townsville which possessed 'qualifications that admirably fit it for being the centre of such observations'.[9] Other schemes had been initiated by various medical men from the southern Universities, who it has been claimed, had 'something to gain from their advocacy, or were trying to persuade various governments to establish posts for them'. The Medical Officer with the Central Board of Health, William Ramsay Smith, believed that Frodsham's national scheme was free from any hint of personal material gain.[10] Thomas Anderson Stuart, founder of the Sydney Medical School and by that time renowned as a competent organizer,[11] recognised that this submission had the attention of the top echelon of British and Australian political authorities and was likely to be adopted. Therefore, his own plans for a similar institute in Sydney were abandoned. However, Anderson Stuart never conceded that Townsville was the ideal location.[12]

Given, as Enid Barclay has revealed, that 'health measures had a low priority in political circles for many decades',[13] it is an indication of Frodsham's influence and determination that he accomplished his goals without acrimony. Anderson Stuart's 'sportsman-like'[14] attitude in abandoning his own plans, although propitious in the short term, was soon to be evidently a leverage point for others to subvert the northern base of tropical medicine in Australia. Political expediency had long been a feature of health management in Australia. Between the 1850s and the turn of the century all States passed public health acts modelled on British legislation largely as a response to infectious diseases.[15] In Queensland, legislation and appointments may be plotted against epidemics and perceived threats of contagion from other racial, ethnic, and social groups. For example, the 1872 smallpox scare brought forth the first Health Act; and typhoid led to the *Public Health Act* of 1884. Non-Europeans were subjected to a variety of Acts in order that white society remained dominant.[16] Exclusion of non-whites from the main hospital wards was standard practice as was the housing together of the insane and criminal.[17] This environment of contingency explains the appointment of the first Commissioner of Public Health for Queensland in 1901 when the bubonic plague struck.[18] By 1910 it was politically opportune to introduce tropical medical science to solve the health problems of a 'working white race' in northern Australia. The dilemma of the new nation was seen as racial – a sort of battle between white man and nature – culminating in *Triumph in the Tropics*.

One of Frodsham's most valued supporters, Gordon Ross, Medical Superintendent of the Townsville Hospital, reasoned –

> ... *if then insect life is so intimately connected with disease it seems evident that the diseases must be studied in their own localities for in these places only can the exact causation be arrived at and the best methods of dealing with outbreaks be discovered.*[19]

But, as researchers at the Schools of Tropical Medicine at London and Liverpool had demonstrated, it was not a prerequisite to have the main laboratory in the tropics. Nevertheless, Ross argued, Townsville which was considered a suitable place for a Base Hospital for the treatment of general diseases should be a centre from which a systematic study of various diseases could be organised. Collection of material from a vast area was envisaged. This was not to eventuate. Studies by the Institute soon demonstrated the comparative absence of disease, due mainly to a small population which was widely dispersed. Calls for the extension of the Institute to Papua where more serious problems existed were ignored.[20] However, the main research problem for Breinl (*Figures 11.2 and 11.3*) and his four staff members was the investigation of all that would hinder a white race from engaging in hard manual labour in this tropical zone.

A need for greater population of the north, fear of 'the yellow peril', and the health of white workers were inter-related. These themes took on a (special linked) social, political, and medical significance. Since Federation various medical gatherings had heard speakers such as John Elkington, Richard Arthur, and Frederick Goldsmith argue for a resolution of problems associated with white settlement of those regions which the popular press labelled as 'unhealthy'.[21] Elkington, Commissioner of Public Health for Queensland, wrote 'The future of tropical Australia appears to lie in the common sense of the people, and of their representatives in the Legislature'. These spokesmen were promulgating a view of racial superiority in harmony with the nationalistic theme. Racism was a big component of Australian nationalism.[22] The 'white Australia policy', embodying the aspirations of the Nation's early national identity, evidenced official expression of attitudes of European cultural and intellectual superiority. Although conventional wisdom of the era[23] suggested that physiologically Europeans were not suited to hard outdoor work in a tropical environment legislation had forbidden entry of non-Europeans and expulsion of those already here. Humanitarianism may have motivated the good Bishop's advocacy of a northern site but it was political reality which justified Commonwealth funding.[24]

**The Australian Institute of Tropical Medicine ceases to be politically relevant.**

The European settlers' view of the Australian continent, differing as it did from that of the Aborigines, was one in which the economic exigencies of Empire, the assumption of the political theory of liberalism, and the development of Australian nationalism led to what one writer has called 'a bifocal understanding of nature and history'.[25] In this mastery of man over nature the valorization of history was a safeguard for progressive thinkers of the first two decades of the twentieth century. The acquiescence of nature in the wake of scientific discoveries highlighted the 'winnable war' over disease. A significant feature of the era was the emergence of an international reform movement – the progressive physicians.[26] Although there was no single stream they were generally committed

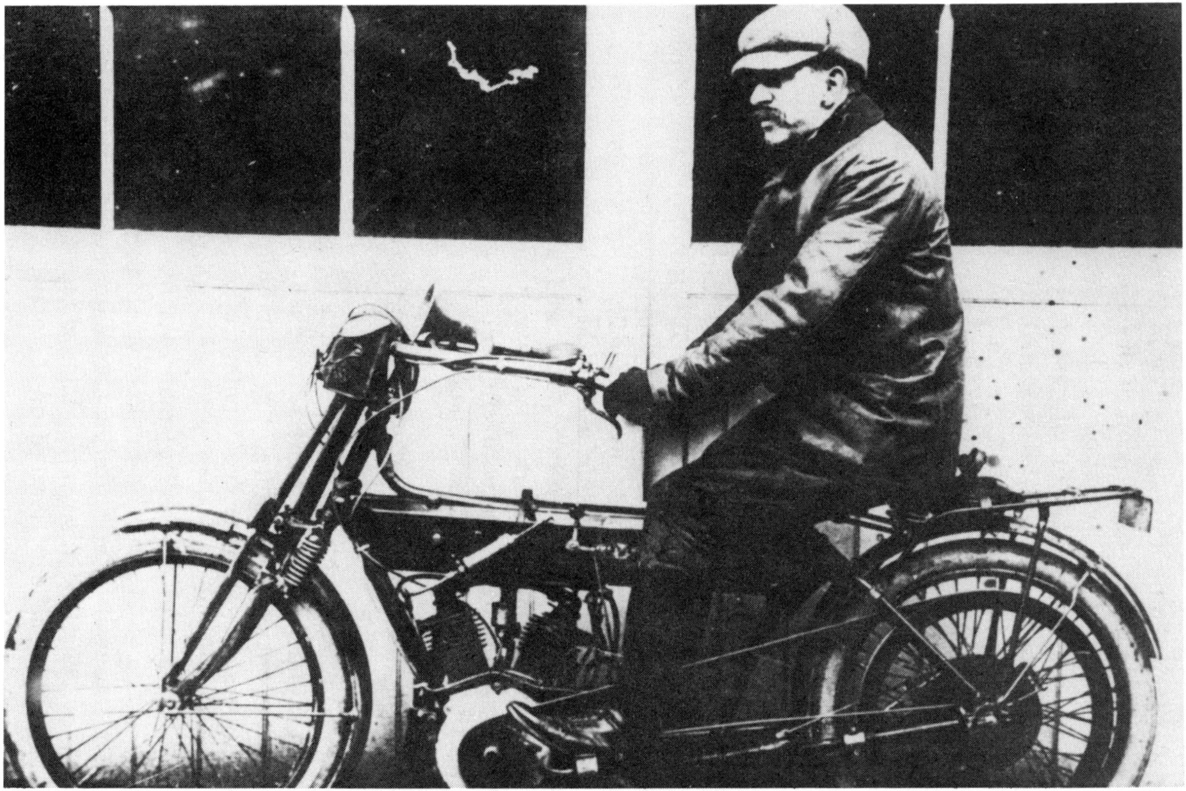

*Figure 11.2:* *Dr Anton Breinl on his motorcycle at Liverpool, England, circa 1908. At the time of this photograph he was Director of the Runcorn Institute, Liverpool. (Courtesy of Dr Robert Douglas AM).*

to political and social reform and were attracted to efficiency and morality. The American version was expressed by Theodore Roosevelt. As Michael Roe explains, the heterogenous nature of progressivism is a problem for historians because within the movement are ambiguities which are bi-polar and contradictory. The progressives believed that 'if bourgeoisie did not redeem society then extremists might take over'.[27] In the story of tropical medicine in Australia the leading medical figures – Cumpston, Elkington and Cilento – applied this philosophy.

At Brisbane on 17 August 1920 the eleventh session of the Australasian Medical Congress heard Breinl's paper on 'Figures and Facts Regarding Health and Disease in Northern Australia influencing its Permanent Settlement by a White Race'.[28] His conclusions were that the incidence of disease in the tropical north did not differ from Central or Southern Queensland. Tropical Diseases with the exception of hookworm infestation were scarce and easily controlled. Moreover, investigations into the physiology of the inhabitants of the coastal areas of North Queensland, when compared with those of a temperate climate showed only a few quantitative but no qualitative changes. On 27 August, the full Congress debated the issue of tropical medicine in Australia which was described as a 'great national question' and applied its energy to solving these 'practical details of any scheme of settlement ... [which presented] no difficulties beyond that of organization, staff, time, and money'. The great national question of the successful development and settlement of Australia they anticipated could be overcome by 'earnest and skilful application of the principles of statecraft'. To this end the doctors resolved to set up a Federal Ministry of Health,[29] a goal achieved in 1921.

The nineteenth century concept in which health initiatives were solely a response to infection and epidemic had given way to a complex interplay of environmental, social, economic, physic and international factors which demanded a multi-perspective approach. Since the First World War the linear relationship between cause and effect had altered. The idea of reality had changed.[30] John H.L. Cumpston, Director General of Health, believed that –

> *...preventative medicine cannot be a success until each medical man in practice is enrolled as an effective and active unit. The medical practitioner cannot escape his responsibilities to the*

> *nation... The first line of defence must be the general practitioner ... under the direction and supervision of the trained central and district staffs, accept the responsibility for all those measures of preventative medicine which can be applied in the home, and must be prepared to accept responsibility for failure to carry out prescribed or obvious measures of prevention.*[31]

After 1921 government involvement in tropical medical research underwent a change. The practical application of funding of public health in areas of larger populations in the south took precedence. Tropical medical research, by providing evidence that the northern regions were safe for Anglo-Saxon settlement, had given strength to the argument that any further research could be performed as well at the southern universities: loss of political justification for the location signified stagnation of the Institute. It was an example of what Ann Mozley Moyal terms 'Government support of medical science for political sake rather than as a deliberate policy for medical science'.[32]

## Southward Orientation of Society

The partiality in Australian society for the south can be assessed statistically in population figures, income per capita, the provision of choice in education, employment, and in opportunity.[33] Not so easy to answer is the question 'Are Queenslanders Different?' However much painters and authors romanticise the bush, the evidence is unassailable that they gravitate, with few exceptions, to the security of the southern power source. In 1979 Humphrey McQueen suggested that inertia was a problem: for the majority of Australians, Queensland was a state of mind which inhibited them from recognising what was wrong in their own states.[34] Similarly, the Northern Territory has been caricatured in Australian historiography as 'a vast iceberg of failure'. As Lenore Coltheart has shown, the early failure of British settlements ignored the attitude to land settlement in the region and undervalued Aboriginal resistance to the British invasion and occupation.[35] However, the 'empty land' syndrome portrayed in Victorian novels began to change public perception of a land controlled by convicts.[36] The battle of man against the tropics was to become entrenched in the national consciousness despite the scientific evidence that no racial degeneration would befall the European inhabitants; nor would they, by the third generation, be victims of jaundice, irritability, nervous disorders, distorted vision, or lunacy. It is interesting to note that the official opening of the Australian Institute of Tropical Medicine planned for December 1913 was changed to the more salubrious month of June.

**Education and Research as Reasons for Removal**

In the years following the formation of the Commonwealth Health Department, pressure from southern universities to include the study of tropical medicine in their curricula was mounting. From its inception, the Institute had been discerned as the starting point to remedy this deficiency. The intention had been to provide a course of three months' duration which included some field and laboratory work. A Certificate was awarded by the Australian Institute of Tropical Medicine and a Diploma was granted for further study by the University of Sydney.[37] Untoward difficulties including the First World War and insufficient staff had made courses impracticable: after cancellation of the first course in 1914, several years elapsed before student interest revived.[38] Rayner L. Bellamy of Papua was, in 1926, the first to gain the Diploma from the Institute.[39]

During the six months to July 1925, the Royal Commission on Health heard evidence against the Institute. Its isolation and the inherent difficulties associated with education and research were emphasised. Some difficulties had been experienced by those who had completed part one of the Diploma in Tropical Medicine at the Universities of Melbourne or Sydney. Instruction in part two was unsatisfactory because of absence of adequate staff after Breinl's departure. The proposal that the whole course be undertaken at Townsville was acceptable to the University of Melbourne, but the University of Sydney 'did not welcome the idea'. Five reasons were advanced as to why objections were raised about the proposal that the entire course be conducted in Townsville. First, the 'difficulty of obtaining an adequate staff'; secondly, the lack of clinical material; thirdly, that 'Townsville did not provide a variety of board and lodgings accommodation and, such as it is, is very poor, or very expensive'; fourthly, the time and cost involved in 'proceeding to and from Townsville'; and lastly, the disadvantage with regard to the supervision of comparative material.[40]

Regarding the desirability of relocating the educational component of the Institute to Sydney, Cumpston, Elkington, and Cilento were in accord. Cilento, the Director of the Institute, was reported to have said it 'would be nearer to the field of action'.[41] Elkington, Director of the Division of Tropical Hygiene in the Commonwealth Department of Health, gave evidence that:

> *...administration of the Islands under control in the Pacific, the necessity is ... the teaching of our medical men modern tropical hygiene. ... it is a truism of tropical administration that the economic or humane control of native races is impossible without a thoroughly efficient medical service. With regard to the suggestion that Sydney is the most appropriate centre for the initiation of such a teaching system, the evidence of the Director-General of Health has already indicated the serious practical difficulties that lie in the path of using Townsville as a teaching centre.*[42]

The reasons are less clear why Ernest S. Jackson of Brisbane objected to Townsville as a site for postgraduate study in tropical medicine. However, it could be argued that his overriding passion for a medical faculty in Brisbane at the University of Queensland may have elicited the harsh comments reported in the *Townsville Daily Bulletin* on 3 October 1927. Elkington in reply used the opportunity to comment that the Institute had long been recognised as too far from the main centres of population. Announcement was made that the Commonwealth Department of Health 'had decided to build and equip a Commonwealth School of Hygiene and Tropical Medicine in connection with the University of Sydney'.[43] Evidence that the centralising forces in Australian society were becoming stronger could hardly be denied.

Following closely on the difficulties experienced during the war years, which greatly interrupted the Institute's educational role and its research work, 1919 heralded a new and disquieting influence. It took the form of censorship of research. As the secretary of the Committee of Management, Atlee Hunt, who was also the permanent head of the Department of Home and Territories, informed Breinl adherence was mandatory. Monthly reports were to be submitted by each scientist and all papers for publication were to be scrutinized by the Committee before publication.[44] This censorship was, in part, later repealed by Elkington, because 'it appeared to show that the staff were not trusted'. Only the Director, or as it was at that time, the Acting Director, was obliged to furnish monthly reports.[45] However, loss of autonomy regarding freedom to publish was to the scientists a cruel blow. It was, for the Institute, a mortal wound. Mapleston, in answer to an editorial in the *Medical Journal of Australia* of 3 December 1921 calling for more money to be spent on research in northern Australia, answered that censorship of scientific papers was 'a strange state of affairs in an institution whose objects are to determine scientific truths and not one calculated to produce the best results'.[46]

No doubt, Cilento was keen on good results when he barred Sundstroem, a Californian physiologist, from publishing at the Institute. Cilento advised Cumpston that Sundstroem wrote in an 'uncouth style' and he possessed an 'unscientific method of expression'.[47] Once Sundstroem realised that the promised equipment was not going to arrive he resigned. In the decade to 1930 resignations were commonplace.[48] Lack of harmony amongst the staff had been mentioned at a Public Works Committee meeting in Melbourne in early June 1928. Breinl, in an interview with the *Brisbane Courier*, denied there had been any discord. Breinl said he resigned because he was annoyed about the appointment of two assistants to the Institute without his knowledge. 'The Department of Health became connected with the Institute long before March 1921'.[49]

What was termed a condemnation of the Institute's research work by Cilento is an observation by Breinl of two facts. Firstly that Mapleston, Breinl's successor, spent most of his time in administrative work, and secondly, the next director, Cilento, published resumés of the work largely performed before his arrival.[50] Certainly under Cilento's directorship a change of emphasis had occurred. No longer was research the main focus. Laboratory examinations had become a dominant part of the work. A glance at the receipts illustrates this. Under Breinl's tenure the revenue was £500 for ten years; by mid 1928 it had increased to £12,000 per annum.[51] Once the *raison d'être* had changed there was little need to maintain the Townsville site for the physiological study of 'a working white race'. More important was the evolution of Australian health care in this period believed by some to be a low point in Australian culture. A culture which was a direct response to nationalistic impulses derived from

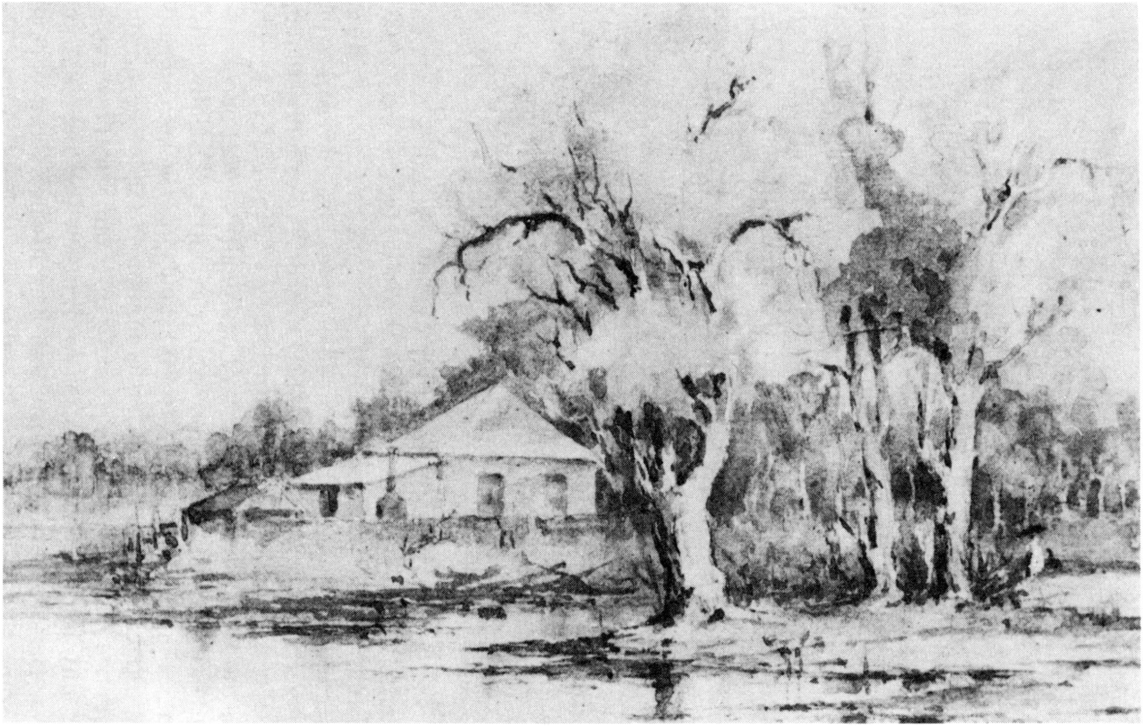

*Figure 11.4: 'House near a Lagoon', near Townsville, circa 1910.*
*Watercolour painting by Miss Gladys Roberts, artist at The Australian Institute of Tropical Medicine, Townsville. (Courtesy of Mr George Roberts.)*

erratic economic growth, increased urbanization and the social democratic style of political government.

As Cumpston did not have any official power over the Institute until 1921, the events preceding that date indicate to some observers that, by a pathway through the Quarantine Department, Cumpston had planned in advance the consolidation of the Commonwealth Health Department. Tropical medicine was one such avenue whereby political power and interest were allied. The assiduous encouragement of Cilento in this branch of public health indicates the importance of the Townsville Institute in the development of centralized health care.[52]

**The People's Attempts to Retain the Institute**

In the north, familiarity with local conditions (*Figure 11.4*) and improvement in diet, housing, and better communications overcame some of the initial problems experienced by the early European settlers. By the second generation, most of the North Queensland newspapers maintained a positive view of tropical living.[53] However the desire for 'independence', according to Bolton, developed 'a sense of community by making habitable a country still regarded by many Australians as remote and inhospitable'.[54] A preoccupation with sickness and disease became a major characteristic of inter-racial contact.[55] The Aborigines were feared as leprosy carriers: the Chinese tended to be suspected of transmitting typhoid and plague. In the decade to 1930 regular plague scares in the local newspaper generated panic. The bubonic plague outbreak of 1921-22 and the associated twenty-one deaths in Townsville caused a public outcry which stalled the translocation of the Institute.[56] Once no further cases of human disease occurred, the Institute was successfully translocated.

Some consolation may have been that the Commonwealth Health Laboratory operated from the same building as the Institute; the transition from a research establishment to a pathological laboratory, providing simply a service function, was unknown to most lay people. Breinl, quite a hero within the community, was in private practice. He remains as one of the founders of the philosophy of modern preventive medicine in this country:

> ... [there is] *another aspect in the settlement of Northern Queensland which hitherto has not received any consideration. Dr Young and myself during our investigations and inquiries have often been*

> *impressed by the influence which general social conditions, environment, etc. exert upon the mental attitude and consequently upon the working capacity of the individual, and our conversations repeatedly turned of* [sic] *the need of inquiry into 'economic conditions'.*[57]

**Conclusion**

The contentious issue regarding the location of the Australian Institute of Tropical Medicine was evident from the start. Anderson Stuart made no secret of his desire to incorporate it within the University of Sydney. Northern medical practitioners, aware of the Institute's *raison d'être*, believed that the best location was in the tropics. Furthermore, it was politically opportune to determine the physiological question of white man's survival in a land in which legislation had proposed exclusion of non-Europeans. This absurd situation, in which European invaders of 'the last continent available for the white man' concentrated totally on the racial welfare of their own cultural tradition illustrates the importance of the Institute in the development of Australian nationalism. The location in the north, then, was politically momentous: equally momentous was its relocation. Not the least significant aspect of the tropical medicine story was the development of the Commonwealth Health Department and the demise of the Institute at Townsville. The need for the tropical location had become redundant once evidence had accumulated (from Breinl's work) that no racially detectable changes were medically important. However, debate about translocation continued for ten years before the Institute was subsumed into the School of Public Health and Tropical Medicine at Sydney in 1930.

Discussion centred upon the role of research and education. Sydney, it was argued, had greater volume of shipping contact with tropical regions, and its larger population guaranteed access to the discipline of tropical medicine by more medical students than could possibly study in Townsville. The complex mix of scientific medicine, government involvement, ideas of progress and nationalism, a tendency for the south to be the physiological centre, and the interaction of personalities all contributed to the ultimate translocation of the Institute from Townsville to Sydney.

# A RAINFOREST PHARMACOPOEIA
## Five Thousand Years of Effective Medicine

**Jeanette Covacevich**
**Tony Irvine**
**George Davis (Nganygabana)**

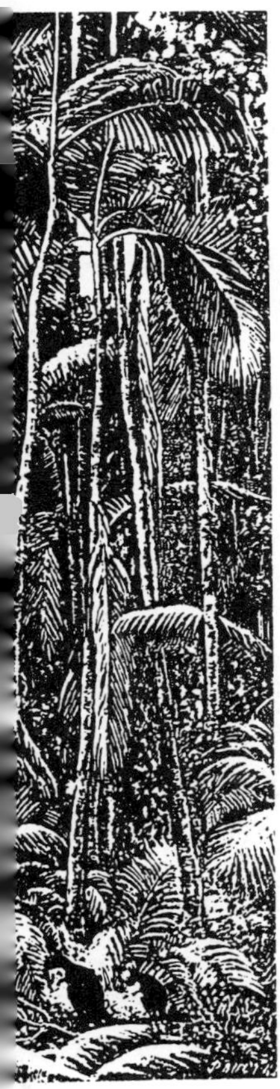

*THE* rainforests which form an almost continuous strip between Ingham and Cooktown, in north-eastern Queensland, are well known for their distinctive, highly diverse species of plants and animals. The substantial botanical and zoological work that has been undertaken in these rainforests has been summarized recently[1] as part of the long-standing conservation battle over their future.

Themes of biogeographic and evolutionary importance, rarity, vulnerability, high endemism, and refugia recur in most of what has been written about them. These themes, or most of them, also characterize the people of the so-called wet tropics. Yet the traditional owners of the rainforests are not well known and they command little of the attention afforded to the plants and animals. At best, it seems, the rainforest people have suffered relative neglect in the 'literature stakes'. At worst, their culture has been ignored and derided. Linguist R.M.W. Dixon has observed –

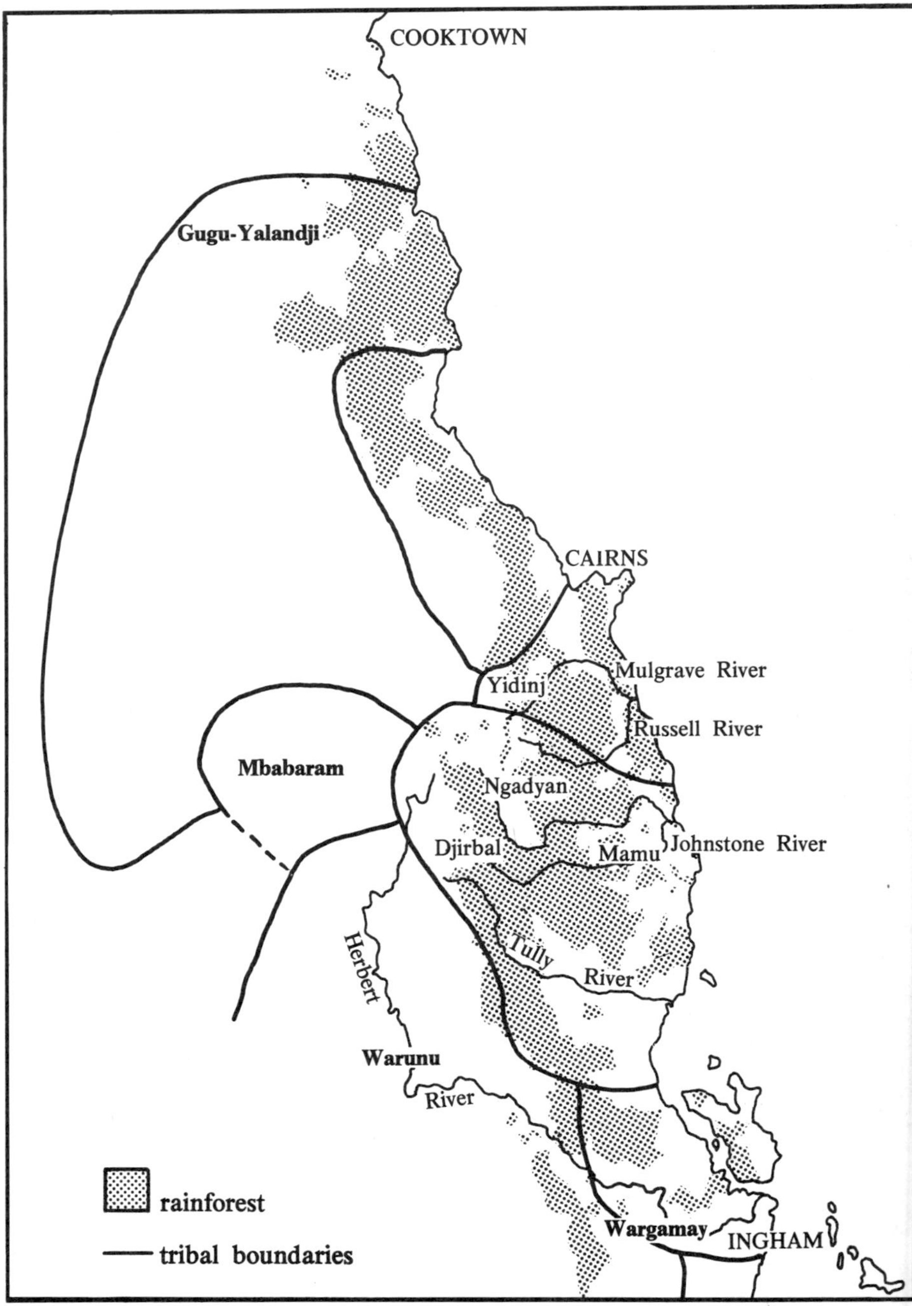


*Figure 12.1: Distribution of rainforest and tribal boundaries in north-eastern Queensland, prior to European settlement.*

> *... they lived in harmony with each other and with their environment. One hundred years ago many of them were shot and poisoned by European invaders. Those allowed to survive have been barely tolerated tenants on their own lands, and have had their beliefs, habits and language held up to ridicule and scorn ... The survivors ... have stood up to these adversities with dignity and humour, fortified by their amusement at the blindness of the invader to the richness of the environment ... .*[2]

The earliest tangible evidence of Aboriginal settlement of the rainforest dates from 5,000 year-old remnants of camps in Jiyer Cave on the Russell River,[3] although it has been proposed[4] that occupation of the area could be 10,000 years old. The distribution[1,5] of both the rainforest and its Aboriginal inhabitants before white use and abuse is well understood (*Figure 12.1*). For many years the small, very dark, curly-haired rainforest people, the so-called 'pygmy races' of North Queensland, were seen as primitive. It had been suggested that their affinities were with the Tasmanians, descendants of another group of allegedly early migrants to Australia who, likewise, had been driven to inhospitable refuges by stronger, 'better' people.

> *Dense wet forests become refuge areas only to be sought by those less fortunate tribes whose mental and physical inferiorities condemn them to the least desirable parts of primitive man's environment.*[7]

The rainforest people[2,6,8] are not linguistically, cranially, karyotypically or electrophoretically markedly different from other Aboriginal Australians from drier areas more characteristic of continental Australia.[2,6,8] Nonetheless, in response to a distinct, but far from 'least desirable' setting, their culture evolved in a way that was, and remains unique.

Contrary to popular belief, the rainforests were extremely rich in resources. They support a wide range of animal foods (e.g. possums, macropodids, birds, lizards, snakes, turtles, fish) and many species of edible plants. These include an array of fruits and nuts which ripen at the onset and in the early part of 'the wet'.[9] Plants were used to make highly characteristic rainforest shelters, tools, and weapons. They also provided staple foods, medicines, and poisons to immobilize fish. High dependence, both daily and seasonally, on very toxic food plants characterized rainforest life. Although Aboriginal people all over Australia use and have used toxic plants as foods, nowhere else is such a large species range of toxic tubers, rhyzomes and nuts used. Food derived from toxic plants is a major dietary component here, another feature which sets people of the rainforests apart from other Aboriginal groups. Use of such plants involves complicated, often lengthy, leaching or heating to destroy or eliminate toxins. Such techniques have evolved to a high degree amongst the rainforest people.[10,11] With these skills came a detailed knowledge of practical preventive medicine and a *materia medica* possibly unsurpassed for millenia.

European knowledge and understanding of Aboriginal medicines have swung from late 19th century ignorance and disregard exemplified by that of Carl Lumholtz, a Swedish adventurer and explorer; through cautious recognition mixed with strong scepticism of the 1950s and 1960s; to current high interest, respect, and recognition that they have worth.

> *The Herbert River blacks have no medicines. The only remedies used are to suck out the blood over a spot where the pain is felt, or to rub the sore place with saliva ...*[12]

> *... native plant remedies deserve systematic compilation and pharmacological screening ... The grotesque and naive uses of some of these plants would be difficult to investigate ... and can only excite scepticism ... the uses of aboriginal drug plants are often clinically vague and absurd ...*[13,14]

> *Aboriginal herbal medicinal knowledge has been gleaned by the best scientific techniques of all ... extensive trial, and presumably error, and observation of results, not on animals in test laboratories but on human patients over thousands of years. Potent cures were recognised and the intricacies of their preparation and uses passed on through generations ... .*[15]

Although the literature on Aboriginal use of plants as medicines and poisons is extensive, very few studies concentrate on either particular tribal groups or on ecological units. Rather, most deal with 'Aboriginal use ...' and record data from widely disparate areas.[13,14,15] Any review of this subject now has been further complicated by loss of information, for the rainforest peoples after over 100 years of contact with Europeans have lost much. With the advent of white men's medicines knowledge of traditional remedies is quickly discredited and lost.

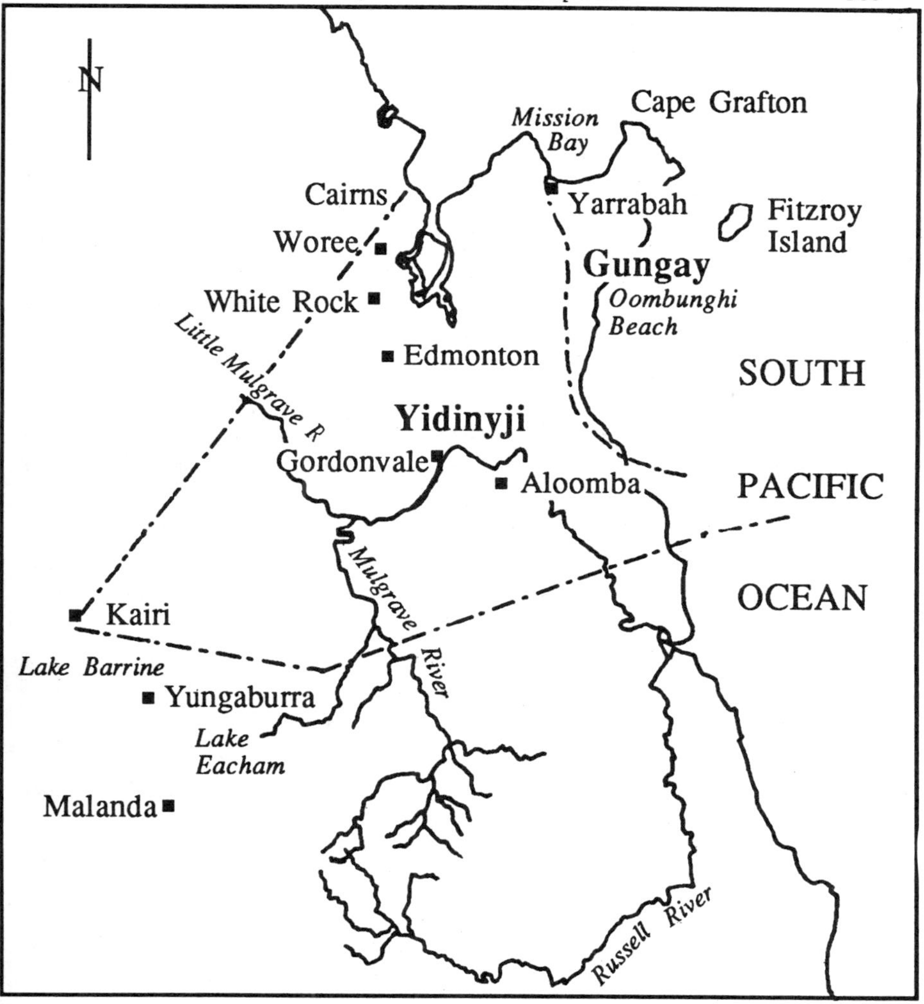


***Figure 12.2:* The Yidinyji territory included most of the rich Mulgrave River catchment.**

> *... as civilization spreads into primitive areas, the first aspect of primitive culture to be lost is knowledge of the use of plants as medicine ... .*[16]

Here we summarize the literature on Aboriginal use of plant medicines in the rainforests between Cooktown and Ingham and provide new, detailed data for the Yidinyji group whose territory ranged from the eastern Tablelands down the Mulgrave River and its tributaries (*Figure 12.2*).

Although there are detailed studies of Aboriginal use of plants from other areas of Australia,[17] the written records of use of rain-forest plants as medicines have hitherto been scant, and they lack detail about precise use. Almost invariably information about quantity, method of preparation, and means and frequency of application is lacking. For example, it is well known that the Cockatoo Tree, *Planchonia careya*, was used for 'medicine',[18] among other things. There is, however, no data about what part of the tree was used or how or why *Planchonia* medicine was administered. There is, therefore, no easy means of testing the efficacy of some of the cures or of identifying any possible curative properties of the rainforest plants. We recognise these deficiencies and have attempted to redress them, but we have often not been successful because so much knowledge of traditional medicine (and other traditional life) has been lost. This is doubly unfortunate. It shows arrogant disregard for Aboriginal culture and it has meant that information on plants potentially useful now, is no longer readily available.

The Yidinyji had a range of beliefs and strategies born out of a nomadic life in the rainforests and adjoining areas. Their means of coping with injuries, ailments and other vicissitudes of life in rain-forests are summarized in Table 12.1. Beliefs in charms, evil spirits, curses, and doctors are really beyond the scope of this paper, but were very elaborate and pervaded all aspects of life.[18]

In assessing the use of any rainforest resource, it is important to realize that many species of rainforest plants are highly specialized and that many do not occur throughout the rainforest, but in isolated pockets in particular communities. Use of a particular plant in one area by a particular tribal or language group does not necessarily mean the plant was used in the same way throughout its range. The nuts of the Candelnut *Aleurites moluccana* (Mamu 'gayga'; Ngjadan 'ngabala'; Dyirbal and Girramay 'gaburra') were eaten by the Mamu people but not by the Ngjadan, yet the species is common and wide-spread throughout the territories of each. Similarly, we have been told[19] that the Matchbox Bean, *Entada phaseoloides,* was used simply as a child's toy rattle in the rainforests near Tully by the Dyirbalan and Girramaygan, yet it was a food item to Aboriginal people elsewhere.[15] To add to the confusion, the use as food in lean times of 'seed kernels from large (*Entada phaseoloides*) beans ...

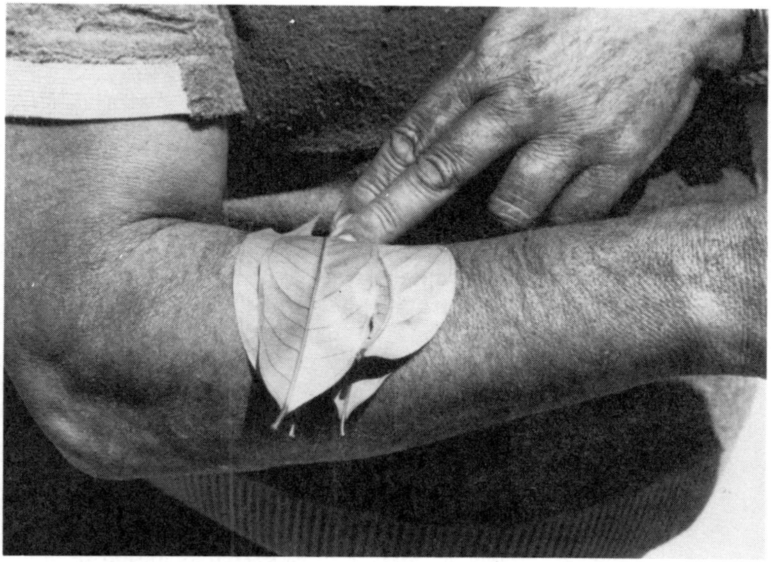

*Plate 12.1:* ***The young leaves of the River Satinash, Syzgium tierneyanum, were heated and then applied as a poultice on boils and other skin lesions by the Yidinyji.***

after special treatment' has been recorded for the Cardwell area, just south of Tully.[20] Wherever possible the people who used particular species have been identified here, although failure to list use by other rainforest people does not necessarily mean that it was not used. It may simply mean that data was not recorded and this precious knowledge is now no longer known for some groups.

The species of plants used by the other major 'tribal' (=?linguistic) groups in the rainforests of the Ingham-Cooktown block are summarized in Table 12.2. Data for groups other than the Yidinyji (*Table 12.1*), Dyirbal and Girramay are from the literature. Data relating to the Yidinyji were gathered on field trips mapping traditional trade routes[21] and recording traditional use of plants, animals and places in both upland and lowland rainforests of Yidinyji territory. Data from Dyirbal and Girramay people have been compiled by one of us (T.I.) with the linguist R.M.W. Dixon from the Australian National University. Table 12.3 summarizes use of plant poisons to collect fish, and Table 12.4 is an Aboriginal herbal of the northern rainforest region.

## TABLE 12.1: Practical Health Care Strategies of the Yidinyji People

### Accidents

*Spear Wounds:* Spears were made of very dense wood (River Gum, *Lophostemon exiliflora* 'bagiram', Beefwood or Golden Wattle, *Rachisperma crassicarpa* 'juwarra'). Essentially the patient gradually recovered or died. Wounds were cleansed in flowing cold water which also eased pain.

*Snakebite:* Assiduously avoided, but if someone was bitten, there was no specific cure. (This contrasts with other places of the north where a variety of 'cures' were used.) It is of interest that although the rainforests of north-eastern Queensland harbour several venomous species of snakes, the highly dangerous species are found in open forests. Snakes are not, generally speaking and despite popular opinion, a hazard of the rainforests.

*Limb fractures:* The people were very careful to avoid fractures and they occurred infrequently. Amongst the Yidinyji there was no understanding or use of splints to set bones. Limbs sometimes healed deformed.

*Poisoning:* Another infrequent accident due to extreme caution of adults, and supervision of children. Sometimes, however, 'porridge' from the fruits of *Cycas media* 'badil', and *Lepidozamia hopei* 'wunu', highly toxic plants, were eaten, incompletely treated and too soon. This resulted in violent vomiting. There was no specific cure and we are not aware of cures for other types of poisoning.

*Blindness:* Caused by the Finger Cherry, *Rhodomyrtus macrocarpus* = 'yaruju' and Tar Tree, *Semecarpus australiensis.* Fruits of the Finger Cherry which grows commonly in and near the rainforests have an attractive, pleasant-smelling, fleshy fruit. When eaten they can cause permanent blindness[20,22] although there are many records of ingestion of these fruits without ill effect and two of us (T.I., G.D.) have eaten the fruits without problems. If the sap of the Tar Tree enters a person's eyes after fruit or broken twigs have been handled, blindness ensues. There were no cures for either.

*Stings:* Generally three types of stings presented problems to the Yidiñyji (and, no doubt, other rainforest people).

Stinging Tree, *Dendrocnide moroides,* 'dungan'. Despite popular European north Queensland beliefs, Cunjevoi, *Alocasia macrorrhiza,* was not used (and is not effective) in alleviating what can be excruciating pain from contact with any part of the Stinging Tree. We can find no local record of the origin of this popular misinformation and are forced to conclude that it may have originated south of our study area. If the sting was large, the area was cut in an effort to inflict a distracting pain. 'Little burns' by Stinging Trees were rubbed briskly with fine, wet sand.

**TABLE 12.1 (contd)**

*Stings: (contd)*

Bullrout, *Notesthes robustus*, and Catfish, *Tandanus* sp., *Arius* sp.. For the painful stings of these species there were three choices – urine applied to sting site, placing the wounded area near a fire, or endure it. It is interesting to note that the first-aid treatment recommended today for stings by Stonefish, Bullrouts and Catfish involves heat, applied by placing the wounded area in hot water.[23] A first-aid remedy which is very effective indeed [Ed.].

**Aches and Pains**

*Toothache:* The sap of the Milky Pine, *Alstonia scholaris* 'jalngun' was applied to a sore tooth or directly into caries to relieve toothache. If it failed, and severe pain continued, a quartz crystal was used to cut the gum near the offending tooth. (This sap was also used for fire sticks and the gum was used as a glue for rafts.)

*Headache:* Swim/rest in cold water. If that failed, a small incision was made on the top of the head with quartz or a piece of glass. This was covered with a leaf and then tapped gently to encourage blood flow. One of us (G.D.) saw a woman nearly bleed to death from this treatment. For more severe cases a sharp tap on the back of the skull with a small grindstone was the next step.

Vine leaves, ? *Ziera smithii*, 'warrwa' (Yidinyji/Mulgrave River). The strong smelling leaves of an unidentified vine were squashed up and used as an inhalent to prevent or reduce headaches.

The leaves of *Clemantis glycinoides* were also effective in the treatment of headache. When rubbed together they release a strong odour. The patient inhales this and the ensuing, sharp, strong smell helps the patient forget the head (or other) ache.

**Gut Problems**

*Diarrhoea:* White clay was eaten. There were two deposits readily available to the Yidinyji, both along Toohey's Creek.

*Constipation:* In lowland (as opposed to Tableland or upland) parts of Yindinyji territory) Green Ants, *Oecophylla smaragdina*, 'jilliburra', and their eggs were squashed together and mixed with water and some ash. The 'mixture' was widely used to cure constipation and to engender a sense of well-being.

Yellow Thorny Mary, *Calamus moti*, 'mudi'. The stalks, particularly when young and fresh, were eaten to cure constipation. They were heated by uplanders but eaten 'straight' by lowlanders. Also used as general food. *(Plate 12.3)*

**TABLE 12.1 (contd)**

**Cicatrices**

After the incisions were made, the wounds were kept open with eel fat to enhance scarring. The leaves of the Sandpaper or Plenty Fig, *Ficus copiosa*, were rubbed into the wounds to keep scabs from forming and this caused large welts.

**Influenza**

This ravaged the Yidinyji communities in early white contact days. The 'cure' was to dive down deep into a cold water hole and lie there until the pressure made the patient's ears 'click', thus clearing the head.

**'Madness'**

There was little tolerance of aberrant behaviour (e.g. a woman walking around with rotten pieces of meat all day). Either people suffering 'bad heads' or 'gone in the head', 'dunguyangan', were driven away to live on their own or they were killed. Prewhite contact Yidinyji people knew of no narcotics or their equivalents (e.g. pituri of arid and semi-arid areas). However, honey from a yellow-flowered tree, 'malibai', had a stupefying effect at the end of the cooler months, August-September.

Fig, *Ficus copiosa*, 'gulugai'. The large leaves of this fig were heated and applied one on top of the other to aching 'rheumatic' joints to relieve aches and pains.

**Boils**

River Satinash, *Syzgium tierneyanum* 'burruburru'. Young leaves are heated and placed as poultices on boils and other skin lesions. *(Plate 12.1)*

**Bleeding**

Red-leafed Fig, *Ficus congesta* 'dagurba'. The bark from young trees is torn into long narrow strips which are then rolled to form a tourniquet to stop bleeding. (Also the plant used by the Yidinyji to make fishing lines). *(Plate 12.2)*

Small leaves; many plants, unidentified. A bundle of small leaves would be forced into a wound to stem bleeding.

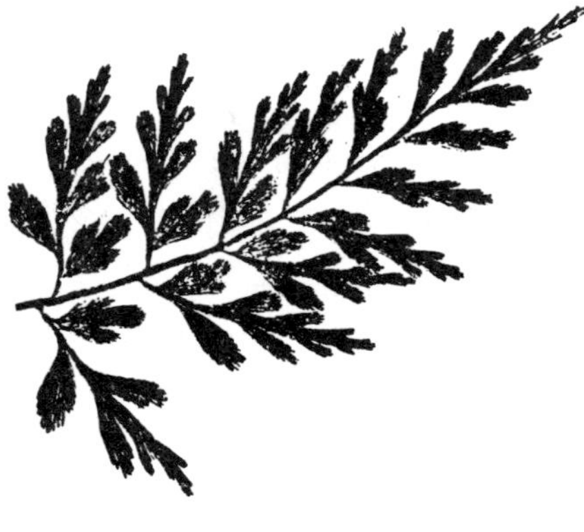

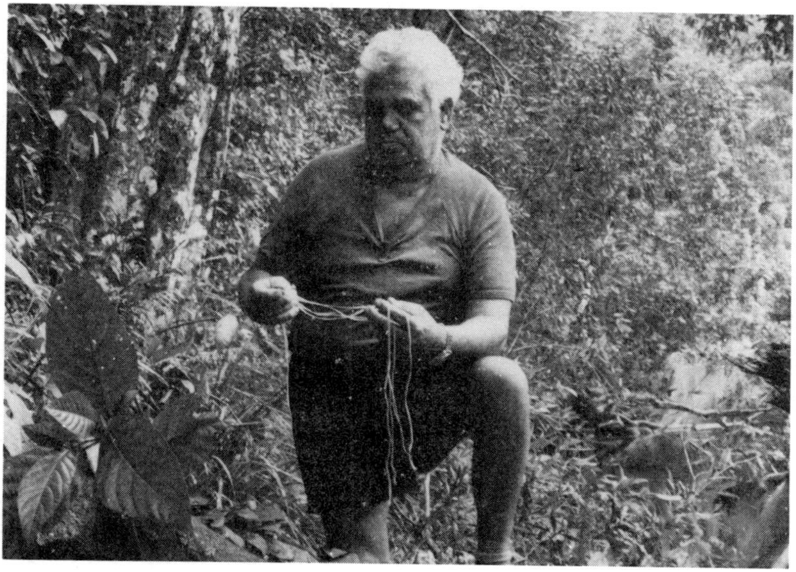

*Plate 12.2: The Red-leafed Fig, Ficus congesta was used extensively by the Yidinyji. Strips of the bark of young trees were rolled to make tourniquets to stop bleeding. Fishing lines were made in the same way from this tree.*

**TABLE 12.2: Medicinal Use of Plants by Aboriginal Groups (Other than the Yidinyji) in the area between Cooktown and Ingham.**

Lawyer Cane or Wait-a-While, *Calamus australis* 'gambay'; *C. moti* 'junggay'; *C. radicalis* 'baygal' (all Dyirbal/Tully River).

Strips used to tie around any painful portion of the limbs.[18] *Calamus* (? sp.) is also used as a 'bandage' for fractures by the people from the Tully River ... 'Numerous superficial longitudinal incisions are made over the situation of the fracture, short pieces of wood or bone are tied along and over the wound, and the whole bandaged up with lawyer-vine (*Calamus*) ... '[18] The Girramay used the young shoots ('gugun') of *C. moti* ('junggay') to relieve biliousness. Shoots were chewed. The shoots were also rubbed on cicatrices. *(Plate 12.3)*

Bladey Grass, *Imperata cylindrica*, 'gulmbinu'? (Girramay, Dyirbal/Tully River).

Strips used to tie around any painful portion of the limbs.[18] Also, a sharp piece of this grass is poked in the nostrils to induce blood flow – to relieve the congestion of headache.[18]

**TABLE 12.2 (contd)**

Tree Fern, *Alsophila australis,* (Dyirbal and Girramay/Tully River)

'The stalks of the young leaves ... are roasted and eaten as a tonic after any form of sickness'.[18] The use of the name *Alsophila australis* is an obvious misidentification, as this species occurs only in southern Queensland, northern New South Wales and Victoria. The species referred to is almost certainly *Cyathea cooperi*, 'galaju'.

Orchid, *Cymbidium albuciflorum*, 'bunggiya' (= *C. madidum*, the current correct name), (Dyirbal/Tully River).

*The bulb of this orchid is chewed for dysentery.*[18]

'bark twine', sp. unidentified, ? (Gugu-yalangi/Bloomfield River).

*... some of the old women, some of the 'doctors', will take a piece of bark twine attached to the one extremity of a spindle-shaped piece of beeswax, the other part being stuck or held on by the patient to that portion of his body which he considers most affected: the operator then takes the free extremity of the string in his mouth and with both his hands rubs it briskly from side to side over the lower lip, behind the teeth, until the blood comes, and then spits it out. He takes some water into his mouth, and after a time expectorates more bloody froth. Sometimes both ends of the string are attached each to a piece of beeswax; in such a case, both ends are held or placed alongside the painful spot by the patient himself, the old woman or the medicine-man 'drawing' the blood with the centre of the string ... .*[18]

*Barringtonia racemosa*, ? (Gugu-yalangi/Bloomfield River)

*... the bark is hammered and dipped into boiling water, and dabbed all over the sick person. Used in non-venereal stricture ... .*[18]

Fish-tail Lawyer Vine or Wait-a-While, *Calamus caryotoides*, ?, (Gugu-yalangi/Bloomfield River).

*... the young shoots, when eaten, are believed to cure head-ache.*[18]

Charcoal, (Gungandji/Cape Grafton)

*... omitting to rub a baby properly over with charcoal after birth ... can be blamed for 'growing pains' or any continued weakness.*[18]

*Calophyllum inophyllum*, 'balburo', (Gungandji/Cape Grafton)

*Nut broken, kernel triturated with red pigment on stone, mixed with water, and then rubbed all over patient's body, especially where pain is ... .*[18]

**TABLE 12.2 (contd)**

*Tabernoemontana* (now = *Ervatamia) orientalis*, ?, (Gungandji/Cape Grafton)

'Fruit rubbed on sores, to heal them ...'[18] This fruit has a milky sap and it is likely that the curative properties were in this.

*Prunus turnerana*, 'dungan' Dyirbal 'dudam' Girramay: 'dunu' Ngadjan

*... ground kernels used fresh for treating toothache by Dyirbal and Girramay people.*[19]

Paper Bark, *Melaleuca quinquenervia*, 'dagay' (Dyirbal/Tully River).

*...Smell the leaves to relieve coughs and colds ... .*[19]

unidentified herb, 'burbaburra' (Girramay/Tully River).

*...Sap is put on sores for healing ... grows in swamps ...* .[19]

Coral? Fern, *Dicranopteris linearis*, 'bundu bundu' (Dyirbal, Girramay/Tully River).

*... Rubbed in hands, produces soap lather, for washing ... .*[19]

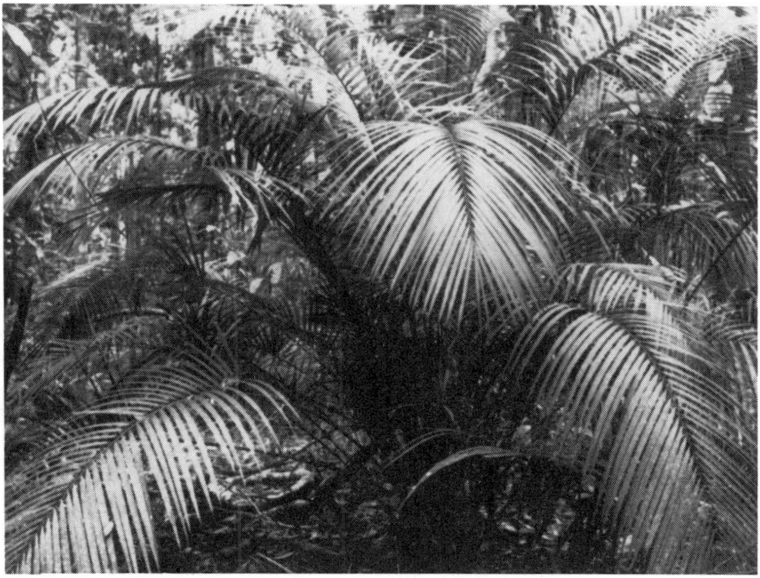

***Plate 12.3: The Yellow Thorny Mary, Calamus moti is very common throughout the rainforest. It was widely used by the rainforest peoples - as a vegetable, to cure constipation, to relieve biliousness, and to enhance scarring for cicatrices.***

**TABLE 12.3: Fish Poisons of Plant Origin of the Rainforest People between Cooktown and Ingham.**

Vine, unidentified, 'girringai', (Yidinyji/Mulgrave River)

The vine was cut into roughly 20 cm pieces. These were pulverised with a stick or stone. A big bundle was then dunked both up and down stream of a suitable fish hole. A milky film is given off. This toxic film forces fish to come to the surface, stunned, and easily captured by hand, spear or in nets. The Bullrout, *Notesthes robustus* = 'bukul', is always first affected. (This species bears spines attached to venom sacs. If handled or stepped on, extremely painful stings result.) The method was also used to clear a proposed swimming/play section of a creek for children.

*Cupaniopsis foveolatus*, 'jilbajin', (Dyirbal/Tully River).

*... scratch bark into still water as fish poison ...* .[19]

*Cupaniopsis flagelliformis,* ?, (Dyirbal/Tully River)

Bark used as fish poison.

Bloodvine, *Austrosteenisia blackii*, 'balibali', (Dyirbal/Tully River), 'ngaway' (Yidinyji/Mulgrave River)

'Used as a fish poison and to varnish boomerangs ...'[19] (for the Dyirbal). Not a fish poison for the Yidinyji, only to varnish boomerangs.

Vine, *Faradaya splendida,* 'janggin' (Dyirbal/Tully River); 'garranggal' (Yidinyji/Mulgrave River).

Used as fish poison by the Dyirbal. When this vine flowers, the Scrub Turkey, *Alectura lathami* is ready to lay its eggs. When it fruits, the Turkey has laid its eggs.[19] Not used as a fish poison by the Yidinyji.

Cocky Apple, *Planchonia careya*, 'majal' (Dyirbal, Girramay/Tully River); 'barjal' (Yidinyji,/Mulgrave River).

'... bark (?) used as a fish poison ...'[19] The Yidinyji placed the bark, leaves and twigs in a hole, covered them with soil and warmed them before use. This method made the poison more effective.

unidentified shrub with yellow flowers, 'malibai' to the Yidinyji..

The honey had a stupefying effect (*Table 12.1*). 'Malibai' was also used as a fish poison.

*We scratched the tree, put it in water* [squeezed it to force liquid out of tree into the water] *and it bit the eyes of the fishes.*

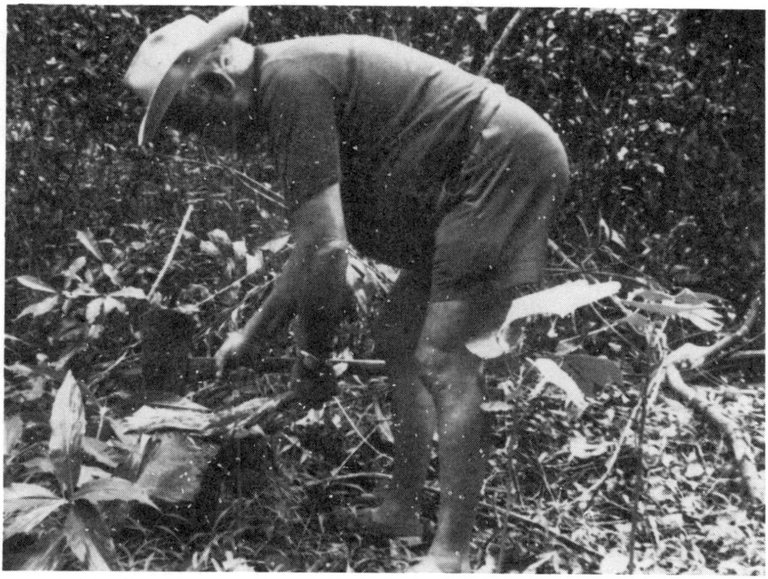

*Plate 12.4: A vine, 'girringai' to the Yidinyji but not yet identified by science, was pulverised and used to stun fish so they could be captured easily.*

**TABLE 12.4: A Rainforest Herbal: List of Plants in Text. (s) Denotes that the name is a junior synonym.**

*Alocasia macrorrhiza* (Araceae)
*Alsophila australis* (s) (Cyatheaceae)
*Alstonia scholaris* (Apocynaceae)
*Austrosteenisia blackii* (Fabaceae)
*Barringtonia racemosa* (Barringtoniaceae)
*Calamus australis* (Arecaceae)
*Calamus caryotoides* (Arecaceae)
*Calamus moti* (Arecaceae)
*Calamus radicalis* (Arecaceae)
*Calophyllum inophyllum* (Guttiferae)
*Cupaniopsis flagelliformis* (Sapindaceae)
*Cupaniopsis foveolatus* (Sapindaceae)
*Cyathea cooperi* (Cyatheaceae)
*Cycas media* (Cycadaceae)
*Cymbidium albuciflorum* (s)(Orchidaceae)
*Cymbidium madidum* (Orchidaceae)
*Dendrocnide moroides* (Urticaceae)
*Dicranopteris linearis*
*Eclipta prostrata* (Asteraceae)
*Ervatamia orientalis* (Apocynaceae)
*Faradaya splendida* (Verbanaceae)
*Ficus congesta* (Moraceae)
*Ficus copiosa* (Moraceae)
*Lepidozamia hopei* (Zamiaceae)
*Lophostemon exiliflora* (Myrtaceae)
*Melaleuca quinquenervia* (Myrtaceae)
*Planchonia careya* (Leycithidaceae)
*Prunus turnerana* (Rosaceae)
*Rhachisperma crassicarpa* (Mimosaceae)
*Rhodomyrtus macrocarpa* (Myrtaceae)
*Semecarpus australiensis* (Anarcardiaceae)
*Scleria levis* (Cyperaceae)
*Syzygium tierneyanum* (Myrtaceae)
*Tabernoemontana orientalis* (s) (Apocynaceae)
*Ziera smithii* (Rutaceae)

The Aboriginal people of the rainforest of north Queensland, like Aboriginal people from other areas, knew their country and its plants and animals intimately. Although early European attitudes to their diverse poisons, potions and life strategies were often cynical and even derisive, their skills and knowledge did not go unrecognised.

> *...The aborigines, being keen observers, knew their botany thoroughly and were well conversant with the properties and practical applications ...* [24]

And, soon after first European contact, the people with whom Lumholtz worked earned grudging respect from him. Of the Herbert River people to the south of Yidinyji territory he observed:[12]

> *... the natives are very kind and sympathetic towards those who are ill, and they carry them from camp to camp ... .*

Product of his time, he continued:

> ***This is the only noble trait that I discovered in the Australian natives ...*** ! [emphasis ours] .

Perhaps the people of the rainforests showed another wisdom. The cynical Lumholtz noted:

> *...the sick* [amongst the north Queensland Aborigines] *are treated by the doctor who, as a rule, is the most cunning man in the tribe and a great humbug ... .*[12]

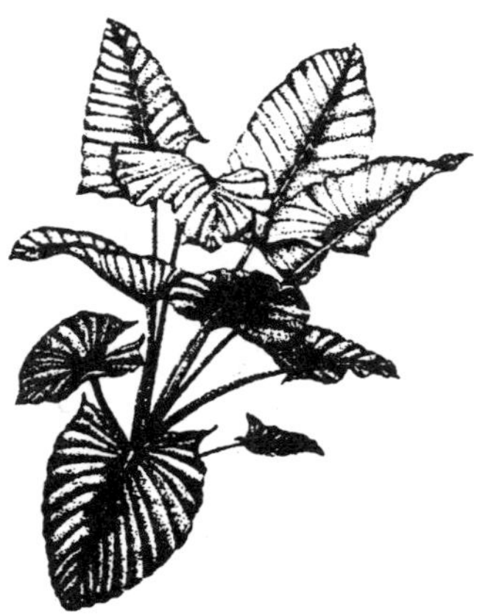

# EARLY HEALTH PROBLEMS IN ABORIGINES

**Dawn May**

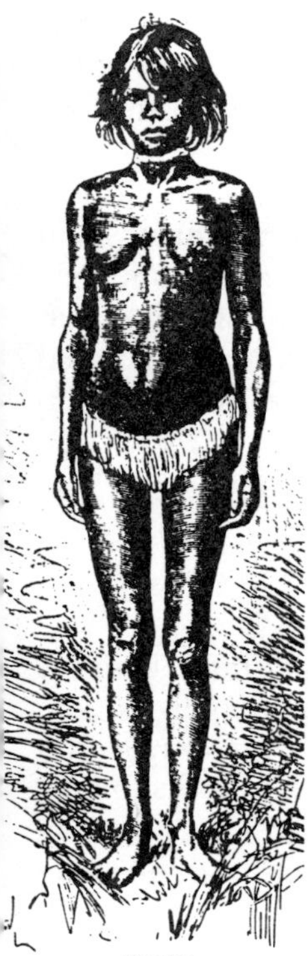

*THE* Aboriginal population has a long history of resisting European medicine, or at best being reluctant participants.[1] For years now signals have been sent that the western medical system is inappropriate for Aboriginal needs. It is only recently, however, that some administrators have been prepared to acknowledge this fact.[2,3] Notwithstanding the extensive survey of the 'health and environmental circumstances of aboriginals' conducted by the National Health and Medical Research Council in the late 1930s, the emphasis has generally been on treatment rather than prevention.[4] This paper will focus on the experiences of Aborigines in outback Queensland hospitals before World War II to show that European medical care clearly caused more problems than it cured.

Country towns typically had a high turnover of medical staff, a factor which was detrimental to both blacks and whites. It was common for doctors and nursing personnel to stay for only a few months. In the interim, hospitals were left for long periods with insufficient staff. Committees were forced to go through, yet again, the time-consuming process of readvertising and selecting new appointees. Even at the Dunbar Australian Inland Mission hospital where nursing staff promised to serve a two year term, there were occasions when trained officials were simply not available.[5] However, with the advent of the Flying Doctor Service, a 'mantle of safety' was provided not only for people living on remote stations, but also for those operating understaffed country hospitals[6] where Aboriginals made up a large proportion of the patients.

Given their primitive living conditions and lack of adequate sanitation, the black population was extremely susceptible to disease (*Figure 13.1*). They were even considered by some authorities to be the 'active agents in the spread of germs'.[7] Predictably their most common ailments were infectious diseases – influenza, venereal diseases, measles, whooping cough, conjunctivitis, hookworm, scabies and malaria. A medical survey of Aboriginal health in North Queensland undertaken by Dr Raphael Cilento in the early 1930s showed that throughout the peninsula 'malaria was more or less endemic although milder forms were often mistaken for Gulf fever or fever and ague'.[8] The State Government in Queensland simply could not turn its back on the sub-optimal physical health of the indigenous population.

In return for subsidies, hospital committees in Queensland were forced to give free treatment to Aborigines referred by medical officers or local Protectors.[9] This led to the common observation that all Aborigines were getting free health care, a fact which generated considerable resentment. The secretary of the Burketown hospital for instance advised the Home Secretary in 1923 that –

> *'the care of the Aboriginals should be borne by somebody other than the handful of whites in this District ... There are only 351 white inhabitants including children in the whole of this huge area.*[10]

In fact those Aborigines who were employed and held banking accounts were responsible for their own medical expenses and an examination of hospital subscription lists clearly shows that Aborigines were amongst their regular contributors.[11] Notwithstanding financial input, hospital committees lacked interest in Aboriginal patients and this was reflected in the appalling accommodation and treatment meted out to them.

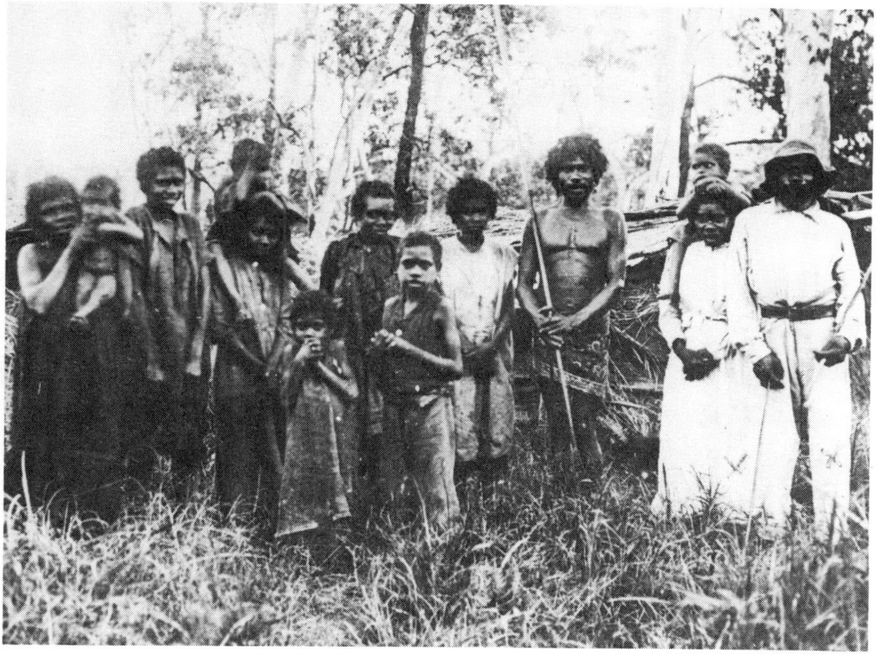

***Figure 13.1:* *The wearing of European clothing often facilitated the spread of disease, particularly as there was no provision for washing in Aboriginal housing before the World War II. (Photograph courtesy of the John Oxley Library, State Library of Queensland)***

Administrators of country hospitals would have preferred not to admit Aboriginal patients. In 1901 Northern Protector Walter Roth noted that 'there was a tendency for certain hospital committees to repudiate or rather, to put obstacles in the way of admission of black patients'.[12] The rules of the Normanton Hospital decreed that 'no aboriginal employed by any resident of the district shall be admitted unless such resident undertakes in writing to pay half the usual hospital charges or furnishes satisfactory evidence that he has not sufficient means to pay same'.[13] At Croydon, where Aboriginal patients were charged an exorbitant 25 shillings[14] they were only allowed on the Hospital verandah![15] Nevertheless this was infinitely better than the situation at Burketown where the regulations of the hospital did not provide for the treatment of Aborigines 'directly or indirectly'[16] a situation which remained

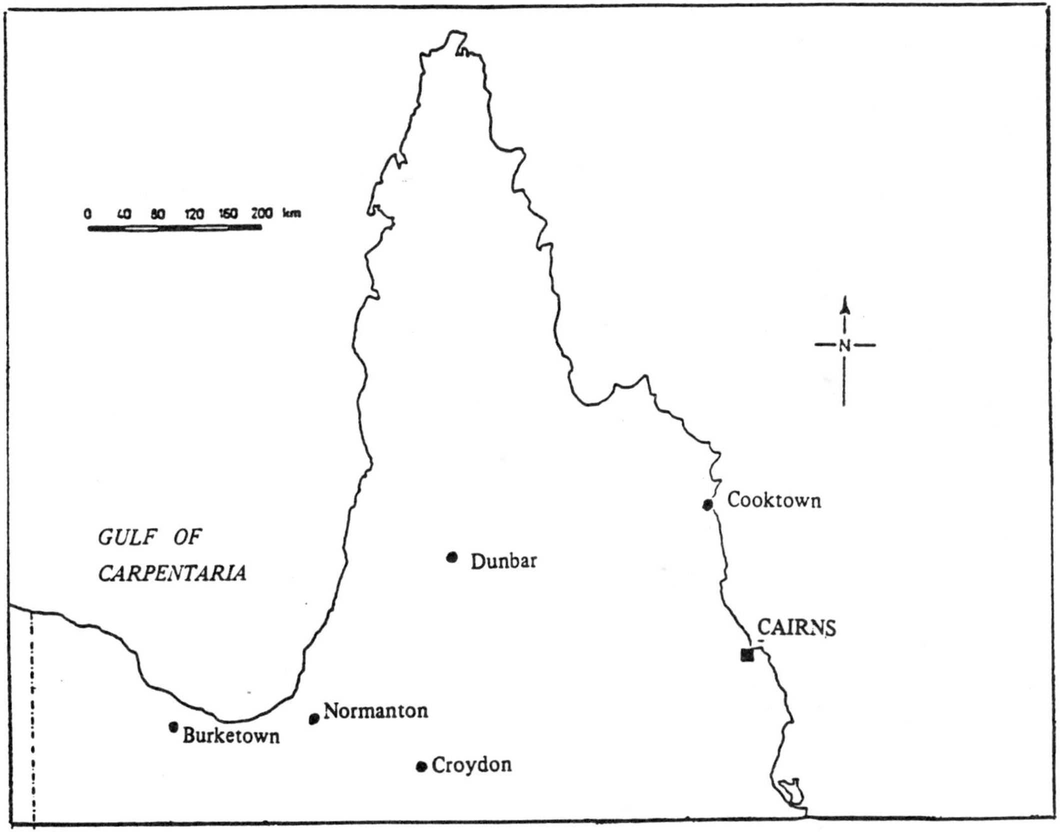


*Figure 13.2: North Queensland, showing the location of Dunbar Hospital, maintained by the Australian Inland Mission.*

unchanged for some years. In 1913 the manager of a large cattle station was angered by the poor treatment one of his employees received at the hospital. He wrote to the Secretary –

> *It is to be conjectured that the Committee considers the treatment of a case by a wardsman is equal to, and worth as much as that by a medical practitioner, also that the charge for an Aborigine camping in the morgue (or as Tiger expresses it, 'in the deadhouse') or on the woodheap, without expense, to the institution for bedding, should be charged for at the same rate as attendance on a white man enjoying the comfort of a more or less well appointed ward.*[17]

On occasions conditions were so bad that protectors took the unusual step of personally communicating with the Minister. For instance in 1923 the Georgetown Protector complained of the poor treatment given to a dying Aboriginal woman at the local hospital.[18]

Aboriginal hospital accommodation was always inadequate and grossly overcrowded. In 1934 the Burketown hospital board asked for a special grant of £115 from the Golden Casket* to extend their Aboriginal quarters. Lack of space had forced administrators to put two patients to a bed, and on other occasions to erect tents to accommodate the surplus.[19] The situation was much the same at Normanton where Aboriginal patients were all crowded into one room – males, females, infectious patients and maternity cases. A 'lean-to' provided two additional rooms; one was used for labour ward and the other to store linen and dressings. The galvanised iron building was located 100 yards from the main wards, a fact which caused great inconvenience to the nursing staff. Matron Hulbert was most dissatisfied with the conditions under which the Aboriginal patients were housed. She described the building as 'little more than a shed with a board floor'. Taking the matter into her own hands, she moved the Aboriginal patients into the isolation building which had been vacant for five years. This was vastly better than the old accommodation as patients could be dispersed between three wards; five beds in one room for women, three in another for men and one in the third for obstetrics. 'Most convenient in every way and near the Hospital proper,' pronounced the Matron. The hospital committee

*The 'Golden Casket' was established as a State lottery, initially to provide funds for Queensland's free Hospital system. [Ed.]

was less enthusiastic and ordered the Aborigines back to their old quarters. The sequel to this saga was that the Matron refused to oblige unless suitable partitioning was installed. She threatened to leave if this was not forthcoming and the committee duly accepted her resignation![20]

Even in institutions with a religious basis, segregated accommodation was the norm. When the Australian Inland Mission (AIM) hospital was established on *Dunbar* Station (*Figure 13.2*) in 1938 it was unlikely that medical care of Aborigines loomed large on the list of priorities. AIM Centres were known as nursing homes rather than hospitals, emphasising the welfare function of such institutions. It was believed that the presence of white women in remote areas would have a moderating effect on those who lived in the district.[21] With an increasing number of Aboriginal patients at the *Dunbar* centre, a decision was made to erect a separate ward for them. The nursing staff was relieved to have them accommodated elsewhere as Europeans generally found Aboriginal personal habits repugnant. 'They cough and spit everywhere despite instructions', an exasperated sister advised her superior.

Many decisions made in relation to Aboriginal health were blatantly racist. At Normanton in 1937, for instance, the hospital committee refused to allow the medical officer to operate on an Aboriginal woman. After lengthy discussion, the motion was carried that:

> *... the committee cannot see its way clear to allow aboriginals and non-whites to be operated on in the theatre nor to receive any surgical after-treatment in the annex to main building.*[22]

Even after the doctor had demonstrated that there was no risk of contamination after sterilization, the committee remained firm in its resolve not to allow the operation to proceed. The only thing for the doctor to do was to arrange to have the woman flown to Cloncurry where the surgery was performed. To avert a repetition of a similar incident, the local Protector recommended that the department build a small hospital in Normanton for local Aborigines with its own operating theatre and sterilising and outpatients' room. While this would have been welcomed by the local white community, the Chief Protector of Aborigines vetoed the suggestion because it would have encouraged similar requests from other country hospitals, the cost of which would have been prohibitive.[23] Poor Aboriginal health clearly exacerbated discrimination and prejudice.[24]

The high incidence of communicable diseases amongst Aborigines was also used to exclude them from both white society and the use of public facilities. There was a marked reluctance to treat Aborigines suffering from venereal disease, a scourge in the Gulf and Peninsula districts throughout the 1920s and 1930s. It was reported in 1923 that there were 'two very filthy cases of syphilis' in the Aboriginal ward at Normanton. The secretary complained that –

> *... the local Protector says we must admit them. My committee are desirous of knowing if such is the case. We admit in these outback places there is no other place to put them. Still, fancy having cases like these within 50 paces of the main ward!*[25]

The disease continued to be the bane of the Hospital Committee which reported a number of years later that two thirds of the patients treated there were Aborigines many with venereal disease. Those infected with granuloma or gonorrhoea were treated as outpatients if suitable isolation could be arranged. As there were no Aboriginal 'lock wards' attached to country hospitals, the local jail was commonly used for this purpose.[26] With the establishment of a Lock Hospital on Fantome Island in 1926 people suffering with syphilis were sent there. Although hospital officials could still not legally refuse treatment to Aborigines, the presence of a specialist institution made it easier to deny medical care to Aborigines with venereal disease.[27]

From an Aboriginal perspective removal from their district often caused cultural difficulties. After two Aborigines sought assistance at *Dunbar* hospital and were sent to Fantome Island for treatment, records show that no further Aborigines with venereal disease went to that centre. A local Protector believed that the complaint was rife amongst bush blacks in the area but they deliberately avoided detection so they would not be removed from their homeland. Subsequent nursing staff at *Dunbar* Hospital were always faced with a dilemma when patients required treatment at a larger hospital such as Cairns. As Margaret Ford recalled –

> *It had become established in the minds of aboriginal folk that once one of their number was taken away in the medical plane*

> *he would never return. This was because so often patients were not brought into our hospital until they were very seriously ill, by which time little could be done for them.*[28]

Removal to hospital often seemed like a sentence of death. If the patient died, the fears of those left behind were confirmed and they quickly lost faith in the European medical system.

At least at *Dunbar* hospital, Aboriginal patients were able to have relatives visit which was an important part of their therapy. Sister Payne recalled that the 'natives [were] a very affectionate race – when one of their number [was] sick the grandmothers, grandfathers, mothers-in-law etc. came from far and near to see Jacky or whoever it may be'.[29] Overcrowding in town hospitals such as Burketown and Normanton precluded the luxury of visitors. At Normanton as many as nine patients were squeezed into space sufficient for three. On occasions this necessitated having three people to a bed. Sick children were put into beds with adult men and or women. Others were rolled in blankets and put on the floor.

Sister Hulbert had worked hard to gain the confidence of Aborigines so they would go freely to the hospital for treatment and she complained bitterly to the Minister of the detrimental effect of 'herding' so many people into the one room. She was obviously aware of the cultural implications writing that 'I leave to your imagination the fears and feelings of superstitious aboriginals under such conditions and our difficulty in getting them to come here to be treated'.[30] Under such circumstances it was not uncommon for patients to abscond after a death in the ward believing that illness would result if the spirit of the dead person were not at rest. This could happen if the proper mourning rituals were not observed; this was particularly difficult when men, women and children were crowded into the one room.

Traditionally, Aborigines believed that most illness and death were caused by 'magical' or 'supernatural' influences. It was accepted that the very old or young could die of natural causes. However sickness could result from direct supernatural intervention. Powerful spirits could cause people to become sick for a variety of reasons. These 'evil spirits' were everywhere and could inflict illness for a breach of Aboriginal law. People could also be stricken with disease by indirect supernatural intervention. The most commonly cited instance of this was of course 'boning' but another form of indirect

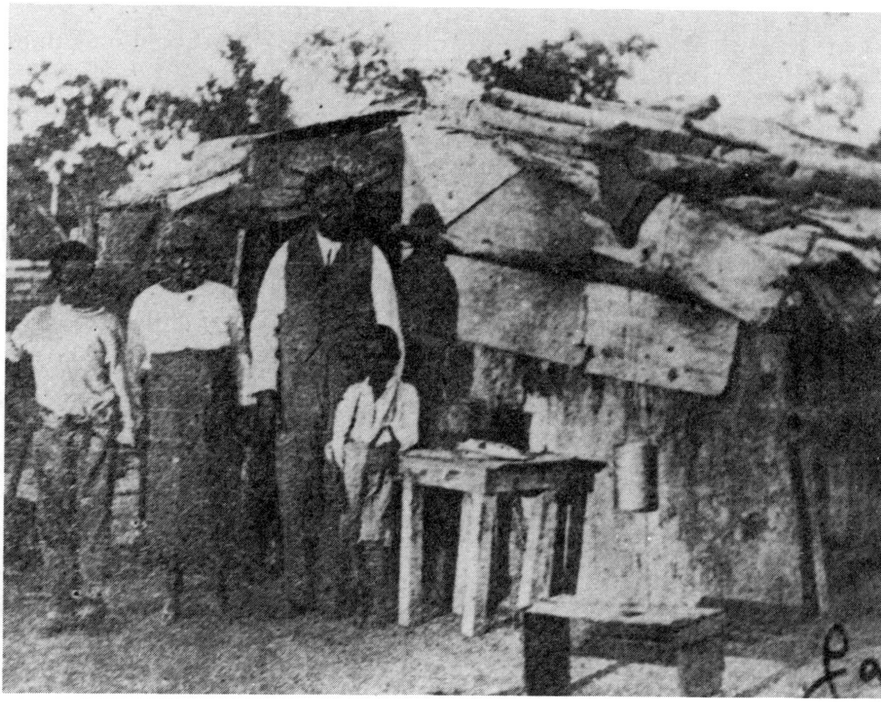

***Figure 13.3:* *'Family Group, Mount Norman, Richmond'.***
***From the North Queensland Register, 10 January 1921.***

supernatural intervention was through the Kadaitcha Man who travelled at night and was often used for 'payback'. Stories abound throughout North Queensland of Kadaitcha's activities and there is still [1988] a strong respect for him evident even amongst urban blacks. In some areas, environmental factors such as the wind and moon could also be agents of illness. For instance, certain winds were blamed for causing diarrhoea.[31]

The durability of the Aboriginal belief in magic has been brilliantly captured by Elizabeth O'Conner in her book *Spirit Man*. This story is based on an actual event which occurred in North Queensland. Believing a curse had been placed on them by an Aboriginal domestic, two men attacked the woman's husband and cut away part of the fat surrounding his kidney.[32] The young European woman left alone to cope with the situation had to keep reminding herself that this was 1934. 'The blacks were civilised,

Christian, their old customs discarded and at least by the young ones forgotten'.[33] It was a completely unnerving experience to discover that in reality the old beliefs lay dormant behind the Aboriginal acceptance of the European practices. Even Herby, a part-Aborigine who had long ago decided that the approval and protection of the white man was more desirable than Aboriginal magic, was affected. When a curse was placed on him, he soon succumbed, developing a high fever and pains in his joints. He remembered the curse and knew that his illness was a result of it. In spite of hospitalisation, Herby surrendered to the powers of Aboriginal magic and quietly passed away.[34]

Some Europeans were well aware that the different Aboriginal perceptions of sickness and death created enormous problems in the delivery of health care. This was reflected in the way they handled black patients. Unfortunately these people were the exception rather than the rule. The high turnover in staff ensured that sympathetic medical officers were regularly replaced with less tolerant counterparts. There tended to be less variation in attitudes to Aborigines from hospital committees drawn from local communities. First hand knowledge of 'disease-ridden' fringe camps tended to reinforce white prejudice which was incorporated into decisions affecting Aboriginal patients. Because they were regarded as second-class citizens, it was acceptable to refuse to treat them or to force them into grossly overcrowded accommodation exacerbating their health disadvantage. Most Aborigines placed a far higher value on traditional remedies and bush doctors. They were usually reluctant patients of the western system forced into it by well-meaning employers or local Protectors. Their experiences served only to confirm their fears of the white system. European medical care clearly caused more problems than it cured.

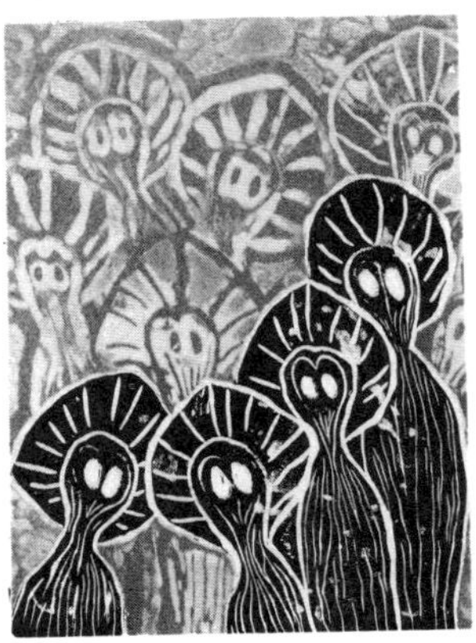

# PART IV

# PIONEERS AND PIONEEERING MEDICINE

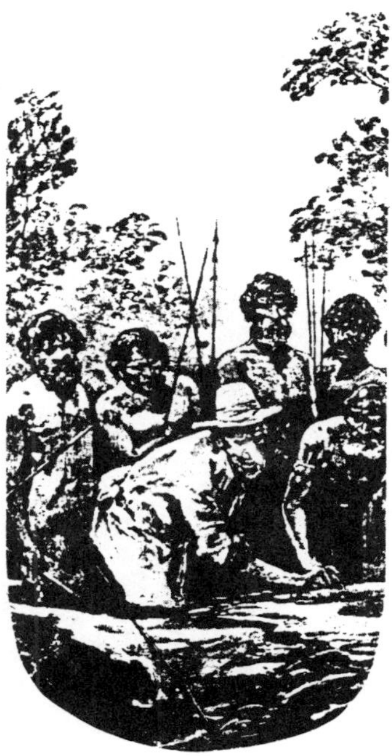

# EARLY DEVELOPMENTS IN AUSTRALIAN OBSTETRICS

**John Campbell**

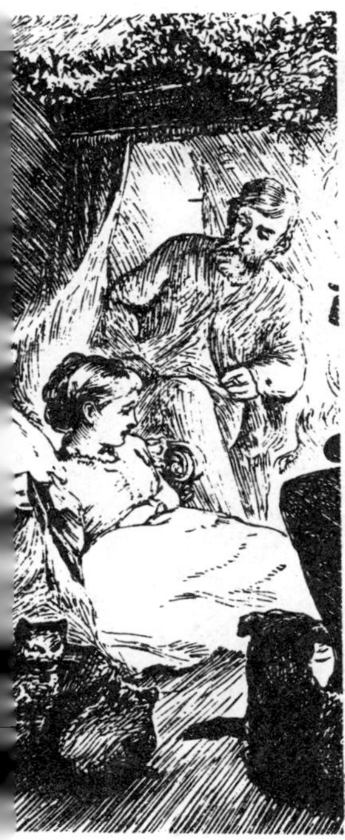

*CHILDBIRTH* is a natural mammalian function. There are significant hazards, of course to mother and child though what the mortality was in the native unaided state will probably never be known. At least 1–2% of the mothers were lost, and depending on circumstances up to 50% of the progeny. To lend a helping hand in this process of childbirth is called midwifery; northern Aborigines had a well developed midwifery service. It was probable that their maternal and perinatal mortality in 1824 was little different from that of their white sisters. Childbirth among the Nation's first inhabitants was more often than not a female and secretive event. Not only were men excluded but the woman and her female attendants moved to a 'a place further than a baby's crying distance' so that male curiosity would not be aroused. The midwives were usually 'blood relatives' and in most cases there were more than one.

Some information concerning the intimate details of aboriginal birth processes has been derived from a description by a Queensland doctor, Jack de Vidas.[1] In 1947 he wrote of his experience in befriending the Aranda tribe. Its members gave him their confidence to such an extent that he was allowed to be a part of their childbirth customs. He obtained exclusive and invaluable clinical knowledge relating to tribal midwifery practice and its associated variations. Two points especially stand out. Firstly, and this is attested by other anthropologists, there was almost no interference whatever with or in the mechanism of childbirth and secondly, though maternal and fetal mortaility was low in normal cases it was quite the opposite when major problems arose. De Vidas describes how he had 'been summoned to native camps only to find the scratched and torn body of a dead child with the head still in the vagina and the attendants and relatives helpless with hysteria'.

The word 'obstetrics' and the word 'midwifery' basically and effectively mean the same. However the term 'obstetrician' is now regarded as referring to a doctor, trained in medicine and surgery

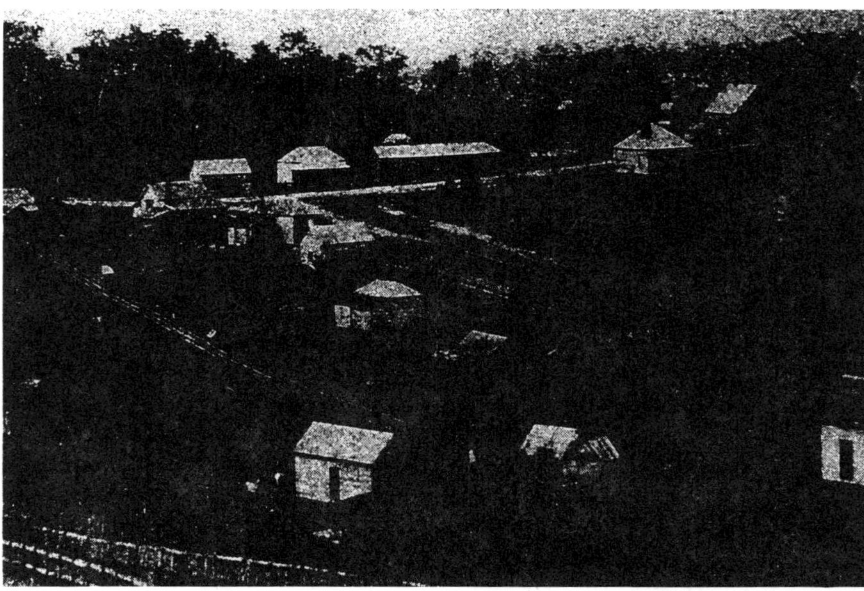

***Figure 14.1:* *An old photograph of Leichhardt Street, Brisbane in 1862. The site of Fairview House – rented premises of The Queensland Lying-In Hospital – is included in this scene, but its exact position remains unknown. (Photo courtesy The Oxley Library, Brisbane)***

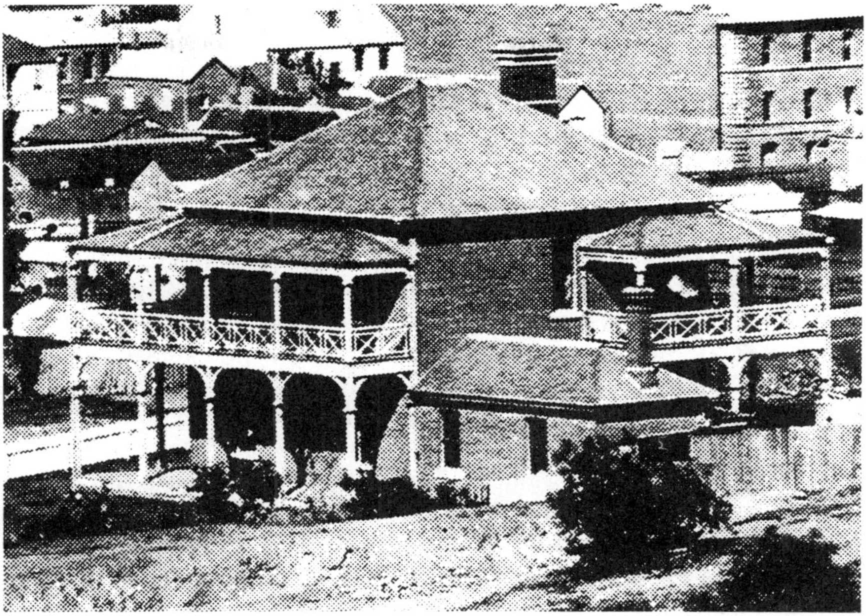

***Figure 14.2: The first Lady Bowen Hospital in Ann Street, Brisbane, opened in 1867. (Photo courtesy of The Oxley Library, Brisbane)***

who is able, and indeed, usually does, undertake major interference in complicated cases. Midwifery is a profession, older than medicine and originally, at any rate, largely female. Midwives still take pride in conducting confinements with minimum interference. When things go wrong in childbirth, as they have from time immemorial, and will continue so to do, there is ample opportunity for the non-interfering midwife and the interfering doctor, when they come together, to engage in mutual and non-productive argument and criticism. Earle Hackett[2] has written of the delightful confrontation of Dr Slop, the man-midwife with the real midwife at the bedside during the birth of Tristram Shandy in Laurence Sterne's wonderful novel. Nevertheless, doctors—whether they were witch-doctors or graduates of world renowned universities – were generally impotent bystanders at childbirth problems until the development of obstetric forceps, caesarean section and more importantly, anaesthesia. Sad to say, even now, in many parts of the world the situation is little different from that which pertained when Mumtaz-I–Mahal, a grand-multipara died in childbirth in the 17th Century – precipitating the erection of the 'world's most beautiful building' which now bears her name. Of it has been said 'it is within more measurable distance of perfection than any other work of man'.

History has not recorded any obstetric adventures of Queensland's first doctor, the surgeon Walter Scott who accompanied Lieutenant Miller in the State's original white Settlement in Moreton Bay on 13th September 1824. Scott's biography recently published by Professor John Pearn[3] is compulsive reading. 'After an atrocious passage of eleven days during which adverse winds almost continuously prevailed' the party landed at Redcliffe. There were thirty convicts, all but one in chains, and at least two pregnant women. Their vessel the *Amity* soon left to return to Sydney and their isolation can only be imagined. The first white boy born in Queensland was Charles Moreton Miller, son of the expedition leader; the first girl was Amity Moreton Thompson – both born at Redcliffe and presumably attended by the wives of the soldiers. The surgeon probably had neither the time nor the equipment to have been much help had his services been required. After some eight months, the settlement moved to Brisbane arriving in May 1825. In August 1825 Dr Henry Cowper – Australia's first medical graduate and a former apprentice of Dr Redfern – was appointed surgeon to the penal settlement. During his tenure of seven years, up to the time of his ignominious dismissal in 1832,[4] Dr Cowper almost certainly acted as consultant to the local practitioners of midwifery. The wife of Captain Logan, the Commandant, was confined during this period and in 1827 the wives and children of male convicts were allowed to enter the Settlement.

It was in 1827 that the 'Female Factory' was established for these wives and children as well as for female convicts at the site of the present General Post Office in Queen Street. It is interesting to speculate on the descent of these 'Female Factories' in penal colonies from the segregated workhouses established in England (Poorhouses in Scotland) from the time of Charles the Second.[5] One recalls that Oliver Twist was born in a workhouse. His mother was attended by the midwife, Mrs Thimgummy – 'a pauper old woman' and 'a parish surgeon who did such matters by contract'. The mother, of course, succumbed shortly after her confinement. It is also interesting to follow the unbroken progression from the 'Female Factory' as it evolved into what is now a great obstetric institution, the Royal Women's Hospital in Brisbane. The 'Factory' in which women lived, worked, gave birth and often died, moved eventually to Eagle Farm* to the site of the old airport, together with its midwives or 'fingersmiths' in convict jargon. These women are believed to have, at times, served the officers' and soldiers' wives in labour.

The closure of this institution when the penal settlement was discontinued in 1839 (and before free settlement commenced in 1842) left a gap. The military hospital accepted free-settlers who paid for their care but paupers were excluded and the plight of destitute pregnant women over the next twenty years must have been appalling. Even among the well-to-do, obstetric cases were only rarely admitted to hospital. Social pressure gradually developed to the point where some provision for services to women in late pregnancy were available.

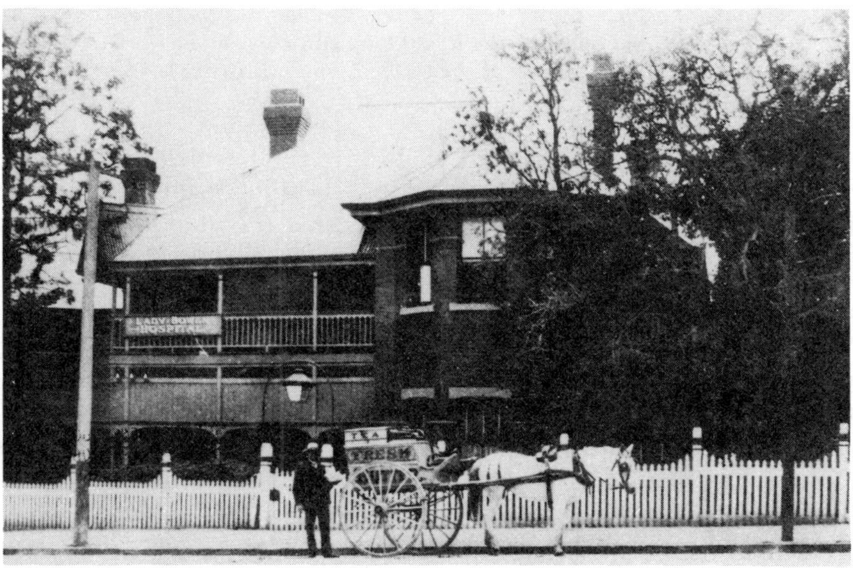

***Figure 14.3: The second Lady Bowen Hospital, Brisbane. This was built on Wickham Terrace in 1889. The Hospital was one daily stop for the tea and butter vendor, shown here with his horse and cart. (Photo courtesy The Oxley Library, Brisbane)***

*'Eagle Farm' was so named in September 1829, being the site selected by Captain Patrick Logan for a maize and rice farm on the banks of the lower Brisbane River. It subsequently became the Female Factory, for recidivist women convicts. It served as Brisbane's commercial airport until 1988.

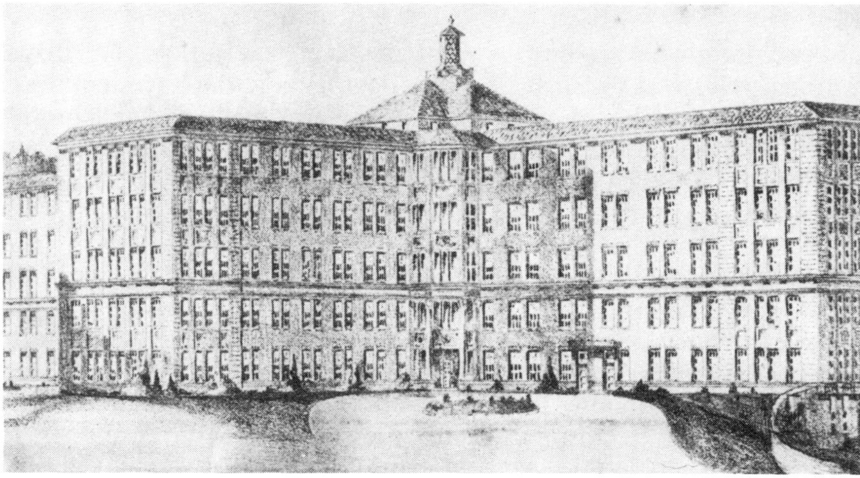

***Figure 14.4: The Women's Hospital in Brisbane. Architects' drawing of proposed hospital, circa 1935. The new hospital was finally opened in 1938, and renamed the Royal Women's Hospital in 1968. (Photo courtesy of the Oxley Library, Brisbane)***

In 1864 the Queensland Lying-In Hospital, which later became the Lady Bowen Hospital, was established in a rented house in Leichhardt Street in Spring Hill in Brisbane (*Figure 14.1*). Women from the lowest socio-economic stratas again received proper care.[6] The Hospital moved to Ann Street in 1867 (*Figure 14.2*) and in 1890 to Wickham Terrace to a building which stands to this day (*Figure 14.3*). Eventually the patients from the Lady Bowen were transferred to the Brisbane Women's Hospital on 26th March 1938 and the hospital on Wickham Terrace closed.[7]

Most of the women in Brisbane, in the early years of this Century, still had their babies at home and most were attended by midwives. The midwives were usually unqualified. Indeed, before training became available in the Lady Bowen after its early days, there were no qualifications to be had. Many local midwives were self-taught, and despite much criticism most were probably kindly and quietly efficient. Around the years of the First World War numbers of 'lying-in homes' or cottage maternity hospitals were established. These were under the management of a midwife who usually had a close working arrangement with the local doctors who referred their patients to these houses. Some of the establishments were in fact adjuncts to small private hospitals. Conditions and patient care in some were of quite high standards; others were mediocre and even dangerous and most were forced to close down with the advent of the Women's Hospital (*Figure 14.4*). It is of interest that in the Bicentennial year small units are now making a comeback and at least three new ones have commenced operation in Brisbane alone in the last three years.

It was natural that education and certification of midwives should commence at the Lady Bowen. In 1870, some seven years after the hospital's opening, two-thirds of confinements in Sydney, and presumably Brisbane, were conducted by midwives, most being untrained. The story of Queensland's midwifery and training has recently been told in a meticulously researched paper by John Thearle and Helen Gregory[8] who show the evolution of the training and the eventual elimination of the uncertified midwife.

With the spread of hospital maternity care throughout the northern parts of Australia and with the assistance of the medical and nursing professions, the training of midwives became widespread. It may be said in this context that not all modern midwives appreciate the interest these two disciplines have shown in their ancient specialty. Nurses have demanded a general nursing training as a prerequisite to midwifery, and doctors have insisted on a significant medical input. Many midwives feel that they have been swamped by well meaning experts who have not fully appreciated their special vocation.

From the days of Henry Cowper, nineteenth century doctors in Australia provided a medical and surgical 'back-up' for midwives; in the last fifty years the medical profession has taken the responsibility for the management of parturition to itself, delegating to midwives the general management of labour, and that of puerperal care. Their medical attendance was then limited to a period which hopefully included the actual birth and variable visits thereafter. Thousands of doctors have carried out these services with great dedication – sadly very few left a detailed account of their work. One exception was Walter Lindsay Richardson of Ballarat, who worked in the 1860s era, and whose story has been told by Frank Forster.[9] Another was the late Paul Hopkins of Mackay who in 1955 published the results of 1500 consecutive and personally confined patients in what he modestly called a 'typical country general practice'.[10] Along with the midwives however, most attending doctors have been unsung and unhonoured.

The story of the development of obstetric teaching throughout the Commonwealth has been ably told by the same Frank Forster, our greatest obstetric historian, in his *Progress in Obstetrics and Gynaecology in Australia in 1967*,[11] a slim volume which still remains an invaluable and interesting reference.

Reduction of maternal mortality to a negligible level in recent years and the dramatic improvement in peri-natal mortality in Australia and in the Western World should not be a cause for complacency. We live in a single world and there are still places where 3% of mothers die in childbirth. We should not forget that among the 777 million people of India, among the 102 million of Pakistan, and among the 103 million of Bangladesh, the benefits of modern obstetrics and midwifery are sadly largely lacking.

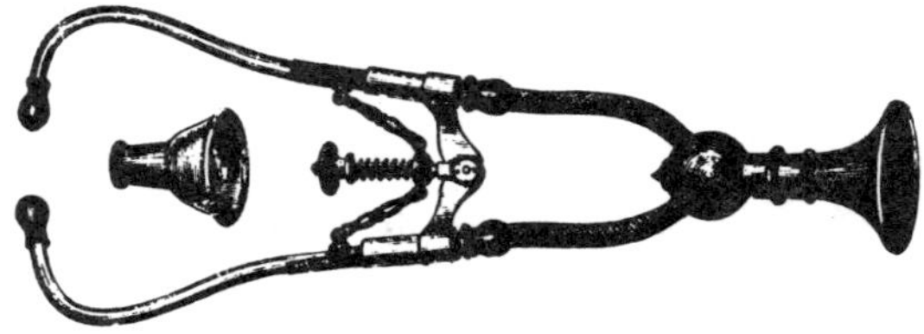

# PIONEER MEDICINE IN AUSTRALIA 15

# AUSTRALIAN MEDICAL GOVERNORS

## Aesculapius and the Vice-Regal Office

**Robert Pearce**

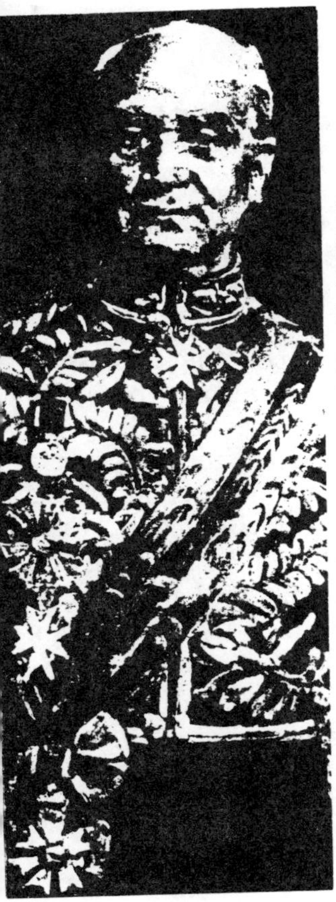

*OUR* colonial and State governors in Australia have most commonly been appointed from the ranks of titled British aristocracy. More recently they have been recruited from the ranks of retired senior service officers, judges and academics. It may seem surprising therefore to find that a small number of governors have been medically qualified.

A precedent was set by Jan Van Riebeeck of the Dutch East India Company who founded Capetown. Having sailed to the Cape in 1652 Doctor Van Riebeeck established the first settlement there and for ten years he was Governor of one of the most important Dutch colonial outposts.[1] Similarly, Cadwallader Colden (1688–1776), Scottish born and qualified MD at Edinburgh University, became Lieutenant Governor of New York State in 1761.

## Dr John Hampton

The first medical governor in Australia was Dr John Stephen Hampton who was appointed to the post in Western Australia on 22nd October, 1861. Hampton qualified in Medicine from the University of Edinburgh in 1828. He was then twenty-two years old and in January 1829 he signed on as Assistant Surgeon aboard the *Brittania.* The following month he transferred to the *Sphynx*. By mid 1832 he was attached to the Plymouth dockyard where he earned high praise for his work in preventing the spread of cholera.[2] Hampton subsequently served on board the *Savage*, the *Firebrand* and the *Portland*. He was promoted to Surgeon in December 1834 and again in March 1843 to Surgeon Superintendent. His was a firm hand.

Having served efficiently on a succession of convict ships to Van Diemen's Land[3] Hampton came to the notice of the Secretary of State for the colonies, W.E. Gladstone. He was offered the appointment as comptroller-general of convicts in Van Diemen's Land in May 1846 and arrived in Hobart Town on 27 October in the same year.

Hampton's eleven years in this post earned for him a reputation of harsh, tyrannical convict administration. Transportation of convicts to Van Diemen's Land ceased at the end of 1852 and Dr Hampton left the colony five years later amid allegations of inhumanity and corruption.[4]

The 1840s had seen a period of serious economic depression in the United Kingdom and there were repeated efforts to resume convict transportation to the eastern colonies. New South Wales, where transportation had ceased in 1840, protested furiously while Western Australia, still dependent on a parliamentary grant for its existence, was in no position to refuse. The first shipment arrived at Fremantle on 1st June, 1850, and by January 1868, nine thousand six hundred and sixty-eight convicts had arrived in Western Australia.[5] On this score Anthony Trollope made the observation that –

> *Western Australia needed population rather than labour and, as free immigrants did not stay, it devoted itself to the custody of compelled immigrants who could be made to come hither where others would not come.*

Until this time the Swan River Colony was considered by many to be a mere backwater of the Empire, and according to Trollope, 'hardly a colonial prize to be proud of'.[6] In 1865, with a total population of only 20,000, it was referred to in an English journal as 'the most sleepy and stagnant of all our colonies'.

Of the three colonial governors who administered Western Australia during nineteen years of convict transportation Hampton's policies and methods aroused the most controversy.[7]

He arrived in Perth on 28 February 1862, to inherit an acutely embarrassed treasury. Within a year he had instituted economies in the private sector by utilizing convict labour in a comprehensive building programme. Road and bridge construction was accelerated, including a new causeway across the Swan River and later an impressive wooden bridge across the river at Fremantle. At noon on 12th November, 1867, he announced –

> *I, John Stephen Hampton, Governor over the Colony of Western Australia, do hereby declare this causeway open ...,*

when another voice called –

> *... and I, John Stephen Maley, do hereby declare that I will be the first person to cross this Perth bridge and causeway.*[8]

The audacious young man galloped across the bridge to the astonishment and applause of the crowd, thus pre-empting the famous action of Captain de Groot who upstaged Premier Lang at the opening of Sydney Harbour Bridge.

Several splendid public buildings were either commenced or completed during Hampton's term of office. These included Government House which was completed in 1864; The Perth Town Hall – for which he laid the foundation stone in 1867; The Pensioner Guards' Barracks – of which there remains today the entrance arch at the top of St George's Terrace; The Supreme Court Building and Fremantle Gaol. A Summer Residence for the Governor was also erected on Rottnest Island.

Convicts were used in large numbers in building roads, some of which comprised sawn sections of tree trunks which were laid like large cobble stones. They were popularly known as 'Hampton's cheeses'.

In his address to the Legislative Council in 1864, he described work in progress –

> *... bridges at North Fremantle, Perth Causeway, Greenough Flats, Beverley and Ferguson River, jetties at Bunbury and Busselton, additions to the poorhouse, Perth, and police stations at Pinjarra, Newcastle, Baylup, Staunton Springs, and the Lakes, and construction of the swamp drain at the back of Perth. Nearly all this is being done by convict labour which not only costs the colony nothing for labour, supervision, maintenance or equipment, but brings in ninety thousand pounds imperial money annually.*

When it was rumoured in 1865 that Transportation would shortly cease, Hampton shrewdly diverted his labour from imperial projects such as prisons and barracks to purely colonial development, offices and schools. Not so shrewd was his handling of public appointments. His 28 year old son, George Essex Hampton was appointed acting comptroller-general of convicts while retaining the offices of private secretary, clerk of Council and member of the Financial Board. G.E. Hampton also continued to receive the comptroller's lodging allowance while residing at Government House. Such acts made both men unpopular.

However, it was Hampton's cruelty to the convicts which most alienated the small parochial community, particularly the hierarchic social and political élite. By his indiscriminate administration of corporal punishment and solitary confinement for minor offences he was probably responsible for the increase in the number of escapes which occurred at that time.

Church-State relations also deteriorated during Hampton's term and by the time his successor, Frederick Weld, arrived in 1869 a revision of the inequitable system of state aid to organised religion and sectarian education was long overdue.

Dr John Hampton was –

> *... the last of the autocrats, the last Governor in nineteenth century Australia to exercise almost unlimited power over both the executive and legislative branches of government, and the last to administer a convict system.*[9,10]

While his dictatorial attitudes made him unpopular with some, his exploitation of the convicts and successful economic management of the colony resulted in an impressive legacy of public works and a balanced budget. To quote Dr Battye, the Western Australian historian –

> *... the benefits he conferred were lasting in nature whilst his mistakes were ephemeral.*[11]

**Dr J.S. Millner**

In the Northern Territory (where self government was proclaimed on 1st July 1978) there have been no State Governors but two doctors have held the position of Acting Government Resident and Administrator at various times. In the year 1870 and again during 1873, Dr J.S. Millner was appointed acting Government Resident at Palmerston for short interim periods. The first Government Resident at Palmerston (later Port Darwin) was George Woodroffe Goyder (1826–1898) who held office from 1869 to 1870. He was the son of Dr David George Goyder, of London.[12] Nicknamed 'Little Energy', G.W. Goyder was reputed to be the ablest administrator and most efficient public servant in the Colony.[13] Another doctor's son who was appointed to vice-regal office was Sir Anthony Musgrave (1828–1888). He was born at Antigua and became governor of South Australia (1873–1877) and subsequently governor of Queensland in 1883 – until his death in 1888.

**Sir William MacGregor**

Queensland can boast of two medical governors. The first of these, William MacGregor, was born in Hillockhead, Aberdeenshire, the son of a crofter. He graduated LFPS from Anderson's Medical School and subsequently MB from Aberdeen University and LRCP from Edinburgh. He was registered on 9 May, 1872 and was initially appointed medical assistant at the Royal Lunatic Asylum in Aberdeen. By the end of the year he had joined the colonial service and arrived at the Seychelles to commence duties as assistant medical officer in February 1873.

Dr William MacGregor (*Figure 15.1*) benefited from a close association with, and mutual respect for, a fellow Scot, Sir Arthur Gordon, also from Aberdeen, who had become Governor of the Seychelles. One followed the other to Mauritius, then to Fiji where MacGregor served from 1875 to 1888, first as Chief Medical Officer then as Receiver-General and later as Colonial Secretary.[13]

He brought a scientific mind to every problem, particularly that of essential medical research. He served at Fiji at a time (1875) when introduced measles killed 40,000 Fijians of an estimated 150,000 population. In 1888 MacGregor was sworn in as Administrator of the newly formed British New Guinea. Here he made efforts to protect Papuan land and labour from exploitation

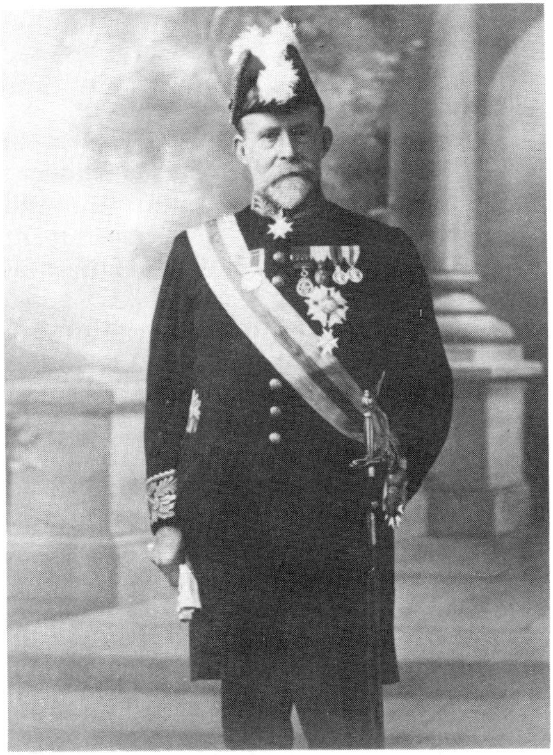

***Figure 15.1:***

***Sir William MacGregor PC, GCMG, CB, LLD, MD. Doctor, and Governor of Queensland, in his Vice-Regal attire. A former Chief Medical Officer in Fiji, he was appointed Governor of Newfoundland, of Lagos, and Administrator of Papua. Photo, courtesy of Archives, University of Queensland.***

and encouraged Papuans to become involved in their own administration and business ventures.

In Lagos, where he was appointed Governor from 1898 to 1902, MacGregor maintained his concern for sanitation and health, assisting Sir Ronald Ross in his scientific work on the transmission of malaria. Ross described him thus –

> *... wise, grave, but humorous, bearded, thickset – his low voice and kindly manner filled all with trust in him ... a mathematician, a practised surveyor, a lapidary, and a master of many arts, but always proud of his medical upbringing and of his nationality.*[13]

Sir William MacGregor (he had been knighted KCMG in 1889) served a term from 1904 to 1909 as Governor of Newfoundland, where many of his ambitions were fulfilled. Here he won his highest compliment from the British Ambassador in Washington, Viscount Bryce, who called him 'a model of what a colonial Governor should be'. MacGregor also received local praise for 'his concern, sympathy and practical aid in combating the 'Great White Plague' (tuberculosis) where he had used his knowledge as a physician and a scientist. He had also helped to found an Anti-Tuberculosis Society.[14]

In 1909, amid political unrest and crisis involving his predecessor Lord Chelmsford, Sir William MacGregor was appointed Governor of Queensland. It was a post for which he had yearned and lobbied for several years. The appointment, at sixty-three years of age, would be his last.

He held office in Queensland from 1909 to 1914 during which time there was a stable conservative government. Although he remained outwardly impartial MacGregor became increasingly critical of labour agitators and socialist union organisers, and said so in his confidential despatches. He also criticised the treatment of Aboriginals and the limited support given to scientific research, particularly in primary industry.

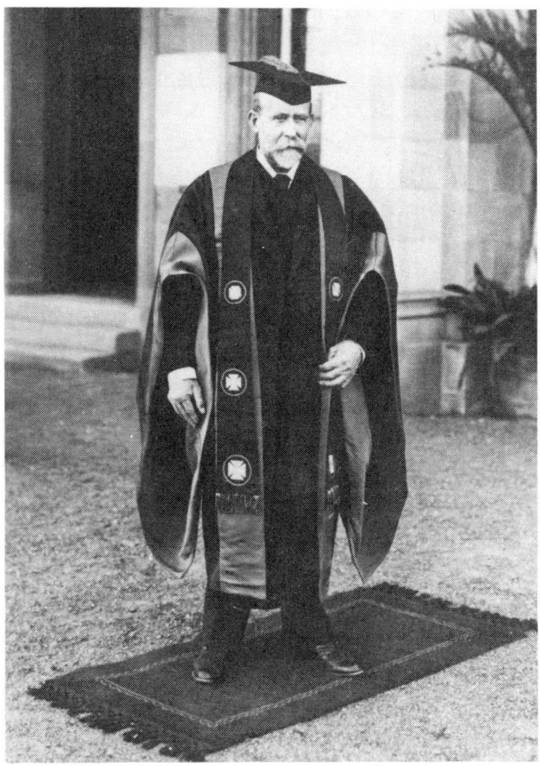

***Figure 15.2:***

***Sir William MacGregor, doctor and Governor of Queensland, in the new academic dress of the University of Queensland. Photographed (so that Vice-Regal shoes would not be scuffed) at the newly established University of Queensland, formerly Government House, The Domain, Brisbane; in his role of the first Chancellor of the University of Queensland. Photo, circa 1912, courtesy of Archives, University of Queensland.***

On 10 December 1909, the fiftieth anniversary of the State's independence, the newly arrived Governor gave his assent to the University of Queensland Bill and formally dedicated Government House to its new purpose of providing a home for the centre of learning.[15]

The University of Queensland received its first student intake in March 1911 and Sir William MacGregor became its first Chancellor (*Figure 15.2*). In this role he influenced decisions regarding matriculation requirements, curricula and academic appointments. Not until 1966 was another Governor, Sir Alan Mansfield, appointed to this academic office.

MacGregor travelled widely and showed continuing concern for the health, education and welfare of indigenous native populations of Queensland and of the Torres Strait Islands. He encouraged all measures to improve the health of school children. He was alarmed to receive a 1911 report which disclosed that 31.7 percent were so physically defective as to affect their educational progress, and that ninety-seven percent had diseased teeth.[14] He officially opened the Institute of Tropical Medicine at Townsville in 1913 (*see Chapter 10*).

MacGregor's scientific interests and expertise extended to Papuan flora and fauna. He made an ethnological collection, specimens of which are housed in the State Museums of Queensland, New South Wales and Victoria. He supported the foundation of the Historical (later Royal Historical) Society of Queensland and became an active president of the Royal Geographical Society of Queensland. Among his many honours, MacGregor received an honorary Doctorate of Laws from Queensland University which subsequently named the Sir William MacGregor School of Physiology in his honour.

Doctor MacGregor retired to Scotland in 1914, and lived through the war years in security. Although occasionally consulted on colonial affairs in the Pacific region, it is reported that he became a lonely, frustrated and embittered man. He died 3rd July, 1919, aged seventy-three years.

## Dr John Gilruth

From 1912 to 1919 Doctor John Anderson Gilruth (1871-1937) held the appointment of Administrator of the Northern Territory, based in Darwin. Commonwealth control of the Territory had been transferred from South Australia in 1911. Within a week of Gilruth's arrival, the Residency, which had recently been occupied by Mr Justice Mitchell, became Government House and its new tenant entertained the local Territorians with a garden party and a lavish banquet.[16] Because of its design this building had become known as 'the house of seven gables'. It provided an essential landmark for brothers Ross and Keith Smith when they landed near Fannie Bay at the end of their epic flight on 10 December 1919.*

Dr Gilruth studied at Glasgow Veterinary College and was admitted to Membership of the Royal College of Veterinary Surgeons, London, in 1892. He also qualified in bacteriology from the Pasteur Institute in Paris and subsequently served with distinction as a pioneer of his profession in New Zealand. In 1900 he was appointed a member of the Royal Commission on Public Health and a year later became pathologist to the newly formed New Zealand Health Department. The New Zealand branch of the British Medical Association elected him an Honorary Member in 1902 and in 1907 he became a Fellow of the Royal Society of Edinburgh.

In 1908 Gilruth accepted appointment to the newly created chair of veterinary pathology at Melbourne University. The following year he was awarded an honorary Doctorate of Veterinary Science.

After investigating the potential of the Northern Territory for economic development (at the request of Prime Minister Andrew Fisher) Dr Gilruth accepted in February 1912 the post of Administrator. Tutored by Baldwin Spencer, he went to Darwin –

> *predisposed to treat the Chinese with reserve, the Aboriginals with heavy-handed paternalism and the white trade unionists with suspicion.*

His term of office extended through the war years but he received neither policies nor powers from the Commonwealth Government to deal with growing industrial discontent in the region. Public disfavour culminated in an angry confrontation between Gilruth and the Darwin townspeople on 17 December, 1918, which became known as the 'Darwin Rebellion'.

As a result of this unrest, Gilruth was recalled in February, 1919. He later joined the newly formed Division of Animal Health within the Council for Scientific and Industrial Research, becoming chief of the Division in 1933. He retired in 1935 and died two years

*Their runway, which marked the end of that historic first flight (28 days) from England to Australia, is now a dual carriageway appropriately named Ross Smith Avenue.

later in Melbourne aged sixty-six. The Gilruth Prize of the Australian Veterinary Association and Gilruth Plains, a research station near Cunnamulla in Queensland commemorate the name of this dedicated scientist and administrator.

**Sir John Goodwin**

The formation of QANTAS in November 1920 directly influenced the inauguration of the Australian Aerial Medical Service, later to become the Royal Flying Doctor Service. In 1927 this service was established in Western Queensland with a plane, pilot and aerodrome facilities provided by QANTAS.[17–19] Lieutenant-General Sir Thomas Herbert John Chapman Goodwin was then Governor of Queensland. Born in Sri Lanka, the eldest son of Surgeon Major John Goodwin, he was educated in England and graduated MRCS, LRCP London in 1892.[20]

Goodwin trained at St Mary's and served in the British Army Medical Service in India, at the Royal Military College, Sandhurst, and saw active service in France during the First World War. He was appointed Director-General of the Army Medical Services in 1918 and later Honorary Surgeon to HM King George V, before retiring from the army in 1923.

Sir John Goodwin (1871–1950) was appointed Governor of Queensland on 19 February, 1927 and arrived in Brisbane on 13 June of that year. Although he served through the years of the great depression, Goodwin faced no constitutional crises during his term of office. The declining economic growth of this period however promoted industrial unrest and insecurity, increasing unemployment and the exploitation of workers.

The new Governor travelled extensively and showed an interest in all aspects of life and industry throughout the State. It is recorded that this medical Governor was particularly concerned for the health of Europeans in the tropics and for the welfare of British migrants generally. His professional interest extended to strong support for establishment of a Medical School within the University of Queensland and for the campaign against eye diseases prevalent in Western Queensland, especially among children and aborigines.

Although a keen shot and a fisherman Sir John Goodwin was a conservationist, sharing with his wife an interest in wildlife preservation.

Regarding the Queensland Medical School, Sir John Goodwin gave official assent to the *University Medical School Act of 1928* after prolonged debate about the proposed site for the new University. The Faculty of Medicine was eventually established in 1936.[21]

The Governor entered into many aspects of Queensland society including horse-racing, rural interests and freemasonry. Goodwin's term of office ended on 7 April, 1932 when he returned to England. He was created KCMG in the same year and was awarded many foreign honours and honorary degrees. A most cherished moment for this medical Governor was when he received the first honorary Fellowship of the newly formed Australasian College of Surgeons. Sir John Goodwin died at Oxford in 1950.

## The Promotion of Health

By virtue of their vice-regal office all state Governors have accepted patronage of numerous medical and charitable organisations including Red Cross, St John Ambulance and the Royal Flying Doctor Service. Through these institutions they have exercised authority and influence on widespread community activities involving the health and safety of all Australians.

A matter of great pride for all Australians is the active role played by the governors' wives, their respective individual patronages and their participation in a wide variety of medical charities. Any doctor's wife will tell you these ladies deserve a history of their own. Among their distinguished number and their numerous honours one might list Lady Helen, (AC) wife of Sir (Arthur) Roden Cutler VC (Governor of New South Wales 1966–81). She was elected an honorary Fellow of the New South Wales College of Nursing in 1981, was Honorary Colonel of the WRAAC (1967–85) and was promoted as Dame in the Order of St John in 1977. Meanwhile her husband received five honorary doctorates from five different Universities. It is of course not uncommon for a state Governor to be honoured in this way. Many however have achieved academic qualifications by their own merits, particularly in Arts and Law, prior to their appointment to Vice-Regal office. Those with non-medical doctorates include –

Sir Mark Oliphant (Governor, South Australia 1971–76) MA, PhD, DSc, LLD, FAA, FTS, a distinguished physicist who was elected a Fellow of the Royal Society;

Professor Gordon Reid (Governor, Western Australia 1984– ) BCom, PhD, HonDLit, FASSA, formerly Professor of Political Science (ANU) and of Politics at UWA where he was Vice-Chancellor 1978–82; and

Rev. Doctor J. Davis McCaughey (Governor, Victoria 1986– ) MA, DD, HonLLD, FACE, a former Deputy Chancellor of Melbourne University and Master of Ormond College.[22]

Our state Governors have frequently been involved in the establishment of hospital facilities. Lachlan Macquarie in October 1811 laid the foundation stone for the Sydney (Rum) Hospital to replace Govenor Phillip's old Colonial Hospital. Earlier this year the present Governor of New South Wales, Sir James Rowland, was involved in a ceremony of rededication of Governor Macquarie's plaque at Sydney Hospital in Macquarie Street.[23]

In Western Australia the central component of the vast Queen Elizabeth II Medical Centre is the Sir Charles Gairdner Hospital, named in honour of retired General and former Governor of Western Australia (1951–63) and of Tasmania (1963–68). The present Governor of Western Australia Professor Gordon Reid officially opened the modern Mount Hospital in Perth in December 1986. In the Nation's first two hundred years the history of Australia has indeed been enhanced by those doctors who have actively participated in state and colonial administration.

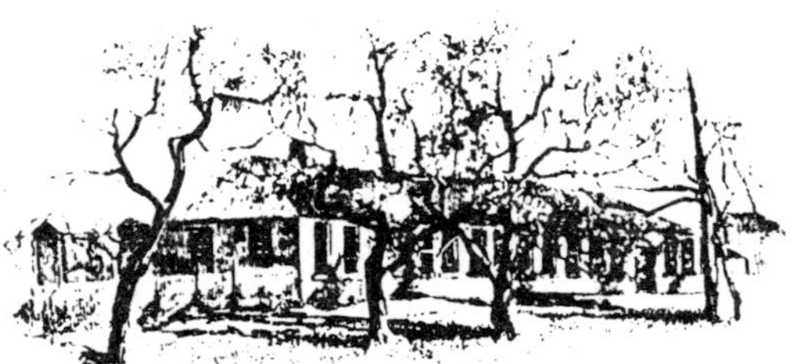

# PIONEER MEDICINE IN AUSTRALIA 16

## THE EARLY DAYS OF THE ROYAL FLYING DOCTOR

**Gary Litherland**
**Max Simkin**

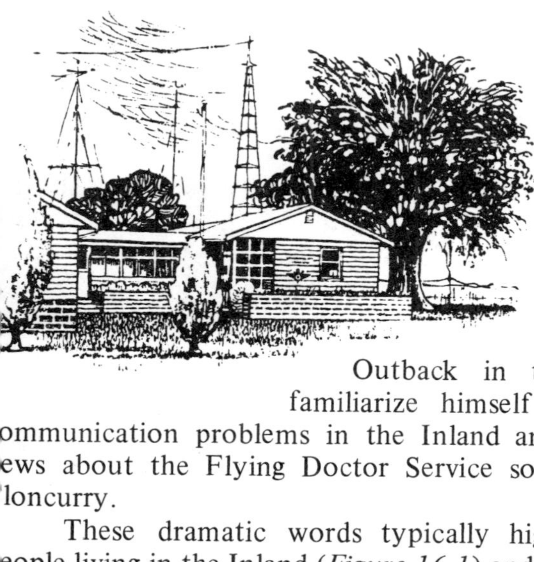

*I had expected a patient but he had not arrived and so after lunch we went out after him. We met him coming in by buggy twelve miles out. He had been three days lying in the buggy ... .*

So wrote Dr George Simpson at Ryans Well on his tour of the Outback in the 1920s in order to familiarize himself with the medical and ommunication problems in the Inland and to spread around the ews about the Flying Doctor Service soon to be established in 'loncurry.

These dramatic words typically highlight the isolation of eople living in the Inland (*Figure 16.1*) and dramatically emphasised ıe need for the introduction of an aerial medical service to vercome the isolation and fear of living in the harsh Outback.

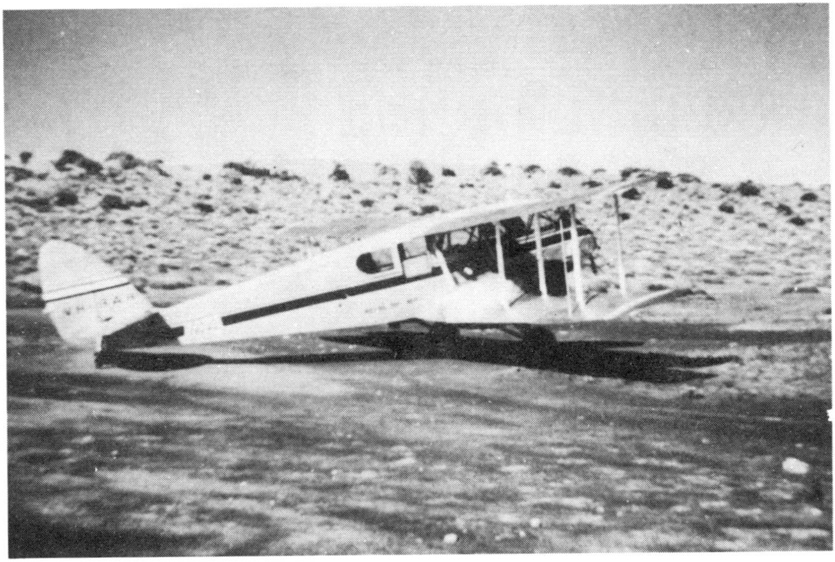

***Figure 16.1: The Isolation of the Australian Outback. The Flying Doctor Dragon, in far western Queensland circa 1944, parked here at the end of a Station property airstrip.***

## Beginnings

The idea of an aerial medical service was originally conceived by a young man named Clifford Peel who was a medical student with a great admiration for the work being done by the Australian Inland Mission under the guidance of John Flynn, its Superintendent. He originally expressed his desire to be a Flying Doctor in 1914.

He enlisted in the Australian Flying Corps during the 1914–1918 war and while sailing for England in the troop ship *Nestor* he wrote to the AIM giving information on air-craft operations and details of flights that could be undertaken if Flying Doctor centres were established at Oodnadatta, Cloncurry or Katherine. Unfortunately he was killed in France just two months before the war ended.

His letter was published in the AIM Journal *The Inlander* in October 1918. From that time John Flynn never let an opportunity pass to press for the establishment of an aerial medical service in which radio was to play an important part.

The Service began because Flynn was impressed and moved by the tragedies which befell his isolated flock. Travelling by horseback and camel over his vast Parish, he found the inland dotted with graves – some marked and some not – largely of people who would not have died if medical aid had been available in time. So he took up Peel's proposal to use an aeroplane to bring medical aid to the people in the Outback, but a doctor with an aeroplane would be of little use unless the isolated people could let the doctor know when they were ill. Flynn suggested radio, cheap, rugged and reliable and so simple it could be operated by bush people, without any technical assistance. Today, radio and aircraft are common, but in 1912 the idea was dismissed by most people as the dream of an impractical visionary. Flynn knew nothing about the technicalities of radio, or aircraft, nor did he know anything about medicine, but he had a flair for getting people to help him, finding, and imbuing with his own enthusiasm, able and devoted technical Lieutenants.

In his publicity campaign Flynn very effectively used the story of Jimmy Darcy to gain advantage in his battle against the twin scourges of the Inland – isolation and fear.

Jimmy Darcy was a stockman badly injured in a mustering accident 100 km from Halls Creek over 3,200 km from Perth. The local Postmaster Mr F. Tuckett sought assistance from Dr J. Holland in Perth after failing to obtain medical assistance from Wyndham and Derby. It rapidly became apparent that the patient would die from a ruptured bladder without surgery, and thus instructions for the necessary surgery were transmitted from one telegraph station to another over the vast distance from Perth to Halls Creek, with Mr Tuckett carrying out Dr Holland's instructions. As each instruction was passed Mr Tuckett carried out the procedure and acknowledged upon completion before further instructions were sent. The operation took seven hours. However following initial improvement he deteriorated and another operation was necessary. Dr Holland then set out for Halls Creek by boat, the only transport available, to Derby and then over terrible roads to Halls Creek. Unfortunately Jimmy Darcy died the day before he arrived.

About 1920, some eight years later, the late Sir Hudson Fysh, founder of QANTAS, was able to tell Flynn that suitable aircraft, such as the De Havilland 50, were available which could carry a doctor and a patient with a stretcher inside the cabin. However, simple inexpensive radio suitable for untrained people was much more difficult to develop. It was not until 1927 that the problem yielded to the genius of Alfred Traeger, a young South Australian Radio Engineer, who invented a self-contained transmitting and receiving set powered by a small generator driven by bicycle pedals – the now world famous 'Pedal Radio'. In this year, 1927, Dr George Simpson, a friend of Flynn made an extensive survey of inland Australia and chose Cloncurry as the most suitable place for the first Flying Doctor Base. It was while this survey was being conducted that the plane – a De Havilland 50 – flew from Cloncurry to Mount Isa to attend to a miner injured when he slipped off a bucket into the Black Star Shaft. His name was Tom O'Brien and the flight took place on 2nd August, 1927. This early flight was taken as proof that the idea of the Flying Doctor was feasible.

Eventually the funds were raised for an experimental year of operations from Cloncurry and it was to prove fortuitous that during Dr Simpson's tour of the Outback in 1927 he literally got the Flying Doctor Service 'off the ground' on August 2nd (*Figure 16.2*). He wrote –

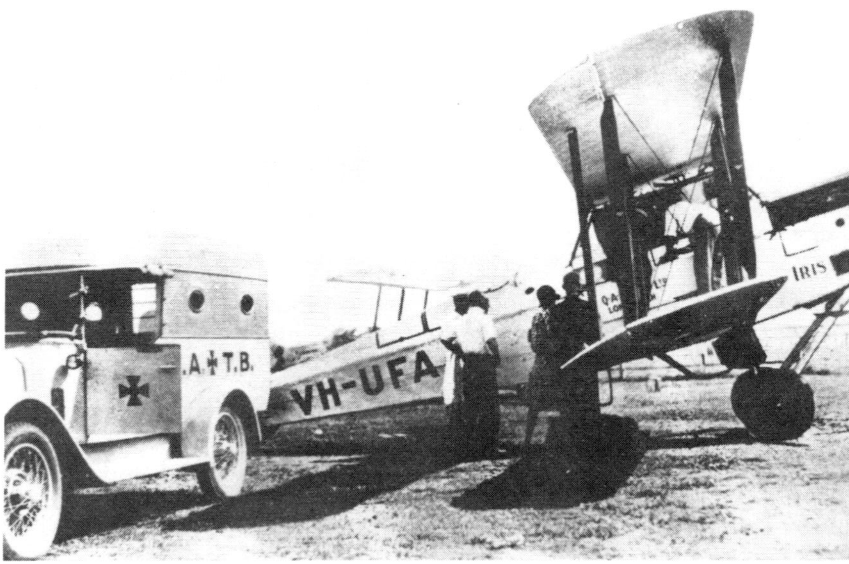


***Figure 16.2:*** ***The earliest Flying Doctor aircraft.***
***Transferring a patient from a Queensland Ambulance Transport Brigade vehicle to the Flying Doctor plane. Cloncurry, circa 1930.***

> *... about midday Mr Evans* [a Qantas pilot] *came across and said he was flying out to Mt Isa to bring in a case of fractured pelvis and spine. I had offered to go with him when the flight was first projected the evening before and he said he would be delighted to take me. We went straight out to the aerodrome and were soon over Cloncurry in the Qantas DH50. The mechanic came with me and we had a most comfortable trip. The return trip was not pleasant as I almost disgraced myself by being airsick. The vibration rather upset our patient so I gave him Morphia ½g and some brandy which he promptly vomited. Evans made a beautiful landing and the aerial medical service of the AIM was an accomplished fact.*

On 30th November 1928 an eighty year old patriarch, 6 ft tall and weighing 200 lbs was badly crushed under a horse on *Squirrel Hills* Station. To raise the alarm at the Flying Doctor Base in Cloncurry his son in law had to ride 65 km to a Station where a vehicle drove the extra 80 km into McKinlay to reach a phone and call the doctor. On top of this the closest landing strip to the patient was on *Blackeye Creek* Station next to *Squirrel Hills.* Due to rugged conditions, four men had to walk 18 miles with an iron framed mattress to get the patient which took 2½ hours and a further 10 gruelling hours to get him back to *Squirrel Hills* arriving at midnight. After the patient was attended to for pain relief he was taken to *Blackeye Creek* by slow car ride and the aircraft departed there for Winton in the early dawn.

On 2nd April 1929, a message was conveyed about an urgent problem at *Koolatah* Station north of Normanton in the Gulf of Carpentaria. It was during the middle of a typical 'wet' and an aboriginal stockman had ridden day and night 110 kms to a nearby Station where a phone message was passed to Normanton and then Cloncurry. The aircraft with Dr Welch aboard departed without delay but on that first day was forced back due to terrible weather. The next day conditions were somewhat better but deteriorated during the four hour flight until the aircraft was skimming the tree tops following the flooded track north. The area is subject to inundation and identifying landmarks under these conditions are non existent; however they were able finally to locate the flooded Mitchell River and from there the property. The patient was taken to Cloncurry that afternoon and recovered but surely would not

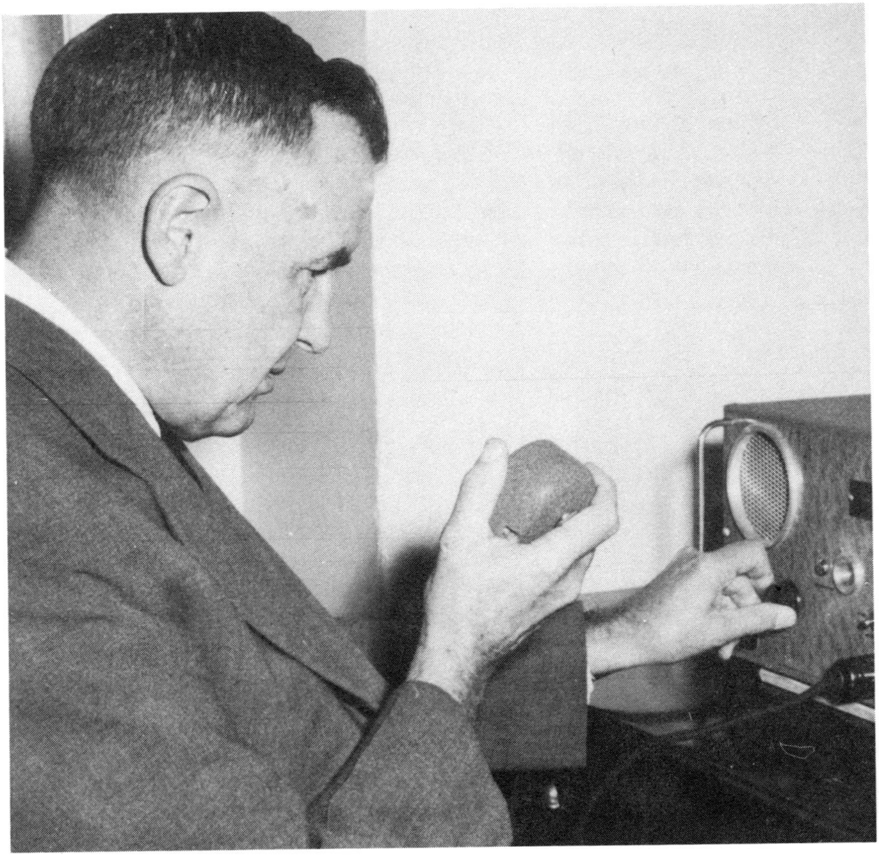

*Figure 16.3: Dr Allan Vickers (1901–1967), former Medical Superintendent of the Royal Flying Doctor Service of Australia (Queensland Section), conducting a Radio Medical, circa 1954.*

have done so had he not been evacuated. Two weeks later Dr Welch returned to New South Wales.

During that first year 255 flights to patients had been undertaken, flying more than 35,000 km, and the Flying Doctor Service had more than proved its worth. Without adequate communications however it became evident that some flights were not necessary, while others were inadvertently delayed.

At the end of this experimental year the AIM decided to continue permanently and Dr Welch was replaced by Dr J. Spalding.

Dr Spalding's year of service was as eventful as that of his colleague and further established the role of the Flying Doctor Service in Outback Australia.

The Base radio station was established in Cloncurry that year. After progressing through morse code, the pedal powered wireless eventually provided two-way communication and gave voice to the Inland.

Dr Alec May succeeded Dr Spalding and continued to uphold the standards set by his predecessors; however he had the misfortune to contract diphtheria shortly after commencing his appointment. His condition was initially diagnosed by the pilot before consulting the local doctor. The pilots often acted, and indeed still act, as 'medical assistants' to help the doctor whenever possible.

Flynn realised that growth would be slow if it were to depend on the resources of the Presbyterian Church alone. He persuaded the Church to make the magnificent gesture of handing over the Service on which it had spent so much labour and money to an 'Organisation of National Character'.

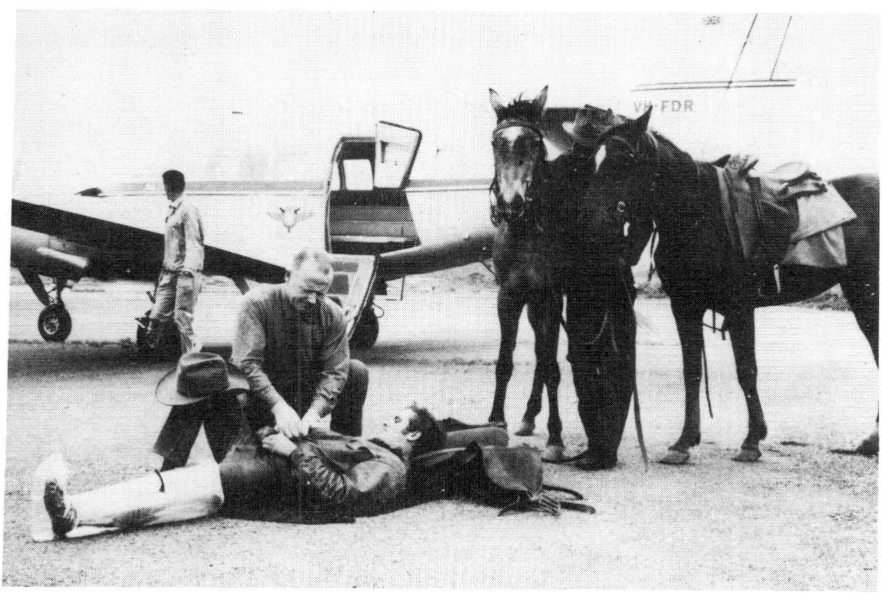


***Figure 16.4: Dr Tim O'Leary tending an injured stockman, beside the RFDS Queenair aircraft 'John Flynn'.***

In 1933, the Australian Aerial Medical Service was established which was shortly to become the Royal Flying Doctor Service as it is known today. It is a non-sectarian organisation. It is not a Government instrument but a philanthropic body on whose directing Councils some of Australia's most eminent business and professional men and women serve in an honorary capacity. It is also a free service – no charges are levied for the aviation or medical assistance provided.

The history of the Service is bound up, so much, with the personalities of its pilots, radio operators, nursing sisters and medical officers. In January 1931 Dr Allan Vickers (*Figure 16.3*) commenced service in Cloncurry. Dr Vickers devoted his working life to the Flying Doctor Service and spent well over thirty years in the Service. His name became synonomous with that of the Flying Doctor. Similarly in 1953 Dr Timothy O'Leary (*Figure 16.4*) started the first of 28 years continuous service in what, in 1955, became the **Royal** Flying Doctor Service.

Dr O'Leary was involved in the only serious aircraft crash in the Service's 60 year history in Queensland when the De Havilland Dragon aircraft crashed on take off from an outback station, killing the pilot and Dr O'Leary's wife of only 6 weeks.[1]

As the Flying Doctor Service expanded, the local small hospital boards did not replace their medical officers as they resigned their posts. The difficulty of attracting medical staff had meant that several of them were not the upright members of society that the local communities desired, or for that matter had trust in. The Flying Doctor Service thus filled the role of medical officers to these small communities, visiting them on rotation for the provision of clinical services.

In 1942 the first of the RFDS Medical Chests were distributed to enable the doctors to not only diagnose the presenting problem but to be able to provide effective local treatment from these kits. They are continuously updated by the homestead as drugs are used or become time expired. Each drug is numbered and prescribed by number and generic name, not trade name, as the cheapest item is usually provided by the distributor.

Radio diagnosis evolved from 1929, when Alfred Traeger developed the practical pedal wireless. Both patients (and their Flying Doctor, often 600 kilometres away) have a chart kept in the

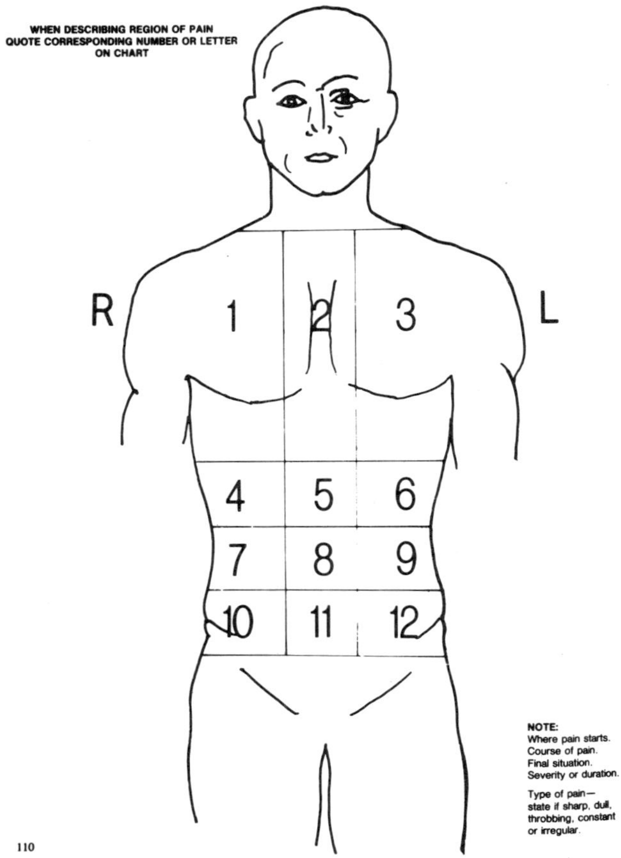


*Figure 16.5:*

*Patient's Diagnostic Chart kept in the RFDS Medical Chest. Pain or other symptoms referable to any part of the body can be described, as part of the Radio Consultation. The Flying Doctor has a similar chart, at the Radio Base.*

RFDS Medicine Chest, which enables a patient or his family to pinpoint parts of the body affected by pain or other symptoms (*Figure 16.5*).

## Current Perspectives

Since its origin in 1927, the RFDS has developed to a stage where it now operates one of the largest high frequency radio networks in the world, all to provide a 'Mantle of Safety' over the Outback.

Throughout Australia today, the Royal Flying Doctor Service operates from some thirteen main bases to over 7,000 transceivers which are located in houses, mines, survey camps, in vehicles and even on horseback, across two thirds of our vast continent – an area of about two million square miles. Over the radio network, people of the Outback talk to each other, link into a national telegram network, educate their children, hold committee meetings, maintain such organisations as Country Women of the Air, Brownies of the Air, Cubs of the Air and School of the Air (*Figure 16.6*), and they keep alive through that network the community spirit that is so important to living in the Outback. Through that network they pass meteorological data to each other and assist in searches for lost people and aircraft. Above all, that radio provides them with the medical advice and assistance without which day-to-day life would be extremely difficult.

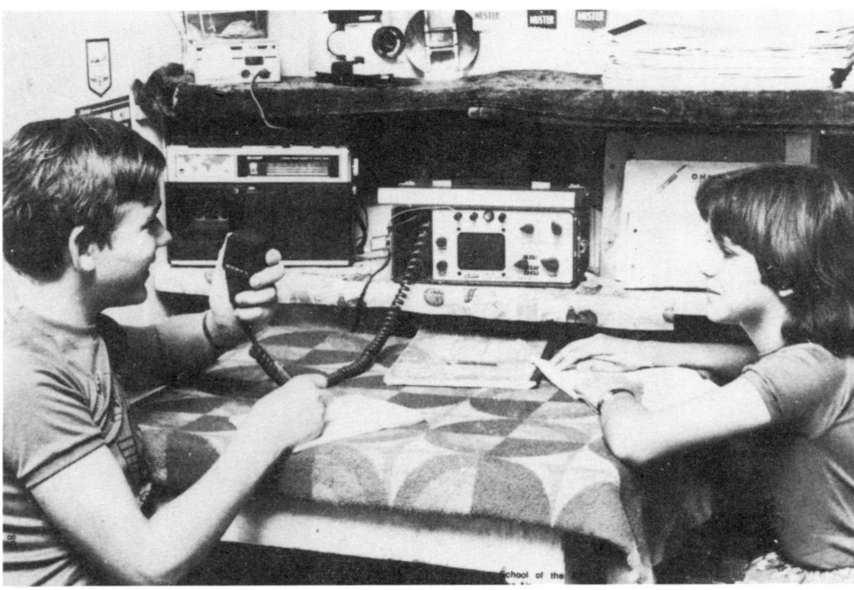

*Figure 16.6: As the history of the Flying Doctor Service evolved, many ancillary services became associated with it. Here children as part of The School of the Air, use the Royal Flying Doctor Service communications for their daily lessons.*

The Service now has faster pressurised turbo prop aircraft, cutting flight times dramatically. From the Cairns Base, for example, the 1 hour 30 minute flight to *Blackeye Creek* now takes 20 minutes, and the 4 hour flight to *Koolatah* now just a few minutes more than an hour. The pressurised cabins can overcome all of the aviation medical aspects associated with critically ill patient transfer and they can fly over the weather rather than through it.[2]

The Service's medical equipment suffices the needs of any mobile intensive care unit and our 24 hour continuous operation ensures prompt and effective treatment as quickly as practicable.

In 1987 we flew –

| | |
|---|---|
| At Cairns Base – | 1546 hours and 253,091 Nm; |
| Queensland Section – | 3165 hours and 497,257 Nm. |

The Royal Flying Doctor Service is a uniquely Australian organization. From its early historical steps, its organization has evolved to provide that 'Mantle of Safety' long dreamed of by Flynn, which would cover the Outback without regard to creed, colour or ability to pay.

At each Base, the Royal Flying Doctor has under his control, a powerful radio control station supervised by a fully qualified radio staff and ambulance aircraft flown by experienced commercial pilots. Near each base there is a well equipped hospital, and around it, some 400 to 500 nautical miles from each Base, a group of small transceivers which are the modern development of Traeger's original pedal set. Thankfully now, though, they are not morse key but Radio Telephone.

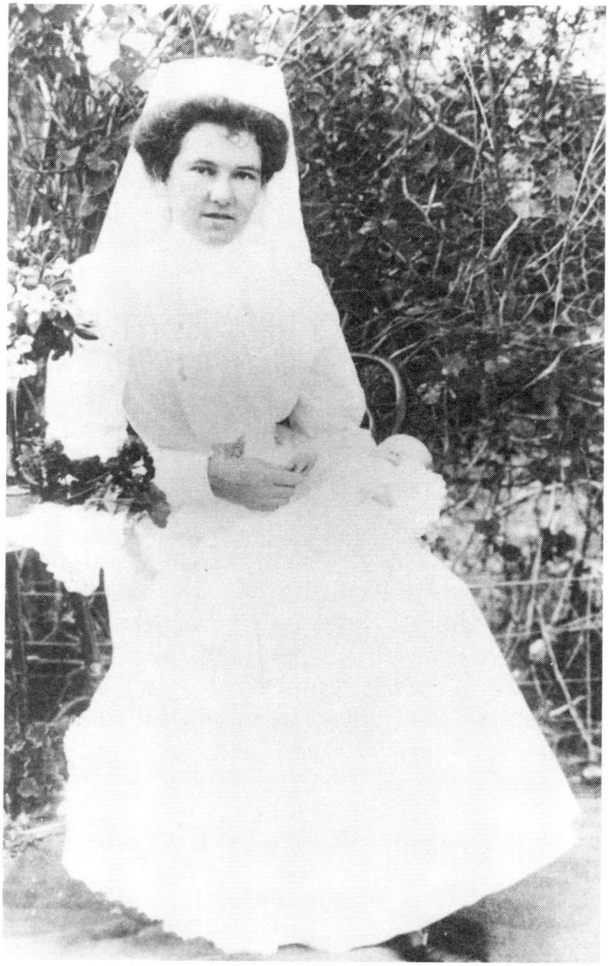

*Figure 17.1: Bush Nurse Elizabeth Kenny at Clifton on the Darling Downs, Queensland (1911); nursing baby Reginald Lewis.*

*Photograph courtesy of Mrs F. Mohr.*

# SISTER ELIZABETH KENNY

## Her Nursing and its Influence on Innovation and Leadership

**John Wilson**
**John Pearn**

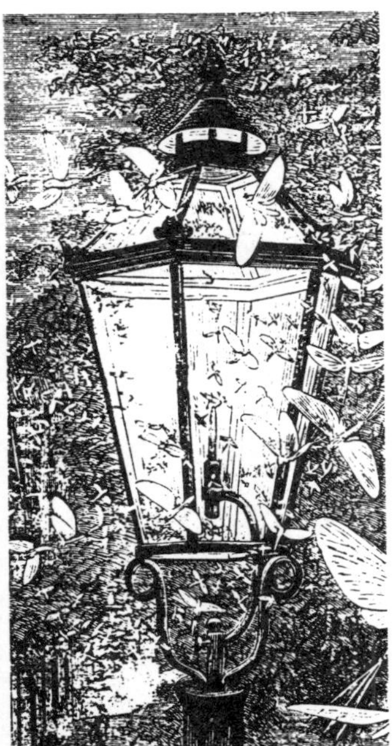

*FOR* several decades, Sister Elizabeth Kenny (1880–1952) led an international campaign which radically altered the nature of rehabilitative medicine. At a time when trained nurses in Australia were struggling to attain professional status, this nurse from Nobby, a small town on Queensland's Darling Downs, came to be recognised as an international authority on poliomyelitis. Dogmatic and controversial, she attracted doctors, nurses and therapists to her clinics in Australia, America and Europe to learn her techniques.

Sister Kenny's achievements are all the more remarkable because she was not formally qualified. Her background as a bush nurse and as an army nurse during the First World War provided the foundation of clinical and organisational skills with which she achieved much in the rehabilitation of patients with neuromuscular disease. Her sense of entrepreneurship, her confidence in decision-making and her capacity to produce innovative solutions to complex medical problems were undaunted by conventional notions of a nurse's 'proper place'. An analysis of her life reveals that had Sister Kenny complied with the established processes of training, examination and registration to become a nurse, the course of rehabilitation history might have been different.

Misrepresented and controversial in life, Sister Kenny remains, to a degree, enigmatic in death. She was adored by Americans who voted her their 'most admired woman'. Yet she was ignored in her own country. Her ideas were openly opposed by members of the medical profession, but all now use the practical guidelines which she introduced against enormous opposition. She demonstrated to nurses that their subordinate role in health care services was not 'pre-ordained', yet she left her nurse trainees feeling isolated and confused. She provoked accusations of 'quackery' when she achieved what were then (1935–1950) regarded as excellent results; and she fed the rumour-mongery by tactless talk.

Now more than 40 years since the last Australian Kenny Clinic quietly closed its doors at Royal North Shore Hospital (Sydney), a review of some aspects of Sister Kenny's nursing career lends additional insight into the development of the Kenny movement.

**Training Options**

At the time when Elizabeth Kenny opened her cottage hospital *St Canise's* in Clifton in 1911 (*Figure 17.1*), the mechanisms for nurse education and registration in Australia had been in place for almost a decade. The Australasian Trained Nurses' Association (ATNA) and the Royal Victorian Trained Nurses Association (RVTNA) had strict rules and regulations aimed at standardising nursing and controlling membership. Reciprocity between the organisations had been agreed upon in 1902. Rule 18 of the ATNA stipulated that all nurses completing training after June 30th 1906 needed to pass an examination.[1]

Fragmentary accounts of Elizabeth Kenny's early nursing exist. She may have had several years of obstetric experience at Nurse Sutherland's lying-in hospital at Guyra in northern New South Wales; and it has been suggested that she also went 'slum-nursing' in Sydney because 'the training was too expensive'.[2] In her

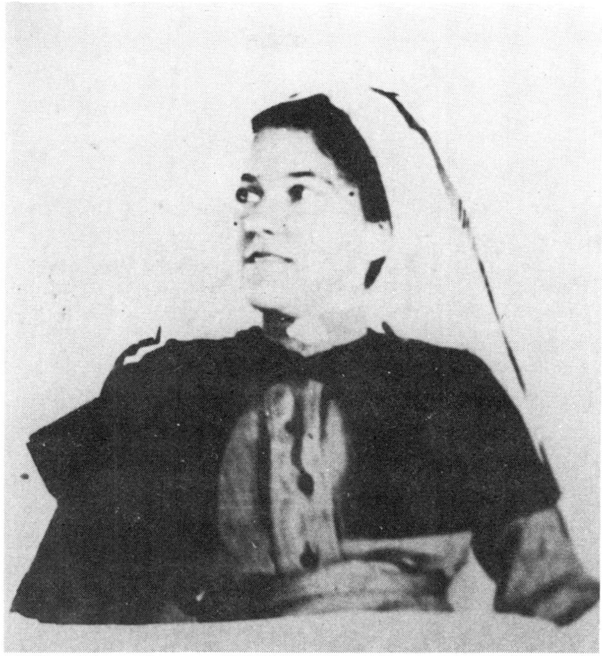

*Figure 17.2:*

*Army Staff Nurse Elizabeth Kenny (1915).*

*Kenny Collection.*

autobiography, Sister Kenny wrote simply that she 'entered a private hospital and began my training'.[3] In some accounts, Elizabeth Kenny began nursing during 1909. Photographic evidence points to her being an independent nurse practitioner in May 1911.[4] Late in her life, Sister Kenny alluded to training at Scotia Private Hospital[5] but no evidence of this institution has come to light. In any event, she was not registered with either the ATNA or the RVTNA.

ATNA rules governing obstetric nurses required that candidates for registration prove that –

> *... (a) prior to December 31st 1906, they had received a six months' course of practical and systematic training at one of the Maternity Hospitals of Australia recognised by the Council, and had passed a satisfactory examination before a competent Board of Examiners;*
> *or (b) that subsequent to December 31st, 1906, they had received a twelve months' course of practical and systematic training at one of the Maternity Hospitals of Australia recognised by the Council, and had passed the final examination of the Association for Obstetric Nurses,*

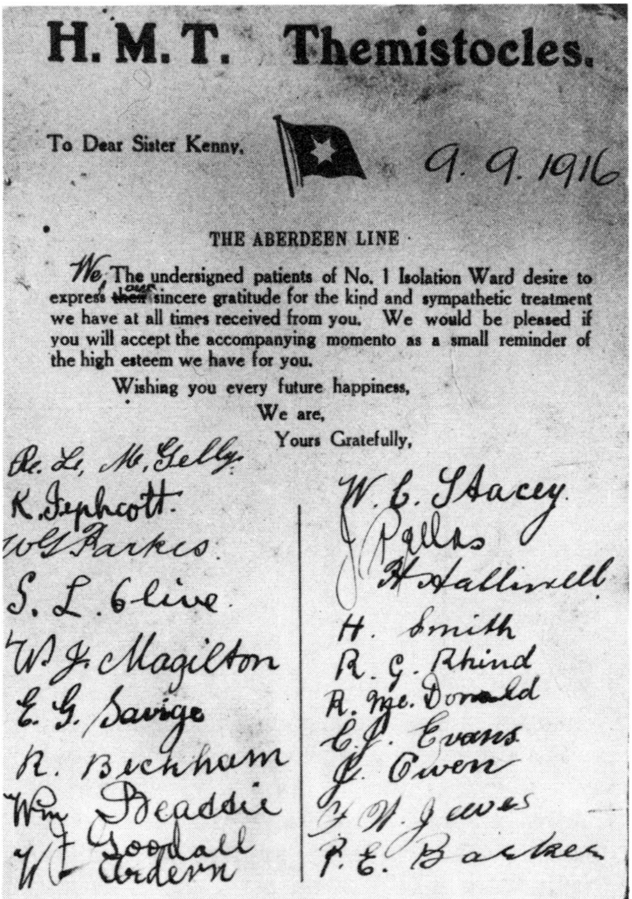
**H. M. T. Themistocles.**

To Dear Sister Kenny, 9. 9. 1916

THE ABERDEEN LINE

We, The undersigned patients of No. 1 Isolation Ward desire to express ~~their~~ our sincere gratitude for the kind and sympathetic treatment we have at all times received from you. We would be pleased if you will accept the accompanying momento as a small reminder of the high esteem we have for you.

Wishing you every future happiness,

We are,

Yours Gratefully,

Ae. Li, McGelly
K. Jephcott.
W. G. Parkes.
S. L. Clive.
W. J. Magilton
E. G. Savige
R. Beckham
Wm Beadsie
W. J. Goodall
W. Ardern
W. C. Stacey.
J. Rallas
H. Halliwell
H. Smith
R. G. Rhind
R. McDonald
C. J. Evans
J. Owen
J. W. Jewes
P. E. Barker

*Figure 17.3: Card to 'Dear Sister Kenny' dated 9.9.1916 from patients of No. 1 Isolation Ward on board the Themistocles en route from England to Australia. 'Sister' Kenny was still Nurse Kenny at that time, serving with the No. 1 Sea Transport Section of the A.I.F.*

*or (c) that, being registered as a general nurse, they had subsequently received a six months' course of practical and systematic training at one of the Maternity Hospitals of Australia and have passed the examination of the Association for Obstetric Nurses.*[6]

Several factors mitigated against compliance with these regulations. Firstly, Elizabeth Kenny was country-born and bred. Opportunities were limited. The nearest maternity hospitals recognised by the ATNA Council in 1910 were a considerable distance away either in Sydney (the Royal Hospital for Women, The Women's Hospital, St Margaret's and the South Sydney Women's Hospital) or in Brisbane (the Lady Bowen Hospital). Another two were situated further north along the Queensland coast at Maryborough (the Lady Musgrave Hospital) and at Rockhampton (the Women's Hospital). Distance from home and family would have been an important consideration, especially knowing that she could have been called upon to care for sick relatives at a moment's notice.

A second factor was finances. As in the United Kingdom, prospective obstetric nurses were generally charged fees to undertake training. Of the seventeen training schools listed in *The Midwives' Pocket Book* (1897), only one, the Jessop Hospital for Women in Sheffield, offered to train midwives free of charge. Fees ranged from £15 to £25 for three months.[7]

It is unlikely that geographic inconvenience and the cost of training were the only two factors which precluded her following the customary training of the day. When Elizabeth Kenny chose to apprentice herself informally to Nurse Sutherland at Guyra, she was choosing also to avoid the disciplined life of general training at one of the hospitals recognised by the ATNA. Toowoomba Hospital, under the supervision of Miss Ella Tolmie since 1897, was the nearest institution to offer a 3 year training course in 1910. Within a radius of several hundred miles, other smaller hospitals at Armidale, Tamworth and Warwick offered training over four years and those at Inverell, Forbes, Grafton, Lismore, Ipswich (*St Mary's*), Toowoomba (*St Denis*) offered a 5 year training course. It is conceivable that tutor-midwife Nurse Sutherland was also unregistered. In the 1910 Obstetric Register, two Sutherlands are noted – one at Bathurst and the other in North Sydney.[8] Doctor John Solomon Harris who is said to have employed Nurse Sutherland and her apprentice at Guyra[9] would not have been unduly concerned either way.

In an attempt to bring unregistered nurses under its jurisdiction in 1909, the ATNA Council approved an amendment to its rules allowing for the registration of resident Queensland nurses who had been practising for a minimum of three years in a recognised hospital, provided they produced certificates of competency and good conduct from at least 3 reputable Medical Practitioners. These were in practice testimonials of 'attainments and repute'.[10]

Lack of a trained nurse's certificate did not disadvantage Elizabeth Kenny in setting up her private cottage hospital at Clifton and in obtaining customers. Nor did it imply nursing incompetence as quite the contrary appears to have been the case. The hospital did not confine itself to the treatment of maternity patients.[11] As proprietress and entrepreneur, self-made Nurse Kenny established a solid reputation in the rural community. That she took on the qualities of a professional 'responsible only to the doctor, the patient and her own conscience'[12] but avoided much of the indoctrination of the contemporary nurse education system which invoked conformity, subordination and unhesitating obedience was an important factor in shaping her attitudes which were to be so influential in her later life.

That she was untrained, however, did force Nurse Kenny to travel to England in order to enlist in the war, as nurse registration in that country was not in place until 1919.[13] Her lack of formal training was without doubt a negative influence when she was assessed by the medical establishment of the day. This was particularly the case with the various medical members of the Queensland Royal Commission which met in 1935–1936 to investigate her unorthodox treatment. One of the Commissioners later wrote:

> *...if Sister Kenny was any good she had three alternatives – to study medicine, nursing or physiotherapy. She did none of these. She got the ear of an Under-Secretary named Charlie Chuter who imposed her on the Government and she never looked back as the Cabinet ignoramuses felt she was good political build-up stuff; the morality of their action was never considered ... If she had gone to a power-house about which she knew as much about polio-myelitis and told the engineer she could build a turbo-generator better than his, she would have been escorted to the looney-bin...*[14]

Unable to join the fledgling Australian Army Nursing Service in her own country because she possessed none of the prerequisite nursing certificates, Elizabeth Kenny presented to the Australian Army Medical Corps in London with testimonials from her family doctor in Toowoomba, Doctor Aeneas McDonnell. Doctor McDonnell was at that time Senior Honorary Surgeon at the Toowoomba General Hospital[15] and a Medical Life Member of the Queensland Branch of ATNA.[16] On the strength of his recommendation, she was taken on as Staff Nurse (*Figure 17.2*) under probation at Southall Military Hospital and appointed to the Australian Infantry Forces in 1915.[17] Assigned to transport ships after being wounded in France (*Figures 17.3 and 17.4*), she was promoted to the rank of

'Sister' in 1916 having by then demonstrated proficiency in nursing the ill and wounded.

In retrospect, it seems fortunate that Sister Kenny avoided the contemporary nurse training system as innovation was not one of its particular strengths. Although subsequent enquiries were to identify a nurse's 'blind uncritical obedience' as an impediment to the profession's growth and standing in the health care industry,[18] a large section of the nursing body of the day were convinced that strict grinding discipline instilled the best qualities and habits in probationers.

Trained nurses instructed in the art of being 'good nurses' were for a long time being told by their medical instructors:

> *...criticism on your part of the treatment by the doctor only renders you ridiculous, since you talk about matters of which you do not know – and cannot know – anything whatever ...*[19]

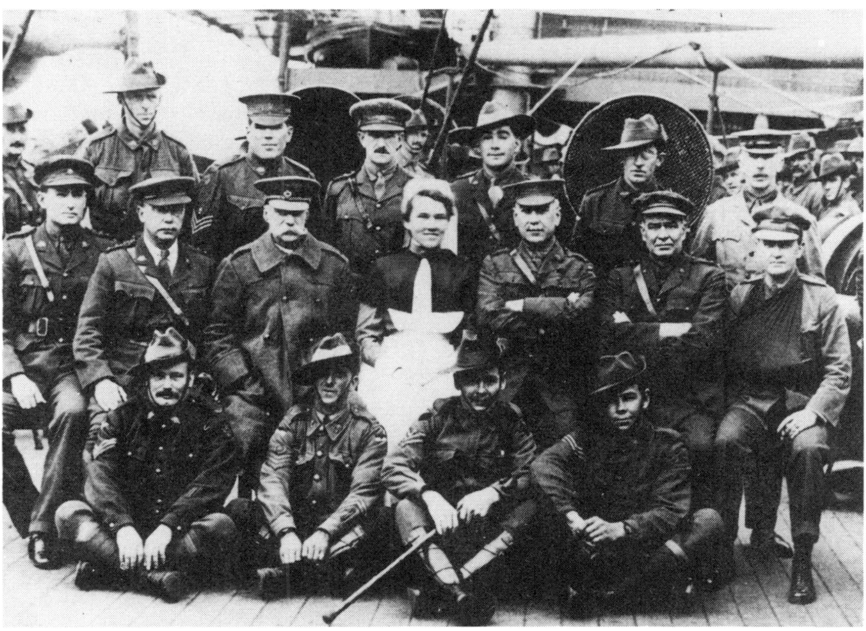

***Figure 17.4:* Postcard showing Sister Kenny with Australian Army Officers and NCOs aboard ship.**
***Nursing Archives of Australia Collection, Tasmania.***

**TABLE 17.1: A Chronology of the Life of Sister Elizabeth Kenny.**

| | |
|---|---|
| **1880** | September 20th – Born at Kelly's Gully, Warialda, N.S.W. |
| **1886–1895** | Schooling at the Ben Venue School, Wetella, N.S.W. |
| **1895–1904** | Farm work at Headington Hill, Darling Downs, Queensland. |
| **1905** | Applied for permission to give Religious Instruction at the Provisional School at Rockfield. Listed occupation as 'Teacher of Music'. |
| **1907–1909** | Lived at Guyra, N.S.W. – sold vegetables on a commission basis as a first business enterprise. |
| **1909–1911** | Began informal nurse training with Guyra midwife, Nurse Sutherland. May also have gone 'slum-nursing' in Sydney. |
| **1911** | Bush nursing. Treated her first cases of infantile paralysis (poliomyelitis). Opened a private hospital at Clifton, Queensland – *St Canice's* – mainly for obstetrics and medical cases. Some surgical. |
| **1915** | Sold hospital and travelled to England to enlist. Documents of the Australian Imperial Force (A.I.F.) show enlistment date as 30th May, but likely to be later. Accepted after month's probation at Southall Australian Military Hospital. Wounded in the left leg at Ypres, France. |
| **1915–1918** | Nursing escort duties on troop ships *Snevic, A32, Orestes, Marathon* and *Thermistocles* travelling between the United Kingdom and Australia. (No. 1 Sea Transport Section of the A.I.F.) Promoted to the rank of Sister on 20th December, 1916. |
| **1919** | January – Discharged medically unfit. Diagnosis of viral myocarditis. Returned to her mother's farm house outside Nobby, on the Darling Downs. |
| **1920–1925** | Organised and became the first President of the Nobby Chapter of the Country Women's Association of Australia (C.W.A.). |
| **1926** | April – adopted Mary Stewart. An active period of full life with her daughter, her activities as a country nurse and her service with the C.W.A.<br>May – accident to Sylvia Kuhn at Nobby. Developed and patented the 'Sylvia Stretcher'. Awarded a Certificate of Membership of the Institute of Patentees. |

**TABLE 17.1 (contd)**

| | |
|---|---|
| **1930–1933** | Rehabilitation of poliomyelitis, spastic paralysis and birth palsy patients in north Queensland. Set up a backyard clinic in Townsville for 17 patients.<br>September – unsuccessfully demonstrated to physiotherapists and doctors at Brisbane Children's Hospital.<br>December – Dr (*later Sir*) Raphael Cilento recommended the opening of an experimental 'Muscle Re-Education Clinic' for 6 months to evaluate her methods. |
| **1934** | February – first nurse trainee Sister Leila Cooper appointed.<br>March 1st – Government sponsored Kenny Clinic opened in the Queen's Hotel, Townsville.<br>June – 'The Elizabeth Kenny Clinic and Training School' opened at George Street, Brisbane.<br>August – treating 50 patients. |
| **1935** | October 26th – the Queensland Government instituted a Royal Commission to investigate the illicit Kenny method and to compare her results with those of orthodox treatment.<br>Kenny Clinic opened at the Royal North Shore Hospital, Sydney. |

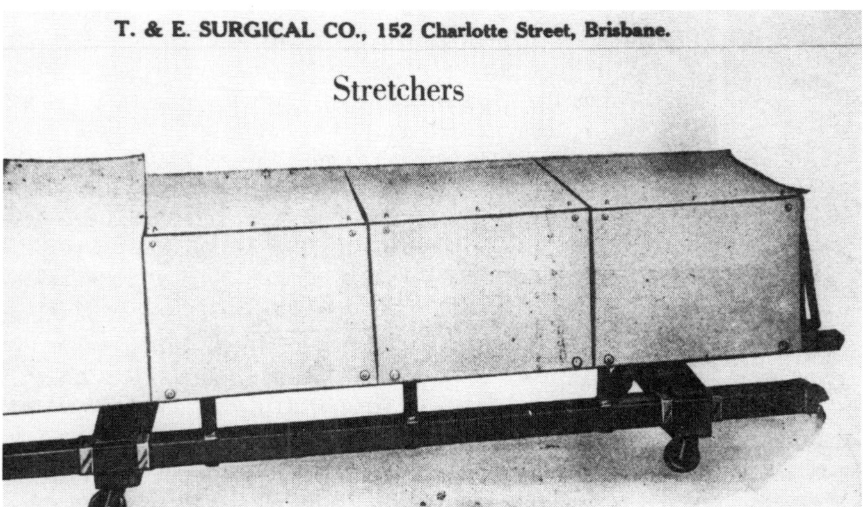


*Figure 17.5: The 'Sylvia Stretcher' invented by Sister Kenny (1926). From the Illustrated Catalogue of Surgical Instruments and Appliances of Taylor and Elliott Surgical Company, Brisbane, 1938 edn., p.B/297.*

**TABLE 17.1 (contd)**

| | |
|---|---|
| **1936** | January – Kenny Clinic opened in Toowoomba.<br>October – treating more than 600 patients. The Kenny Clinics at Brisbane, Townsville, Toowoomba and Sydney are staffed by 3 full-time medical officers and 48 attendants (40 of whom are trained nurses). |
| **1937** | Published her first textbook *Infantile Paralysis and Cerebral Diplegia*. Kenny Clinic opened at Newcastle, N.S.W.<br>Travelled to London. Kenny Unit opened at Queen Mary's Hospital for Children, Carshalton. Favourable review of method appeared in *Journal of the Chartered Society of Massage and Medical Gymnastics.* |
| **1938** | January 6th – Report of Royal Commission critical of Sister Kenny's methods, the Commission finding that her claims were unproven. Despite controversy, Kenny Clinics are opened at Cairns (Qld) and Hobart (Tas.). Moves are also made to introduce Kenny methods at Hampton (Vic.). |
| **1939** | March – Kenny treatment is made available to patients in public hospitals at Cairns, Rockhampton and Brisbane.<br>A group of six eminent Queensland doctors (Drs Nye, Pye, Arden, Fryberg, Lee and Professor Wilkinson) confirm that in a significant number of cases, the rehabilitation of poliomyelitis victims was advanced by the Kenny methods of treatment – 'It is our belief that she has made an important contribution'. The doctors recommend to the Queensland Premier (Mr Forgan Smith) that Sister Kenny's fare be paid to the United States, and that introductions be facilitated to enable her methods and teachings to be pursued in that country. It was hoped that assessment of her methods would be possible without the early controversy that surrounded management of poliomyelitis victims in Australia. |
| **1940** | March – Sister Kenny travelled to the United States with her adopted daughter. At Minneapolis General Hospital, she stayed to treat patients. Minneapolis doctors (Drs Cole, Pohl and Knapp) became clinical patrons. Returned briefly to Australia. |
| **1941** | Allocated a 17 bed ward at the University of Minnesota Hospital and beds at Minneapolis General Hospital. Favourable clinical articles on the Kenny Method appeared in the *Journal of the American Medical Association, The Americal Weekly* and the *Readers' Digest.* |

**TABLE 17.1 (contd)**

| | |
|---|---|
| **1941** | December 4th – the National Foundation for Infantile Paralysis publicly endorsed Kenny treatment, urging the widespread use of the Kenny technique and suggesting that State and city health departments take steps toward training personnel in Kenny Method. Sister Kenny publishes her major textbook *The Treatment of Infantile Paralysis in the acute Stage.* |
| **1942** | Widespread acceptance of the Kenny treatment of 'heat and activity' which replaced the former universal methods of 'splints and inactivity' for the management of acute polio cases.<br>December 17th – the Elizabeth Kenny Institute is endowed and opened at Minneapolis. The *New York Sun* names Sister Kenny as the world's 'Outstanding Woman of the Year'. |
| **1943** | The Elizabeth Kenny Foundation is established. Sister Kenny publishes another textbook (written collaboratively with Dr John Pohl) – *The Kenny Concept of Infantile Paralysis and Its Treatment.*<br>Widespread recognition by Americans – Guest of Honour at the President's Ball; Honorary Doctorate of Science at University of Rochester; Honorary degrees at Rutgers University and New York University.<br>September – published her autobiography (written in collaboration with Martha Ostenso) – *And They Shall Walk.* |
| **1944** | The American Medical Association rejects Sister Kenny's claims. |
| **1945** | Returned to Australia via England. Kenny Clinics still operating (but on a very reduced scale) at Brisbane and Sydney. |
| **1946** | New poliomyelitis epidemic sweeps through the United States of America. Sister Kenny returned to Minneapolis to supervise the treatment of cases.<br>September 27th – World Premiere of the film *Sister Kenny* starring Rosalind Russell. A huge crowd (in excess of 20,000 persons) gathered in Times Square, New York to see Sister Kenny at the Premiere of the film. |
| **1947** | Lecture tour to Soviet Russia and Eastern European block.<br>A private audience with Pope Pius XII. Australian Premiere of the film *Sister Kenny* at Regent Theatre, Brisbane – panned by critics.<br>Last Australian Kenny Clinic closes its doors in Sydney. |
| **1948** | New Kenny Centre with 100 beds opened in New York City.<br>Other Kenny Clinics opened at Buffalo (Pontiac) and Centralia – 65 beds. |

**TABLE 17.1 (contd)**

| | |
|---|---|
| **1949** | Sister Kenny retired from the Kenny Foundation (U.S.A.) after 9 years in America. Returned to Toowoomba. Resides at the corner of Range Road and Fairholme Street – *Struan.* |
| **1950** | January – returns to the U.S.A. The Joint Congressional Committee of the United States' Congress and Senate passed a Joint Congressional Resolution awarding her the rare honour of 'Visa and Free Passage Across the Borders of the United States of America'.* Sister Kenny presented with Florence Nightingale's prayer book and stand from the Crimean War.<br>New Kenny Clinic opened at El Monte (Los Angeles). |
| **1951** | Returned home. Ill with Parkinson's Disease.<br>Received the 'Brith Sholom's Humanitarian Award' and is voted by Gallup Poll as Americans' 'Most Admired Woman'.<br>August – Despite illness, moved to establish an 'International Organisation for Combatting Poliomyelitis'.<br>Held public meetings in Toowoomba. |
| **1952** | Wrote a second autobiographic work (published posthumously in 1955) – *My Battle and Victory.*<br>November 30th – Sister Kenny died at Toowoomba. Buried in the Nobby Cemetery next to her mother's grave. A guard of honour of the Schoolchildren of Nobby and special tributes from the Country Women's Association and the American Consul were paid as last respects before interment. *Sydney Morning Herald* obituary noted the –<br>... *loss of one of our great ones, perhaps one of the greatest.* |

★

## An Innovation Patented

In 1926 Sister Kenny designed and patented a sophisticated casualty stretcher for use in transporting orthopaedic patients in open ambulances over rough rural roads.[20] Known as the 'Sylvia Stretcher', it incorporated a solid plywood base, springs to reduce shock, retractable handles, a partitioned hood to protect the patient from the weather, and pockets for hot water bottles (*Figure 17.5*). Although subsequent trials proved that the new stretcher was too

*This honour has been bestowed on two occasions only. The other recipient was General Lafayette.

complicated, too cumbersome and difficult to clean, and although closed ambulance cars were already in use (ensuring its early redundancy) the surgical supply company Elliott Brothers were persuaded by Sister Kenny to contract for commercial production.

The royalties paid to Sister Kenny amounted to a not inconsiderable sum of £3 per week. Together with her war pension, these royalties provided Sister Kenny with sufficient independent means to allow her to concentrate on her poliomyelitis work. Described by its suppliers as 'the best community stretcher ... recommended to communities by the Country Women's Association and Bush Nurses' Association',[21] fewer than 200 of these stretchers were sold and it seems that none survive.

Its contemporary success, however, was a personal milestone of achievement and gave her confidence in the international area. In 1926 she was awarded a Certificate of Merit by the Institute of Patentees of London, for this invention.

**The Teacher and the Teachings**

Her methods were empirical at the outset, and probably developed from her robust common sense, and belief in her own 'hands-on' experience. In response to early criticism and innuendo that her muscle rehabilitation techniques were dependent on 'hypnotism, religious fever and emotional stimulus',[22] Sister Kenny purposefully withdrew from day-to-day patient therapy so that the results of treatment at her clinics could reflect the students' application of her methods.

The question of whether or not she could pass on the principles of her treatment was a difficult one. Empirical results demanded a theoretic base. This involved finding new language, defining new terms such as 'spasm' and 'alienation', establishing a comprehensive system of muscle-testing and charting, organising patient-centred programmes and setting graduated objectives.

In the process of teaching, Sister Kenny continued to learn from her own experience. Moreover, in the light of orthodox argument and evidence continually being presented to her, she elaborated the early theories and developed ideas based on her empiric observations. These did not really find final expression until 1942.[23] Teaching was central to the success of the Kenny movement. As early as 1934, Doctor Rae Dungan, a regular visitor to the Muscle

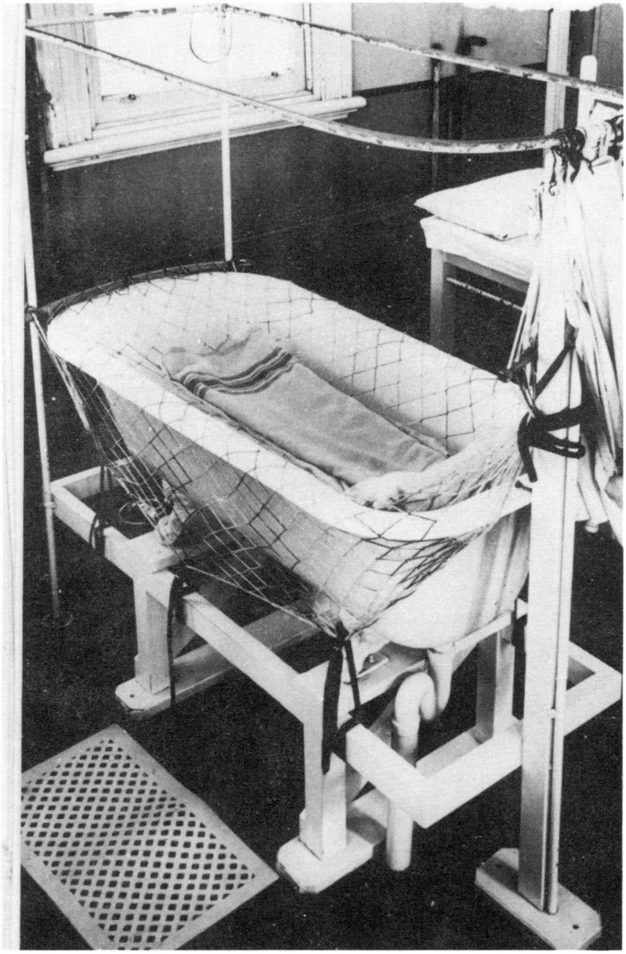

*Figure 17.6:*

*A treatment bath for paralysed poliomyelitis victims at the Sister Kenny Clinic in Townsville (1935).*

*Department of Agriculture and Stock.*

*Kenny Collection.*

Re-Education Clinic in Queen's Hotel, Townsville (*Figure 17.6*) stated his belief that the Kenny method could be taught to others because 'the whole method can be worked out on a psychological and physiological basis'.[24] But there were teething troubles. Sister Kenny's first 'painful' attempts to lecture to masseuses and doctors at the Royal Brisbane Children's Hospital met with 'obvious disgust'[25] and hostility. Doctor James Duhig, Professor of Pathology at the University of Queensland and Director of Brisbane Hospital Pathology Department, recalled that Sister Kenny 'definitely told us when she first came down she had no knowledge of anatomy whatever'.[26]

Resistance to her ideas varied. As Sister Kenny noted about her first trainees in Townsville – Nurses Cooper, Steele, Swann and Eales:

> *... the students have to an extent absorbed the idea and to the same extent could apply it in cases of paralysis other than spastic, but owing to their rigid training in other branches of the profession, they cannot see their way clear to accept the theory as taught by me ... I cannot see my way clear to waste further time with these students or any other until a text is written and submitted to the right quarters for approval ...* [27]

The first Kenny textbook (1937) elicited a mixed response. Persuaded by Doctor James Guinane, the son of the proprietress of the Queen's Hotel, to avoid aspects which had the potential to arouse contention, Sister Kenny set out a detailed document of remedial exercises based on five broad principles. Only one of these principles, the 'avoidance of generally accepted methods of immobilisation'[28] contravened accepted medical practice. History, however, has shown that she was correct.

Her book was scorned by medical reviewers. Doctor Lennox Teece wrote that 'she does not profess to offer any new principles of treatment whatever',[29] and Doctor Max Hertz publicly espoused 'the principles set down are good and new: only the good ones are not new, and the new ones are not good'.[30]

Not surprisingly, the textbook was nonetheless well accepted by many of her trainees. At the time of the book's release, there were 40 trained nurses, 5 lay persons and 3 masseuses training at the Kenny clinics (*Figure 17.7*). Only a few trainees failed to learn. Sister Kenny felt obliged to dismiss one masseuse who 'kept introducing methods in which she had faith and for which I do not blame her' and two nurses who 'would have been satisfactory, but they were subject to undue influence'.[31] Senior Kenny nurse, Sister Jean Hansen, often thumbed through her copy of the text and used it in conjunction with lecture notes from Doctor Jean Rountree, the Clinic's Government Medical Officer.[32]

Reaction to the textbook from most orthodox quarters was antagonistic. The Queensland Director General of Health and Medical Services, Sir Raphael Cilento, told the Royal Commission of his suspicions that the work was plagiarised from a 1913 book by Sister Wilhemina Wright.[33] This claim was not substantiated.[34] However

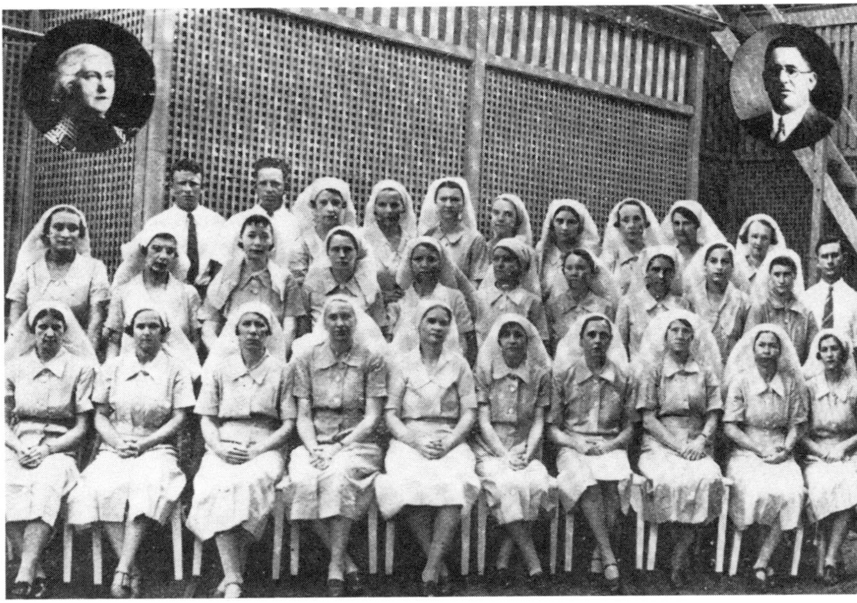

*Figure 17.7: Staff at the Elizabeth Kenny Clinic and Training School, George Street, Brisbane (1937).*

*(Left to Right)*
*Front: Sisters Norris, McNally, Mason, Jenson, Lynch, Parker, Cooper, Pengally, Andrews, McPherson.*
*Middle: Sisters Kippling (?), Chuter, McCauley, Squires, Stirling, n.k., Harvey, Keyes, Coles, Redman.*
*Back: Mr McLaughton, Mr Tutin, Sisters Davis, Hansen, Farquhason, Keyes, Barnett, Worden, Greuber, Rountree, n.k.*
*Inserts: Mrs McCrae, Dr A. Fryberg.*

*Frontispiece to Kenny E., 1937, 'Infantile Paralysis and Cerebral Diplegia', Angus and Robertson Ltd., Sydney.*

the suspicion itself was used to discredit the Kenny movement in Australia and to attempt to remove Sister Kenny from directorship of the clinics. As she complained to the Royal Commissioners:

> *...Sir Raphael Cilento informed me that it was the Minister's wish that I should be got rid of, giving for one of his reasons a statement that the Minister had understood that I had gone to America and as it were, stolen a method which was in operation by a certain Sister Wright ...* [35]

In view of her earlier humiliations, it is not surprising that Sister Kenny attempted to develop a comprehensive curriculum for training therapists. For instance, between the months of June 1939 and January 1940, she delivered 18 lectures and demonstrations at the Brisbane General Hospital to senior medical officers[36] and forwarded a copy of these to the Home Secretary.

Although Sister Kenny expressed the opinion in 1936 that she needed two years to train a nurse in the Kenny Method,[37] when her training began in America in late 1941, short courses had to be introduced to cope with the enormous demand from a wide range of health workers from around the country. By 1950 however, the training of Kenny therapists at the Sister Kenny Institute was based on an intensive two year course. A further twelve month enrolment was offered to qualified nurse graduates at accredited schools of physical therapy.[38]

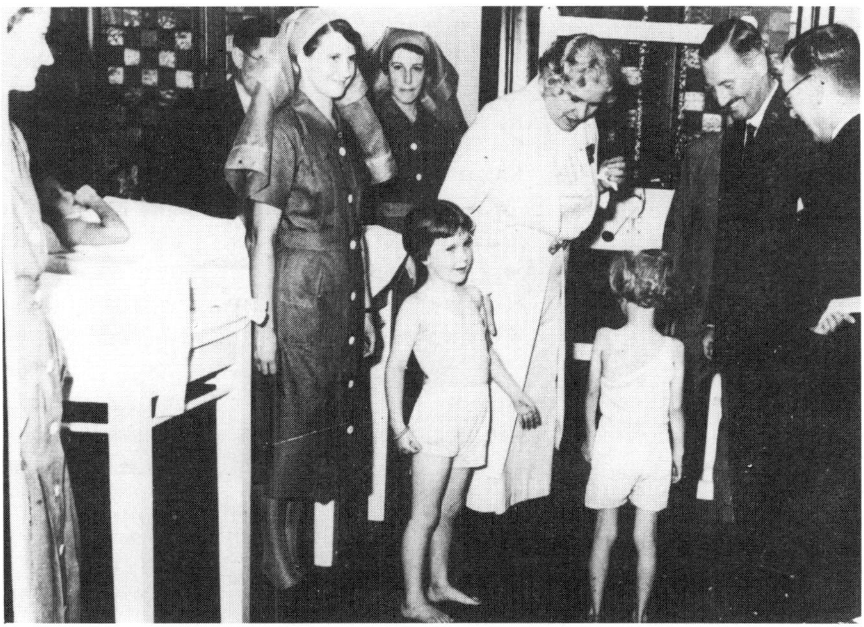

***Figure 17.8: A visit of the Governor and Minister for Health to the Kenny Clinic in Brisbane (1937).***
***(Left to Right) Sr Redman, Dr Fryberg (partly obscured), Sr Greuber, Sr Davis, Sr Kenny, Governor Sir Leslie Wilson, Minister for Health Mr Hanlon.***
***Photograph courtesy of Mrs Smith.***

**Relationships with Doctors**

Sister Kenny's confrontation with members of the Queensland Royal Commission and the well-publicised adverse findings of the Commission have established a public perception in Australia that her relationships with the medical fraternity were irreconcilable. However, the reality outweighs the perception (*Figure 17.8*). Support from members of the medical profession has been essential to the positive impact of the Kenny movement. Doctors played a vital role in the infrastructure and function of the Kenny movement.

Dr Jean Rountree was one of the first to enthusiastically promote the Kenny method. To the Home Secretary, she wrote:

> *I am happy to say that the work is giving satisfactory results without exception. I have no hesitation in saying that each case of the total 225 has shown definite improvement and in many cases outstanding improvement is shown. Several cases who showed no signs of walking for years before admission here have made such promising progress that we have every confidence in the expectation that these cases will be able to release their parents of the burden of total crippledom* [sic] ... [39]

Other Australian doctors showed consistent support. Professor Herbert John Wilkinson, Dean of the Faculty of Medicine at the University of Queensland, was an early confidante and mentor. In the foreword of her textbook, Professor Wilkinson described Sister Kenny as a 'woman of exceptional personality'.[40] Later, along with Doctors Nye, Pye, Lee, Arden and Fryberg, he was instrumental in persuading the Queensland Government to send her to America.[41]

A number of doctors in New South Wales – including Doctors Little, Fletcher and Roberts, were won over not on the basis of fully understanding her ideas but because they were impressed by the evidence.[42] The same thing happened in the United States (*Figure 17.9*). To Sister Kenny, the conservative nature of medical practitioners was a frequent target for chastisement. Kenny as an individual was just as stubborn as the collective medical profession was conservative. Both parties saw the other as dogmatic and unyielding on the key issue of movement and warmth for paralysed limbs. Just prior to her death, she was reported as saying:

> *' I'm sorry that I haven't always been able to see the doctors' point of view. In the thick of the fight, when the comfort, the health, the very lives of countless polio victims hung in the balance it was very difficult to condone what seemed to be unreasoning stubborness.* [43]

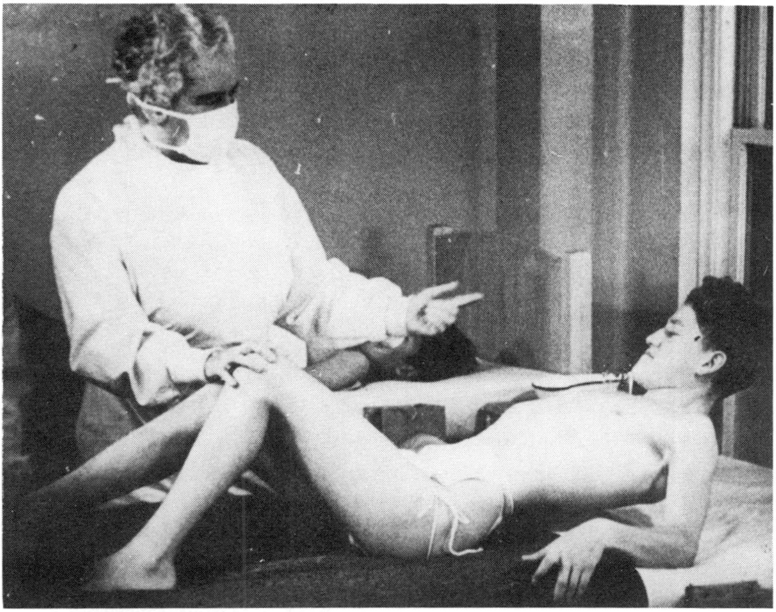

*Figure 17.9: Poliomyelitis patient Mr Wally Bienecke (1943). After 16 months of orthodox treatment, he could not sit up or feed himself. Over the ensuing 16 months of Kenny treatment, he made a good recovery. A single frame from Documentary Film (1946) 'The Kenny Concept of Infantile Paralysis: Early Diagnosis and How to Prevent Deformities'. Kenny Collection.*

Behaviour which she perceived as 'intransigence' on the part of many doctors was, to a large extent, the result of enormous frustration at being unable to prevent crippling deformities in their patients with poliomyelitis, regardless of the effort put into treatment. Among doctors there was also a despondent philosophic view towards the effects of polio. This had evolved alongside their collective feelings of ineffectiveness and futility. As Sir Raphael Cilento explained:

> *...it is doubtful whether it is worthwhile either to the patient or to the public, to transfer a physically low-grade potential person into a physically high-grade potential person, none the less dependent ...*[44]

Sensationalism in the press was a further cause of conflict. Many media releases distorted claims and counterclaims. As a whole, the press clippings collected by Sister Kenny show that medical resistance to her ideas featured prominently in her life's work. In an interview with *The Digest of World Reading*, she stated:

> *During my stay in America, I personally worked with approximately 7,000 victims of Infantile Paralysis. I have had the great satisfaction of seeing most of them get up and walk after many of them had been condemned to lifelong crippling. I knew from the outset that the only way I could convince the world of the soundness of my system was by actual work and accomplishment, not by indulging in theoretical discussions and arguments.*[45]

Regardless of conflict, there was underlying mutual respect. Doctor Abe Fryberg, asked to compose an obituary for Sister Kenny in the *Medical Journal of Australia,* speculated charitably:

> *... whether Miss Kenny's contribution would have been greater or less if early in her career, her gifts of patience, pertinacity and attention to detail had been co-opted by those of us working in Australia for the same objectives ...*[46]

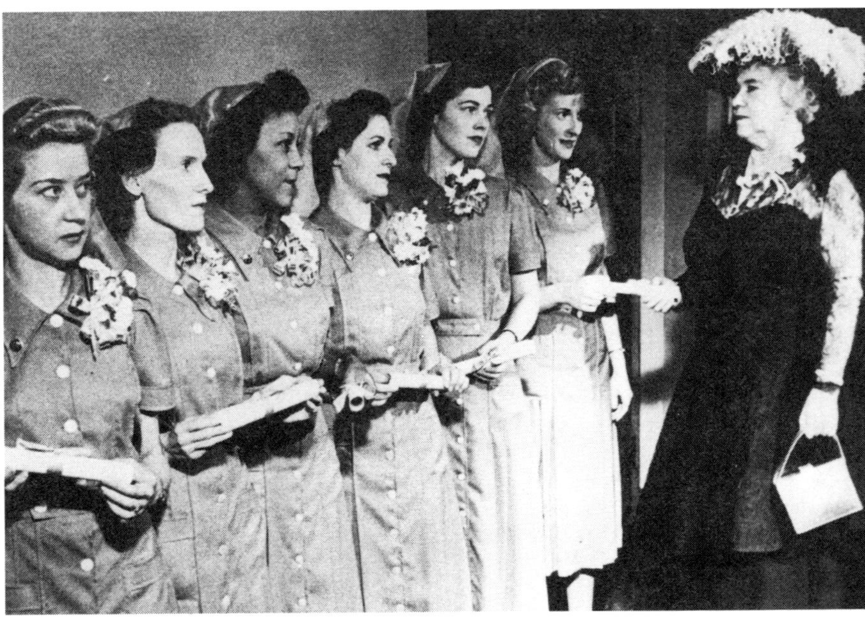

***Figure 17.10: Sister Kenny congratulates graduates of the Kenny Therapists' Course at the Elizabeth Kenny Institute, Minneapolis (1951). Kenny Collection.***

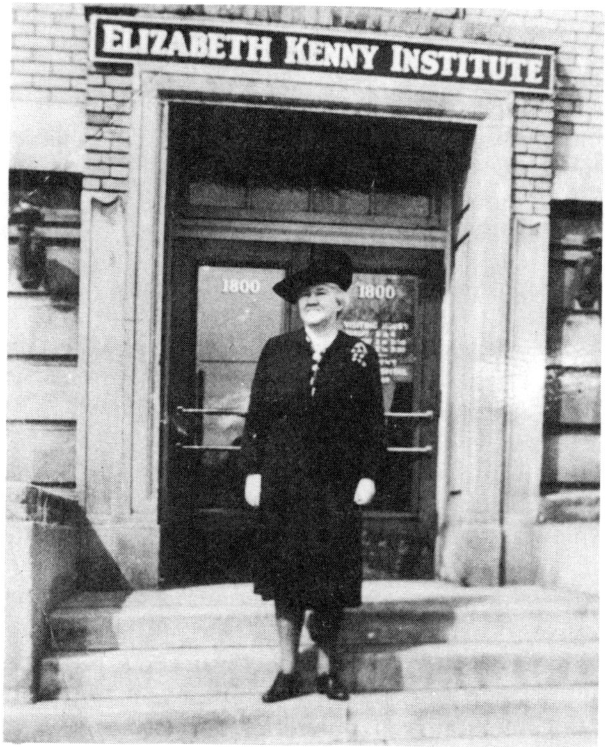


*Figure 17.11:*
***Sister Elizabeth Kenny outside the Elizabeth Kenny Institute, Minneapolis, Minnesota, USA. (1950).***

***From – The Kenny Collection which is held privately.***

**The Kenny Legacy**

On December 4th, 1941, the National Foundation for Infantile Paralysis announced its endorsement of Sister Kenny's treatment and on the following day in New York City, it issued a statement urging the widespread adoption of the Kenny techniques and training of State and City personnel in the Kenny Method. Many felt that the stage was set for rapid and effective reversal of the effects of poliomyelitis by new treatment and rehabilitation (*Figure 17.10*). Doctor Miland Knapp, Director of the Sister Kenny Institute in 1955, observed that the influence of Sister Kenny's ideas was so pervasive in the United States that 'those who are now treating the disease have forgotten they ever employed prolonged immobilisation'.[47]

Today, the Sister Kenny Institute at the Minneapolis Medical Centre offers one of America's most energetic rehabilitation services. In modern premises adjoining the Abbott-Northwestern Medical Campus, the Institute maintains comprehensive in-patient and outpatient rehabilitation programmes for a wide range of problems including polio, CVA, spinal cord injury, muscular dystrophy, low back pain. chronic pain, amputation, cardiac problems and multiple sclerosis.[48] In 1984, the Institute employed 5 specialist physicians and more than 250 support staff in treating 500 in-patients and an out-patient population of approximately 10,000 patients. In 1978, Albertson wrote that:

> *Just as America's Space Program has developed a technology which is used in thousands of non-related products and systems, the knowledge gained in the treatment of polio was applied to many remaining causes of paralysis and disability ... It would be virtually impossible to receive any physical therapy anywhere in the world without embracing concepts which have been developed at the Sister Kenny Institute.*[49]

**Conclusion**

Sister Kenny's nursing career was unusual in many respects. She was untrained, but she led nurses, doctors and lay therapists in an intensive innovative campaign aiming to alleviate and prevent iatrogenic deformities. She focused on the care of cripples for whom conventional medicine could do nothing more, and she gave them hope. To many of them, she returned some degree of muscle function and a chance to regain a useful life. When denied treatment facilities for her patients at public hospitals, she set up a group of clinics outside the public health system (*Figure 17.11*). To health workers she offered an alternative to doctor-leadership. She was a pioneer in demonstrating the capacity of nurse-practitioners to help in the diagnostic role, and to care independently for patients.[50]

Seen from the perspective of a new generation, her career highlights many of the professional polemic issues facing Australian nurses and doctors today.

**Acknowledgements**

We thank Mr & Mrs H.F. Farquharson, Mrs J. Hansen, Mrs F. Mohr, Sister Una Salmon, and Miss M. Stirling, of Queensland; Mr & Mrs J. Kenny of New South Wales, and Mrs A. Smith of Tasmania. Special thanks are also due to Mr Stewart and Mrs Mary McCracken (née Kenny) for much help in the compilation of the chronology of Sister Kenny's life. Many of the illustrations are from the Kenny Collection (held privately) whose kindness in providing these figures is gratefully acknowledged.

# PIONEER MEDICINE IN AUSTRALIA 18

## FRANK BUCKLAND, AUSTRALIA AND ITS FISH

**Christopher Gardner-Thorpe**

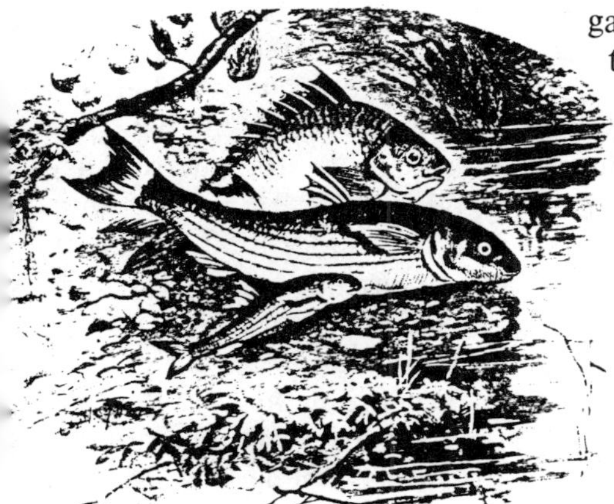

*MANY* medical pioneers gave much to Australia beyond their clinical specialties. One outstanding name in this band of doctor-naturalists was Dr Frank Buckland, whose contributions led to the trout and salmon industries in Australia.

A career military surgeon, he served in the Life Guards until 1863; a geologist and botanist, he had a flair for natural history, a fascinating personality, he was engaged by the great to accompany them on adventures; but it was as an ichthyologist that his name is remembered across the world.

In conjunction with the Australian Acclimatisation Society, Frank Buckland introduced salmon and trout ova to Australia and Tasmania. Attempts had been made intermittently since 1841, but each had failed when the ice supply had run short on board ship. Buckland shipped 100,000 salmon eggs from the Dovey, Ribble,

Hodder, Severn and Tweed Rivers and 1,000 brown trout eggs from the Itchen. The eggs were conveyed by the steamer *Norfolk* which sailed from London Docks on 21 January 1864 on an eighty-four day journey to Melbourne. They arrived on 19 April and it is to Buckland's efforts that brown trout in Australia and Tasmania now owe their existence.

**Early Life**

Frank Buckland was born the son of Professor William Buckland and Mary Buckland at Christchurch College in Oxford on 17 December 1826. His family was steeped in achievement, and in natural history. William Buckland had been appointed (in 1819) to the first Chair of Geology at Oxford, the year after his election to Fellowship of the Royal Society.

The young Frank was keen on natural history from the age of two and half years and it is said that he had a photographic memory. Some of the letters which he wrote in childhood are preserved in the Royal College of Surgeons in London, and give a graphic account of his vivid appreciation of the colourful life of England in the first decades of the nineteenth century. He was educated at Blundell's school for a year. In 1837 he went to his uncle's school at Laleham near Staines and there he was branded for life when his hand was injured by a round ruler. He developed a fearless strong personality, and in July of 1839 became a scholar at Winchester. He was the most popular boy in the school, often laughed and had a loud voice, and was overweight. His diet was peculiar and included squirrels, mice and other unusual animals; no doubt he developed this interest from his father who once expressed an interest in eating his way through the whole animal kingdom but had problems with the blue-bottle and the mole. Nevertheless his dinner parties were memorable; the dishes included horse, tongue, alligator, mouse, hedgehog, tortoise, ostrich, rat, frog, snails and, it was put about at the time, 'part of the embalmed heart of King Louis XIV of France'. No doubt it was from the remains of these dinner parties that a collection of bones was formed and bequeathed to Frank in 1842.

At Winchester Frank was taught by Charles Wordsworth nephew of the poet, who eventually became Bishop of St Andrews, Dunkeld and Dunblane. It was while he was at Winchester that the youth decided to become a surgeon. Instead of the more usual book of poems Frank chose Graham's *Domestic Medicine* as a parting gift from his tutor. He visited the patients in Winchester Hospital and paid some of his schoolfellows sixpence to allow him to practise bleeding on them.

His University days were as frenetic as those at school. He studied at Christchurch in Oxford from 1844 to 1848. In his room there he kept various animals including a bear, a jackal and adders. He obtained his degree of Bachelor of Arts in May of 1848 and went to St George's Hospital in London.

**Medical Training**

The young medical student studied at St George's Hospital from 1848. In 1849 he went to Paris to study cholera and practised surgery on corpses there. His natural history interests continued and on 12 October he heard Mantell's lecture on corals which he described as 'amusing and instructive'; on 4 November he saw the bones of the New Zealand lizard which Mantell had found. One of Frank's contemporaries was Francis Day, born in 1827 and educated at Shrewsbury, who had enrolled as a surgical student in September of 1848; he became a famous ichthyologist, lived in India and died in 1889 at the age of sixty-one. In 1850 the youthful medical student visited Guernsey with Huxley, a fellow student at St George's.

In 1851, the year of the Great Exhibition, Frank and his father carried out Foucauld's experiment by suspending a pendulum from the roof of the nave of Westminster Abbey opposite the entrance to the Deanery. This experiment, which had first been carried out in France in 1845, demonstrated the rotation of the Earth and can be seen today in the Science Museum in London. Frank Buckland used to show visitors around Westminster Abbey where his father had been appointed Dean after his Oxford geology post. On one occasion he was locked in so he tolled the bells to draw attention to his predicament. On another occasion he extracted a dead cat from an organ pipe which was playing flat. His widespread rambles in natural history did not disturb his studies unduly for he passed the examination of the College of Surgeons on 9 May 1851 and from May 1852 until 1853 he was House Surgeon at St George's Hospital.

**Marriage and Personal Life**

In 1850 Frank had met Hannah Papps who was probably the daughter of a coachman. Their son, Francis John, was born on

23 August 1851 at 18 Pulford Street in Pimlico. The birth was registered by Hannah on 3 October 1851 in the District of St George at Hanover Square. Frank and Hannah married on 11 August 1853 at the church of St Mary Magdalen in Munster Square. At about this time Frank became deeply religious and worshipped there. He believed in a single act of Creation, perhaps partly due to his strong family history of religion. The young couple lived at 37 Albany Street, Regent's Park, in a house which had belonged to Mr Hogarth, father-in-law of Charles Dickens.

The animals which Frank kept at home had the run of the house with the exception of the dining room although occasionally they went there too. After death the animals were stuffed and kept in the dining room or else buried in the garden which soon became overcrowded.

In November 1858 Frank was invited to go to Egypt with the great Brunel as his medical attendant. Brunel suffered from Bright's Disease and had been seen by Brodie from whom the suggestion may have arisen that Frank accompany Brunel in search of the sun. The journey was planned from 4 December 1858 until the following March with a fee of a guinea a day plus expenses. Brunel wanted an amiable companion who had wide interests, not least to occupy his son.

Frank Buckland was much impressed by the work of John Hunter, the great anatomist who had been buried at St Martin-in-the-Field's Church in London in 1790. Frank attended a centenary dinner in honour of Hunter in 1856 at St George's Hospital. In January 1859 Frank read in *The Times* a reference to the ceilings and crypts and catacombs of St Martin-in-the-Field's and wanted to search for Hunter's coffin. He took with him a man who had remembered moving the coffin in 1832. They spent two weeks searching and it was a very smelly business. On 22 February they found Hunter's coffin, the bottom one in the last tier but one. The brass plate read –

*'John Hunter Esq died October 16th 1793 aged 64'.*

Frank had an unpleasant illness after all of this. Hunter's coffin was buried in Westminster Abbey on 28 March. This increased Frank's prestige and he was given a silver medal by the Leeds School of Medicine. Frank described the search for Hunter's coffin in the fourth series of *Curiosities of Natural History*, published by Bentley.

**Early Medical Work**

The young Dr Buckland left St George's Hospital in 1853. He used to go on holiday to the old family rectory at Islip and treated several patients in the rectory kitchen. In 1854 Frank became Assistant Surgeon to the Second Life Guards and in the same year became a member of the Athenaeum at the early age of twenty-seven years. He remained in the Guards until 1863 and lived for much of the time in cavalry barracks in London at Knightsbridge, and at Windsor.

During this early medical work his natural history interests were still to the forefront, for he started making casts of fish for the South Kensington Museum. He had a mishap in October of 1853 after feeding a rat to a cobra. He dissected the rat and whilst scraping at the rat's skin with his fingernails he became poisoned. He treated himself with ammonia and brandy which he believed may have saved his life. He experimented with chloroform as an anaesthetic for animals. In 1853 he gave his first lecture entitled 'The house we live in'.

He was a popular man. In 1857 he met Hans Christian Andersen, saw the *Leviathan* launched at Millwall and inspected fossil trees and birds' nests at Portland. In 1858 he met Dr Livingstone, Lord Palmerston and George Stephenson. He often visited the College of Surgeons.

Frank's father gave him some pieces of skin from a mammoth. His father had also obtained some hair from the head of King Henry IV when the tomb in Canterbury Cathedral had been opened, and he presented his collection of skulls to the Museum of the College of Surgeons shortly before he died.

**Fishing**

Frank's interest in fishing started in August of 1861 when he first fished for salmon, and in the same year he pioneered the artificial hatching of perch and salmon so that fish-rearing rapidly attracted attention.

The English Acclimatisation Society sought to introduce new animals for food; sometimes animals destined for the Society were delivered to the London Zoo by mistake. The Society aimed to improve freshwater fisheries and encourage the restocking of rivers. The salmon fisheries in England had declined severely by 1860 and a Commission was set up in that year. In 1861 the *Salmon Fisheries Act* was passed and two Inspectors of Fisheries of England and Wales were appointed. The result of all this activity was that salmon increased dramatically.

In 1863 Surgeon Buckland resigned his Commission in the Life Guards to devote himself to the promotion of food production, particularly fish culture. He wrote letters to *The Times* on fish hatching and demonstrated the technique to the Prince of Wales. He published a book in 1863 entitled *Fish Hatching*. He loved the hard work involved in the cold and tiring techniques needed to collect trout and salmon eggs and he used a diving suit. He described in detail the collection of ova from spawning fish. In 1864 he became interested in oyster culture.

The South Kensington Museum was funded by profits from the 1851 Great Exhibition. Frank had seen plaster casts of fish in the museum of the Royal Society of Dublin in 1864 and in 1865 he transferred part of his museum of fish and oyster culture to the South Kensington Museum where he was appointed Scientific Referee. He surveyed an oyster bed in Exeter on 15 February of 1865, and in the same year was appointed Fish Culturist to Queen Victoria. He set up hatching boxes at Windsor and also advised on the deer in Windsor Park.

Frank wrote for *The Field*. On 27 January 1866 the new publication *Land and Water* appeared and it survived until the 1920s when it was absorbed into *The Field*. Frank edited the Fishery and Natural History columns and he recorded some of Darwin's observations from *The Descent of Man*. He used to write when travelling by train.

**Inspector of Salmon Fisheries**

In February of 1867 Walpole appointed Dr Frank Buckland Inspector of Salmon Fisheries. In the same year he was appointed Superintendent of the Museum of Economic Fish Culture in South Kensington. He hoped his museum would assume equal importance with that of the Hunterian Museum, and would rival the Bucklandian Museum in the University of Oxford which contained his father's geological collection. Queen Victoria visited the doctor's museum in 1876.

Frank was excited by his appointment as Inspector. The rivers were overfished, netted, and polluted with the products of public sanitation and industrial waste. Mill dams obstructed the river and prevented the migration of salmon upstream to spawn. Fish were stranded below the dams. Pound locks and weirs were obstructed and the rising levels of water produced deep and sluggish weedy streams which encouraged the growth of coarse fish. Buckland pointed out the folly of trying to legislate for the welfare of fish when their life histories and habits were not known.

He travelled extensively to learn more about fish. He went to Devon to lecture to the Naturalists' Club of Exeter and to inspect the Exe. He described the system of fishing in tidal waters which was called 'fixed engines' and this was used below Trew's Weir at Exeter; bait was thrown into the water and then the nets were pulled in. He laid down guidelines for the construction of salmon ladders on the rivers Taw and Torridge where there were seventy weirs and over forty miles of spawning ground. He sent salmon and trout eggs to New Zealand in 1868. In 1869 when the Serpentine in Hyde Park was being cleaned he helped move the fish to the Round Pond in Kensington Gardens.

He still experimented with alternative foods at this time. He attended a dinner of horse flesh at the Langham Hotel in London on 6 February 1868. Hippocreas was not pleasant and hippophagy did not catch on.

In 1870 he suggested that the pollutants of rivers and sewage could be used to fertilise the land and help increase food production. He believed the aquaria which were being set up around the country should be used for research and he took parties around the aquarium in Brighton. He enjoyed helping to arrange aquaria. He went to Margate on holiday and described the shrimping industry there.

**Natural History Interests**

This singular doctor and naturalist continued to study all his life. He described a mole and a new spider monkey in 1870. He suggested that children should not wear shoes since walking on shoe leather makes it thinner whereas walking on human leather makes it thicker.

In 1871 Frank saw siamese twins (Chang and Eng) joined by a cartilaginous band from sternum to sternum, and Christine-Millie joined at the sacrum by cartilage, and perhaps bone, whom he named

'The two-headed Nightingale'. He also saw a giant and giantess at whose marriage in due course the two-headed Nightingale acted as bridesmaids. In the Devon Record Office and Exeter Diocesan Records is a handbill calling attention to Senor Joachim Eleizegui, the Spanish giant; Frank Buckland's writing is on the handbill. Frank described the confusion in the Canterbury Museum where fossils were mixed with other objects. He raised money for a blind man and his dog. He described many of the animals in the zoological gardens and described the birth of a hippopotamus on 5 November 1873, named 'Guy Fawkes' although a female.

His personal museum continued to grow. Legends of sea monsters clasping ships were rife, and in 1873 Frank described a monster cuttlefish with arms thirty-five feet in length which had been caught off Newfoundland.

He continued to write to demonstrate the design and skill manifest in all created things, as his father had done before him. He wrote to *The Times* in March 1875 to describe the cruelty to seals hunted in the Arctic. He described the shell of a tortoise as composed of ribs and likened the human skull to a tortoise shell in that the denticulated joints which formed the sutures helped prevent a fracture from spreading from one bone to another. He drew the analogy of the wood in a window frame which prevents the fracture of one pane of glass from spreading to another.

Frank became interested in bell-ringing at Ross-on-Wye in 1874 and in the same year made a pie from part of the old rhinocerous which had died at the Zoo. He treated Jemmy, his prairie dog, for convulsions by putting the dog's feet in hot water, slitting the ear and giving a dose of calomel. Unfortunately the dog died.

Frank pointed out that often he saw unusual objects in multiples, for example a crippled boy or a red-haired girl. He liked to go to the sideshows to see waxworks, monsters and an indiarubber man. In 1876 he bought, for a penny, a telephone consisting of two rings of tin covered with parchment and connected by six or eight yards of cotton.

He became a corresponding member of the Zoological Society of Philadelphia and an honorary member of the Chester Society of Natural History. He attended soirées at the Royal Society and the College of Surgeons. In 1878 he described jackdaws' nests around the towers of Exeter Cathedral, rooks' nests along the railway line from

Taunton to Paddington and doormouse nests in Lord Porthsmouth's woods at Eggesford. He continued to write extensively on birds and their migration and believed the shape of birds' eggs prevented them rolling away which showed evidence of design by The Creator; he remarked on the monkey as Darwin going backwards.

**Trout for the Antipodes**

Frank Buckland continued to send trout eggs to Australia and New Zealand, from 1864. The brown trout in particular flourished in the cold streams of New Zealand, Tasmania, and the southern parts of Australia. He attempted to send eggs of other species, especially salmon (from 1864), but it is doubtful if his early consignments of this latter species survived.

One of his last attempts to stock Australia with salmon was in 1879 when he packed salmon eggs in ice on board SS *Durham* which was bound for Australia. These were the last eggs he collected and a few days later he developed pneumonia which recurred throughout the year. He prepared another revised edition of White's *Natural History of Selborne* (he was an admirer of Gilbert White). His last fishery report was presented on 31 March 1880. He left his house for the last time on 21 August 1880 to see an orang-outang from Malacca.

Dr Buckland was of very large girth and four and a half feet in height. He suffered from asthma and smoked a pipe. He developed dropsy and died on 19 December 1880, two days before his fifty-fourth birthday. He may have died from tuberculosis but his death certificate reads '...hepatic disease about two years. Bronchitis'. He was buried on 24 December in Brompton Cemetery in London, in the same grave as his son Francis John ('Physie'). An obituary appeared in *The Scotsman.*

The Buckland Museum containing four hundred fish casts was given to the nation and put in store. Much of the museum was damaged in the 1939–45 war and some of the contents were moved to The Fisheries Museum at Anstruther in Scotland. It is not thought that anything has survived. Thomas Huxley succeeded Buckland as Inspector of Salmon Fisheries. A Trust Fund known as the Buckland Foundation was set up in 1926 under the terms of his Will. The first Buckland Professor of Economic Fish Culture, Professor Walter Garstang, delivered the annual lecture in 1930.

Australia has owed much to the work of doctor–naturalists. Surgeon General John White, Surgeon Dennis Considen, and Surgeon Bowes Smyth (all of the First Fleet) set this pattern. Sir J.B. Cleland, Dr Hugo Flecker, and Dr Jack Barnes continued in this theme, in the twentieth century. Dr Frank Buckland stands with individuals such as these, but with an influence from across the world. He was only four feet six inches in height, was grossly overweight, was warm and congenial, energetic and kind. These traits, together with his insatiable curiosity and enthusiasm for natural history, make his colourful biography an enriching one for all with a love of the history of Australian fauna.

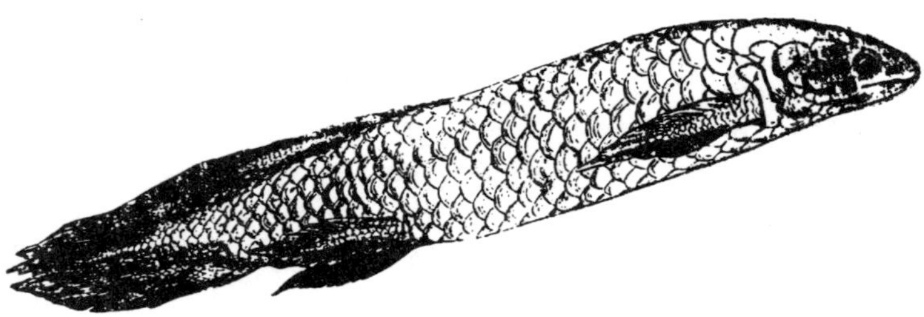

# WHO KNEW JACK BARNES?
## A Short Bioglraphy of Dr John Handyside Barnes Pioneer Medical Toxinologist

**Jennifer Roberts**
**Barbara Kinsey**

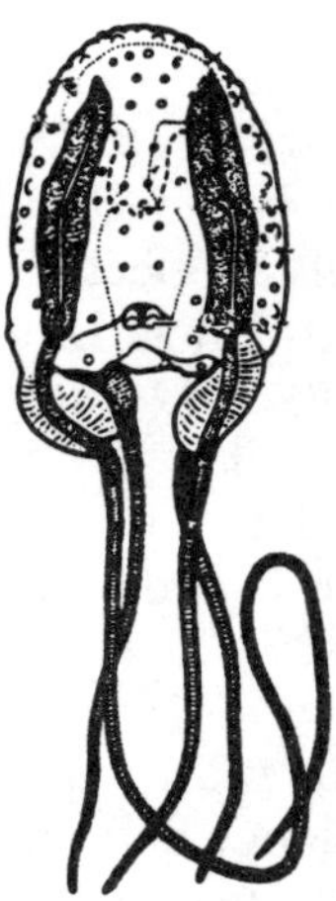

*AUSTRALIA'S* medical pioneers have worked in diverse fields. In Northern Australian waters lives the box jellyfish, the world's most venomous animal (*Figure 19.1*). Responsible for the recorded deaths of some seventy victims, the majority of whom have been children, the box jellyfish has undoubtedly killed many thousands of the first inhabitants of this Continent. Three early workers did much to elucidate the puzzle of marine stingers in Northern Australian waters – Hugo Flecker, Ron Southcott and Jack Barnes. Of these, Jack Barnes went on to discover the cause of the enigmatic 'Irukandji Syndrome'; it is about this latter pioneer that this short biography is written.

John Handyside ('Jack') Barnes was born in Charleville, Western Queensland on April 2, 1922. His father, Henry Edward Barnes, was a pharmacist and son of a Toowoomba family. His mother, Vera Adeline, was the daughter of pastoralist G.T. East whose family home was in Warwick. They had one other child, Joy, four years older who is still working part-time as a Barrister in Melbourne. For most of Jack's childhood the family lived in the

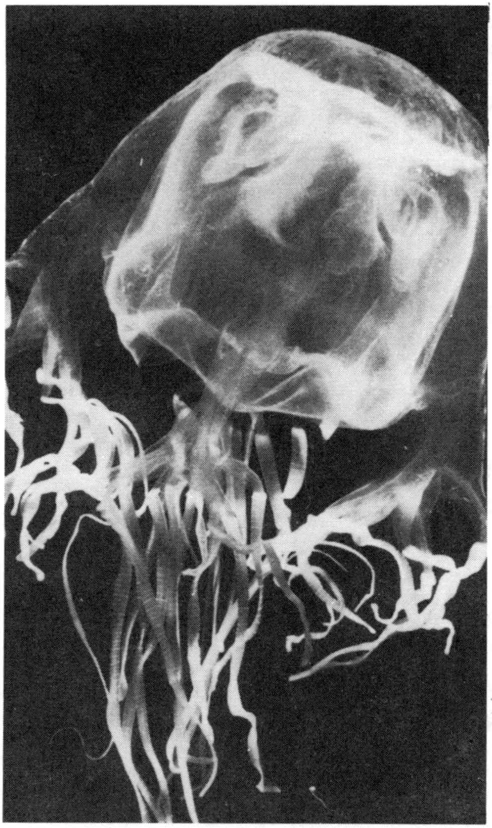

***Figure 19.1: The box jellyfish, Chironex fleckeri, the world's most venomous creature. A specimen collected by Dr Jack Barnes, circa 1960.***

homestead of *Dungiven* Station which was a sheep property owned by his mother.

The family lived briefly at Southport. Jack was always an individualist, a trait manifested early in life when he was expelled from St Hilda's Kindergarten for swearing. Joy remained at St Hilda's school and when the family returned to *Dungiven,* Jack did his school work by correspondence. For a short time he stayed at an hostel in Charleville to attend school. It was there, however, that one of the other pupil-boarders died from scarlet fever, and Jack believed he had been cruelly neglected. He walked to his Uncle Eric East's Station *Maxvale,* some twelve miles from Charleville. There he borrowed a horse and rode the rest of the 100 miles home to *Dungiven.* He was then 7 or 8 years old.

From then on he became a pupil of the Correspondence School. He would spend Sunday mornings doing his school work, finishing in time to give it to the mailman by lunchtime and receive his package for the next week. So he had six and a half clear days to roam, to work with the workmen on the sheep station, and to listen to their stories.

His mother managed the Station with the help of two men, one of whom, Mac Sutton, became Jack's mentor, encouraging his interest in radio and all things mechanical. The boy was at home wandering the vast countryside with only his horse and dog for company. At an early age he developed an empathy with his environment and was an observant and keen naturalist. His mother was a very experienced and successful show rider; to her horror and great disappointment, Jack insisted on riding relaxed with long stirrups, and rode slumped in the saddle in the manner of a boundary rider. She taught the young boy to shoot. These lessons were not wasted, as he became an expert marksman and was well-known for taking meticulous care of his equipment. Every weekend he was given five bullets to provide for Sunday's meal. He developed great patience and his familiarity with the tracks and habits of animals helped him. It became a matter of personal pride to use as few bullets as possible and hoard those remaining for times when game was scarce. This, together with living through the Depression, formed the basis for his habit of keeping anything that could be useful in the future.

He attended Brisbane Grammar School for four years of secondary schooling (*Figure 19.2*) and found it was THE mark of

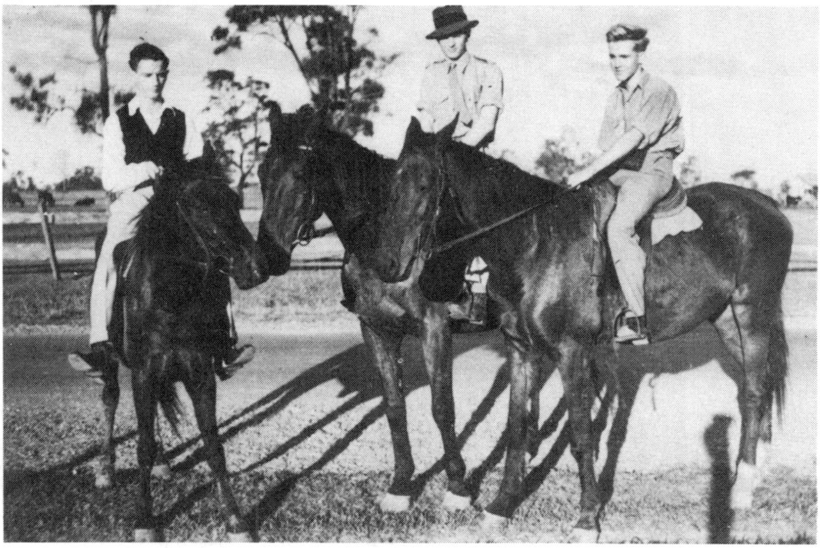

***Figure 19.2: School days. Maurice Dingle (left), Rud Crosier (centre) and Jack Barnes (right) – 'a day at Zillmere, Brisbane', as final year high school students at Brisbane Grammar School. Photo, 1939.***

success to have a sporting 'pocket'. Knowing nothing of team sports, and being limited by his size, he was made coxswain of the rowing crew but to his chagrin the crew did not win. He joined the School Cadet Corps which he enjoyed; when he found 'pockets' were given for shooting, he made sure of his! His hobbies at this time were photography and radio. He earned money by photographing people at country shows, then developing and printing orders. He won several competitions and developed expertise which was to be a great help to him in his later work on jellyfish. Radio was also a lifelong interest. He had a 'true ear' and in Cairns was often called by amateurs to tune their homemade stereo sets.

In 1940 as a seventeen year old youth, Jack Barnes started a Medical Course at the University of Queensland. After the war broke

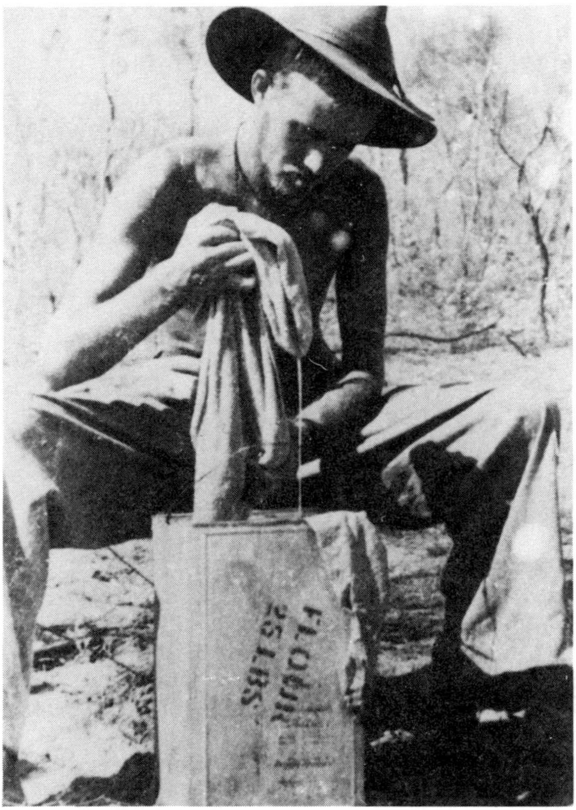

***Figure 19.3:***

***Jack Barnes, former medical student, as a Private of The 2/4th Independent Company, an Australian Commando Unit of the A.I.F.***

***Photo showing a necessary part of field training; Vanderlin, Sir Edward Pellew islands, Gulf of Carpentaria, 1942.***

out the Medical Course was classified as an 'essential service'. Most students decided it was more important to become doctors, while others decided more immediate action was necessary. At the end of his second year of Medicine, Jack Barnes went with his best friend, Rud Crosier (*Figure 19.2*) to join the Air Force. Rud was accepted but Jack was refused as it was found he was 'blue-green' colour blind. Later in the war the Air Force traced all these men in an effort to recruit them as it had been learned that this disorder enabled them to detect camouflage better than those with 'normal sight'.

On the 12th December, 1941 he enlisted in the Army in Brisbane at a time when middle stage medical students had to remain and complete their course. He volunteered for the 2/4th Independent Company, a Commando Unit. They trained at Wilson's Promontory and were then stationed outside Katherine and on the Roper River in the Northern Territory (*Figure 19.3*). His father and the University had the Armed Services trace him. One afternoon the unit Major sent for Jack and told him of the letter he had received that day instructing that he be returned to the University of Queensland forthwith. The Major said he could postpone receiving the letter until the next day, but that it was for Jack to decide. Jack realised some action must be taking place, (a confirmation of rumours), so asked that the letter be held over. The next day they moved out to board a destroyer bound for Timor.

The expedition was ill planned from the start. The ship ran aground, alerting the Japanese to the arrival of the replacement troops. The Japanese opened fire on the beaches while they were still landing and the men had to scatter in their sub-section groups to seek cover. They fought in groups of seven and had to have complete trust in one another to survive. The physical strain of malnutrition, malaria and other infectious diseases and wounds affected Jack's health permanently. Never a large person, he weighed only 28 kgs on his return to Australia. While recovering in Greenslopes Repatriation Hospital, he began a 'Pelmanism Course' in memory training. This was enormously important for the studies he was about to resume, and of continuing benefit in all aspects of his professional life. He was discharged on the 24th April, 1943.

Jack returned to the University of Queensland and there was some doubt whether he should repeat second year or be allowed to proceed. With third year already in full swing, the Dean (Errol

Solomon Meyers) said he could sit for the third year exams and if he passed he could go on to fourth year. With great application, together with the assistance of his fellow students, he passed third year. In May 1945 he married a second year Physiotherapy student, Loma Mavis Hudson. Jack graduated in May 1946 and their first daughter, Anne, was born in September of that year. Loma graduated at the end of that academic year.

His residency was undertaken at the Mater Misericordiae Hospital in Brisbane from May 1946 until May 1947. At that time doctors being discharged from the Army were being given refresher courses in Obstetrics and Child Care, so at some hospitals it was difficult to be assigned terms in these areas. The Mater rotated residents through the children's wards, paid £50 a year more than Royal Brisbane Hospital and the food was excellent by any standard, so there was no other choice for Jack.

He was appointed Superintendent of Thursday Island Hospital and took up his duties in July 1947, wise in the ways of the world at the age of twenty-five years. His medical practice included all the Torres Strait Islands, the northern section of Cape York Peninsula, and the mission stations and islands in the Gulf of Carpentaria. Three of Jack and Loma's children were born on the island – Jennifer (October 1948), Catherine (July 1950) and Nicholas (August 1951). The civilian population had been evacuated from 'T.I.' during the war but many of them had returned. Pearling had started again and all Government Departments had been re-established. Jack was the first post-war doctor. There was a tremendous backlog of medical work to be completed for the Islanders and Aboriginals. From his first outpatient session Jack insisted that sick people be seen first, irrespective of the colour of their skin. This had a price, and it was some time before he realised that he and his family had become social outcasts of the white community. Pre-war, all white patients had been seen first, then others, regardless of presenting symptoms. He never could understand this point of view and ignored it. Fortunately for his family the matriarch of an old pearling family and her daughter had been to the same school as Loma and became her firm friends. Also newcomers to the Island, and those transferees serving a term there, were disinterested in such pettiness.

The Hospital Dispensary was still in the state in which it had been left when evacuation took place. The Army had used it, and their leavings were there also. It took many weeks to sort and clean equipment. Jack worked until midnight when the powerhouse shut down, and no further electricity would be made available until the following day. New supplies were slow to arrive, aggravated by transport difficulties. Every morning he was available to give advice by radio to questions from other islands and mission stations, and visited these places in times of trouble. Once he spent four weeks on Darnley Island when there was a severe outbreak of malaria. Similarly he spent a week at a mission on the east coast of Cape York where he found all the children suffering from hookworm (*see Chapter 6*).

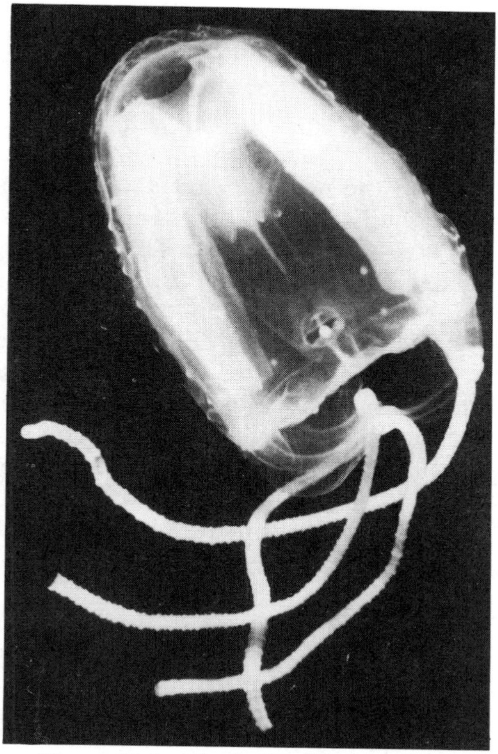

***Figure 19.4: The Irukandji, a small box jellyfish; named Carukia barnesi, after Dr Jack Barnes, who established its causal role in the severe 'Irukandji Syndrome' by personally subjecting himself and volunteer colleagues to its sting.***

Historically, in the Torres Strait a woman had a baby before marriage to prove her fertility and this baby was adopted by a family from another Island. Then tribal custom allowed the couple three children. There was great pressure for any ensuing pregnancies to be aborted, the methods sometimes killing the mother. Early missionaries and general acceptance of Christianity had stamped out these practices but adoption of the 'extra' babies remained very common. This way of life made the compilation of records of genetic family and adopted family very difficult. The young doctor spent a great deal of time trying to perfect these and left them in excellent order.

There was a very high incidence of venereal disease throughout Torres Strait but this was completely overshadowed by the numbers of patients with tuberculosis. The problem of treatment became enormous because of the lack of hospital beds, equipment and staff. Jack trained one of the nursing sisters to take chest x-rays and perform the necessary tests to establish the diagnosis of tuberculosis. Until the time he left the problem was accelerating. A second hospital, the *Waiben*, was opened for recovering patients. Later a hostel was opened for the use of visiting Islanders who came to have medical checks or short term treatment. Jack's records were of great importance in the continuing checking of patients and their contacts.

For about two years he was completely alone as the only doctor for a vast area of Australia. Then at times he had an assistant, once even two, briefly. Isolation made him self-sufficient, and practice enabled him to handle a crisis calmly and with common sense as well as skill. In one such crisis a rhesus–negative baby required a blood transfusion and Brisbane was unable to supply matching blood. The only member of the family with suitable blood was the baby's five year old sister. Jack was able to give enough of the sister's blood to save the baby and the five year old, somewhat weak, was given a sojourn in hospital to rebuild her strength.

Conditions were difficult. In T.I. Hospital, surgery was performed on an examination couch that the wardsmen tilted with bricks. The only anaesthetic available was spinal. Later an Oxford Vapouriser arrived which the Matron was trained to use. This made an immeasurable improvement in conditions for the staff and the patients. It distressed Jack that no pressure chamber was available anywhere in North Queensland for the treatment of pearl divers suffering the effects of 'the bends' (*see Chapter 9*).

During the periods when Dr Barnes had an assistant he relaxed by sailing and fishing. He had the hull, the outriggers and the sweep oar of a New Guinea canoe towed from the Fly River in Papua New Guinea to Thursday Island. He worked on the canoe and calculated mathematically the distance the outriggers should be from the hull. After estimating the sizes and shapes of the sails they were made to his patterns. The boat required a minimum crew of three men; one on the oar, one on the sails and one on the outrigger poles. When possible, Loma worked as an outrigger boy. The other men involved eventually left T.I. and Jack could not find replacement crew for this vigorous and hair-raising sport. He then bought a small motor boat and developed a love of fishing. The family used the boat for picnics on neighbouring islands. Friday Island was their favourite because of the deer, wallaby, sandy beaches, and fresh water; and the presence of lovely shade trees growing to the water's edge.

Wherever Jack Barnes lived he made a garden. It was while he relaxed in this way that he did his deepest thinking. Vegetables were particularly important on Thursday Island. In the 1940s and 1950s T.I. was serviced by only one ship a month from Cairns. Because of strikes and absconding seamen (the ship was not allowed to sail without its full crew), it rarely kept to its schedule and was often a week or two late. Fruit and vegetables were carried as deck cargo. Later refrigerators were installed. The planes from Cairns were too small to carry cargo other than mail. Later, when DC-3s were put on the run, they brought limited fresh supplies from Cairns. As T.I. has no topsoil, Jack's early efforts involved borrowing a small boat, puttering to Prince of Wales Island, filling bags with soil and bringing them home. The soil was placed in two rounds cut from an old domestic water tank and so he made his beds. The encroaching tree roots and lack of water made this method impractical.

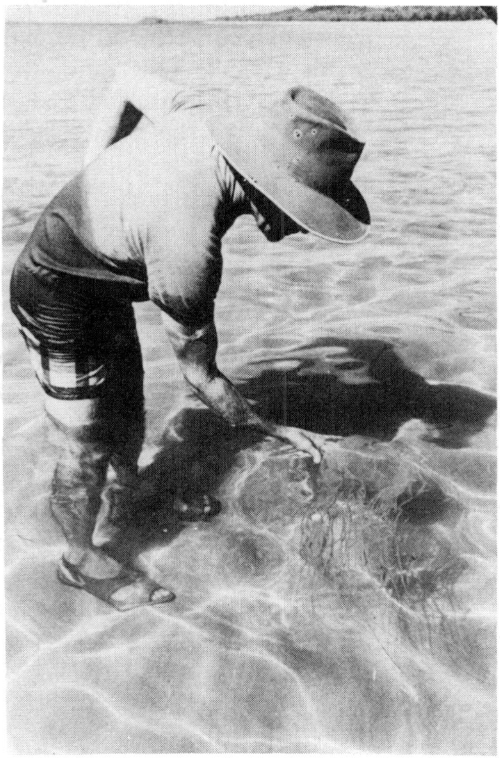

***Figure 19.5:* *Dr Jack Barnes about to lift a trapped Chironex from the sea at Mission Beach, North Queensland. Photo, circa 1972, courtesy of John Carnemolla.***

His next venture was hydroponics. He successfully grew crops such as

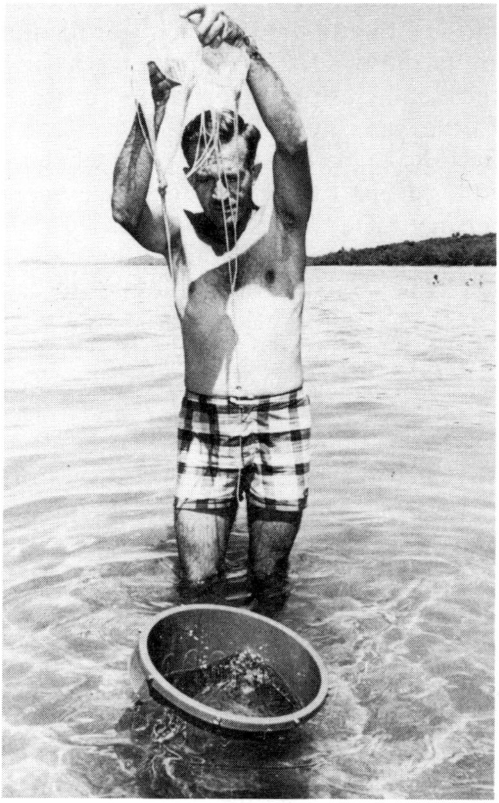

*Figure 19.6: Dr Jack Barnes holding aloft a box jellyfish, Chironex fleckeri, at Mission Beach, North Queensland. Photo, circa 1972, courtesy of John Carnemolla.*

lettuce, silver beet, tomatoes beans, carrots, radish and eschallots. He made three terraces on the backyard hill slope. On these he placed three rows of corrugated iron guttering, half rounds about 30–45 cm diameter joined together. At the bottom of the hill in a shaded old dry well shaft, he placed an old square ship's tank. This tank held the nutrient solution. It was pumped to the highest level and allowed to trickle back down to the tank. The pH was adjusted daily. It was the perfect solution for that environment, though the searing climate meant that crops could only be grown for a short time of the year. When he moved to Cairns to live he reverted to soil gardening. In the last couple of years of his life, when he could no longer work hard in his garden, he reverted to hydroponics. This allowed him to have the pleasure of growing vegetables and flowers with the minimum of effort, even to using a comfortable stool of convenient height.

The young doctor accumulated a large collection of Torres Strait and Cape York orchids. He built an orchid house and treasured them greatly. Disaster struck when one year a plague of rats ate all growing shoots and roots from his plants; all were destroyed. While walking around Weipa he found a ground orchid he had seen nowhere else. He brought home specimens and sent both plants and pressed flowers away to be classified. The man who did the classification now has an orchid named for himself. He did write to Jack telling him that it belonged to a Malaysian family that had never before been found in Australia!

The complete difference in the music of the Torres Strait Islanders fascinated him. He recorded this on wire and had forever in his memory the dramatisation of their history and way of life in their Dance.

The family left Thursday Island in January 1953 and moved to Cairns where Jack set up in general practice. He kept abreast of medical advances and filled a great need in North Queensland by developing an expertise in the use of the newer techniques of anaesthesia. Over the next few years his medical practice grew quickly, though his personal life was marred by tragedy. Four of his five children were affected by a progressive neurological disorder. His eldest daughter Anne died in June 1954. His son, Nicholas, lost most of his sight in November 1957 and his daughter Catherine died in November 1959. Rudyard was born in Cairns, October 1964 and lost most of his sight in January 1982.

During his early years in Cairns, Jack had met Dr Hugo Flecker, a keen naturalist who had compiled a Registry of Injuries due to Plants and Animals. Flecker had, in collaboration with Dr Ronald Southcott of Adelaide, discovered the role of *Chironex fleckeri* in fatal stingings (*Figure 19.1*). Jack's interest in marine stingers dated back to Thursday Island where his practice had brought him into contact with jellyfish stings and with the toxic effects associated with the ingestion of certain marine foods. Two children had been fatally stung at Weipa and Jack was shown the jellyfish that the local Aboriginals believed responsible. He did not keep the specimen, assuming that this knowledge was general. Recounting this story to Flecker years later he discovered his mistake.

Hugo Flecker died in June 1957, and his Register of Injuries was lost. In 1958 Jack was asked by the local branch of the British Medical Association to continue Flecker's work. Jack Barnes was intrigued, as was Flecker before him, by a presumed marine stinger syndrome first described by Flecker in 1945.[1] This syndrome is characterised by intense bachache, agonizing abdominal and joint pains, and vomiting with recovery over several days. The actual contact can be so mild that people are often unaware of the sting.

There is only a slight redness at the site and onset of symptoms is normally delayed 10 to 20 minutes. Victims had even been subjected to unnecessary appendectomies. Flecker always believed a specific, and as yet unrecognised, marine stinger was responsible. Southcott had termed this a 'Type A Stinging'[2] and Flecker had coined the term 'Irukandji'. Most of the stingings occurred between the Mobray River to the north of Cairns and Trinity Inlet to the south. This coastal region had formerly been inhabited by the Irukandji tribe. Hence the name. Flecker and Southcott had made strenuous efforts to establish the causative agent of this syndrome. Flecker had arranged for lifesavers, ambulance men and the bathing public to join the search by providing specimens, but these had never been found.

Feeling that his own zoological knowledge was inadequate for the task ahead, Jack Barnes established contact with Southcott. A most productive partnership developed. Jack would supply raw information and specimens and Southcott would identify these or organise the appropriate literature. It was a long haul so far from access to the libraries and texts so freely available these days for city dwellers. Cairns in the early 1950s was a long way from such luxury.

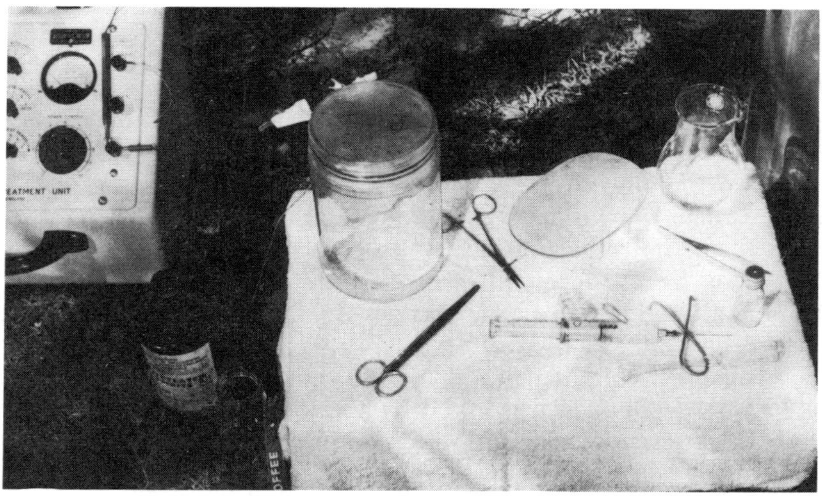

*Figure 19.7: The venom research kit of Dr Jack Barnes. The bottle is covered by a human amnion membrane, a technique for venom collection pioneered by Jack Barnes, in North Queensland. Photo, circa 1962.*

Jack had learned something of teamwork in the Army but nothing prepared him for the effort entailed in continuing Flecker's research. He had to establish an information network within the community. Hundreds of people left specimens of a great variety of marine life with the Cairns Ambulance or Life Savers in various centres. These all reached Jack. The animals were described, catalogued, and sent off for identification. Dr Southcott and Professor Paul Kramp in Copenhagen were of enormous assistance in this regard. Jack perfected a method of preservation whereby the specimens were unstressed and appeared lifelike. Many were photographed. Duplicate specimens were kept and labelled, providing the nucleus of a reference collection.

While much valuable information came out of the collection, it was a further three years before the agent responsible for the Irukandji syndrome was identified (*Figure 19.4*). Its discovery was a tribute to Jack's perseverance and ingenuity. He surmised that the organism was small but not microscopic, transparent and highly motile. It would most likely be found in shallow water or the top 45 cm of deeper water, and at times occurred in large numbers.

Many nights were spent suspending lights above or just below the water mark. Devices were constructed to manipulate the light and background in the hope that the organism might be detected. Efforts were concentrated at Palm Beach where most stings had been reported. Stings were also more prevalent when winds blew steadily from the north, and during these conditions an obvious stream of clear oceanic water is to be seen about half a mile off shore, beyond the more murky coastal water. This oceanic water travels southwards and is split by the presence of Double Island and an 'arm' of faster flowing clear water is diverted shoreward, toward Palm and Ellis Beaches. The proximity of this stream to the beach is affected by the state of the tide and wind strength. This phenomenon was described in Jack Barnes' paper on 'Cause and Effect in Irukandji Stingings'.[3] At the convergence of the two streams there is a tendency for marine life near the surface to congregate and therefore concentrate.

Eventually (following reports of stings at Palm Beach) success came in December 1961. Jack was using SCUBA gear and one of his home made 'catchers'. With his hand held before his face to provide the right lighting conditions, Jack discovered the first small carybdeid known to have been obtained in these waters. This was in water 4 ft

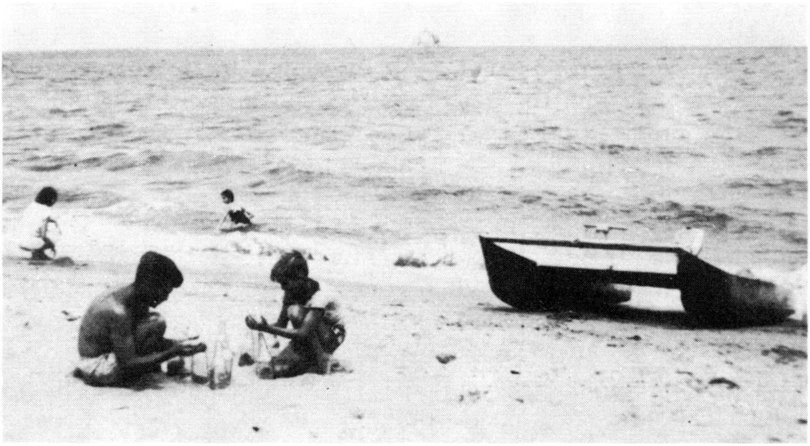

***Figure 19.8:*** ***Preparing drift bottles for the detection of sea current movements and the migration of the box jellyfish, Chironex. Foreground (left) is Dr Jack Barnes, with his son, Nicholas. Photo, on a beach near Cairns, circa 1960.***

deep just in front of the Beach Patrol tower. The lifesavers inspected the specimen and donned facemasks to look for further specimens. Another was found because it had captured a small fish and this was being dragged through the water in an unnatural manner. This prompted a lifesaver to dive in to investigate, whereupon he discovered the carybdeid jellyfish to which it was attached.

The two specimens were compared, they appeared identical, and were of similar size. Sections of tentacle were then applied to the upper inner forearm of Jack, his nine year old son Nicholas, and a young lifesaver. The onset of typical symptoms over the next 25 minutes meant that Barnes had at last found his elusive stinger. Dr Graham Cossins, as always, was on hand to offer medical assistance. It was reassuring to Jack, and even more so to his family, to know that Graham would be unsparing with his time and efforts to assist in every way possible. The volunteers were treated with pethidine hydrochloride, administered through indwelling intravenous needles. Jack claimed the effect to be dramatic.[4] Symptoms returned after about 20 minutes and further pethidine and later aspirin were required. The truest medical pioneering spirit!

The Irukandji stinger was given the name *Carukia barnesi* by Dr Ron Southcott as a tribute to Jack Barnes' work. It appeared as a small translucent box jellyfish about the size of the end of a man's finger (*Figure 19.4*). It swims by muscular contractions of the bell, which allow it to manoeuvre by directing a jet of water from the bell. It possesses simple eyes, carried in a fold on each of the four sides of the animal. There are four tentacles varying in length from 5 cm to 1.2 metres long, when extended in their search for prey. Beads on the tentacles and body of the jellyfish are aggregations of quite small but potent nematocysts. Even in transient contact, fluid from these can be transferred to the tissue of the victim. Other carybdeids were found which did not have the virulence of the originals. This caused a great deal of confusion. It was important that the identified cause of the disease be published, but there were still fine details which Jack would have preferred resolved. As a true scientist he delayed publication until 1964 in the hope that he could find the clues to the differences between stings from apparently identical carybdeids.

Because deaths and severe stings continued to occur from the box jellyfish *Chironex fleckeri*, Jack spent more and more of his time familiarising himself with the behaviour and lifecycle of this creature (*Figures 19.5 and 19.6*). Recognising the need for pure *Chironex* venom, Jack set about the task of 'milking' the tentacles, ascertaining a way to extract as pure a venom as possible from its source. He reasoned that if the tentacle was presented with a membrane which would appear to approximate a food source to its sensory receptors, then the nematocysts could probably be induced to discharge their venom. Furthermore, if this membrane was of an appropriate thickness, then the venom would be discharged onto, and could be collected from, the far surface, eliminating much extraneous material from the tentacle itself in the process. After trial and error, he settled on amniotic membrane (*Figure 19.7*) as an appropriate lure.[4] Only small amounts of toxin could be collected. The work was arduous and involved his family (*Figure 19.8*) and volunteers, and a supply of amniotic membrane from the maternity wards of the Base Hospital.

Collecting began at first light while the sea was calm enough to observe shadows on the bottom through the clear water. After spotting and marking the positions of the box jellyfish, Jack entered the water and herded them into large plastic rubbish bins. Several of these were returned to the milking site at a time. The weather was hot and humid, and as individual tentacles had to be removed and transferred to the membrane, the work had to be done away from any breezes. The jellyfish were kept cool and milking continued through the day. Then the equipment had to be cleaned, the toxin stored and the jellyfish buried. The need for clear water meant this could not be done in the immediate Cairns area. There was considerable personal expense involved in the exercise, but many local people were very generous with their help. With time, modifications in his milking methods occurred which allowed greater amounts of higher quality venom to be collected. The venom so extracted was used for the production of the currently used box jellyfish anti-venom.

The realisation that *Chironex* was stimulated to sting only by living tissues which it recognised as food or danger, led to the use of synthetic stockings as protection (*Figure 19.9*). The lifesavers, always at risk and often stung, were very reluctant to use pantyhose. Abashed as they were at first, it was not long before they were striding around in them with great confidence. These have been replaced by the present day stinger suits.

Jack Barnes made other significant contributions to marine biology, both before and after the identification of *Carukia barnesi.* In 1960 the *Medical Journal of Australia* published his paper which clarified differences between the nematocysts of *Physalia, Cyanea, Chironex,* and *Chiropsalmus* and his description of the different clinical appearances of these stings.[5] Also by 1960 he was starting to develop his ideas on the differences in gonad development between *Chironex* and *Chiropsalmus.* This research together with his breakthrough discovery about the shape of the canal which leads from the bell to the tentacles, culminated in his paper, '*Chironex fleckeri* and *Chiropsalmus quadrigatus* – Morphological Distinctions'.[6] In 1964 he published a joint paper with Dr Robert Endean on the Crown of Thorns Starfish.[7] He followed this in 1966 with another in which he detailed the occurrence of an outbreak of Crown of Thorns in plague numbers on Green Island.[8] His records also noted the presence of stings from a diverse assemblage of marine organisms; *Cyanea* – (the 'snottie' or hair jelly), stonefish, stingrays, *Physalia* – (bluebottle, Portuguese Man O'War), anemone, bullrout, stinging hydroids, siphonophores[9,10] and a variety of other jellyfish.

In retrospect, an early pattern emerged in Jack Barnes' research. The initial 'grab bag' of information and specimens was very quickly refined to specific pathways. His curiosity and keen

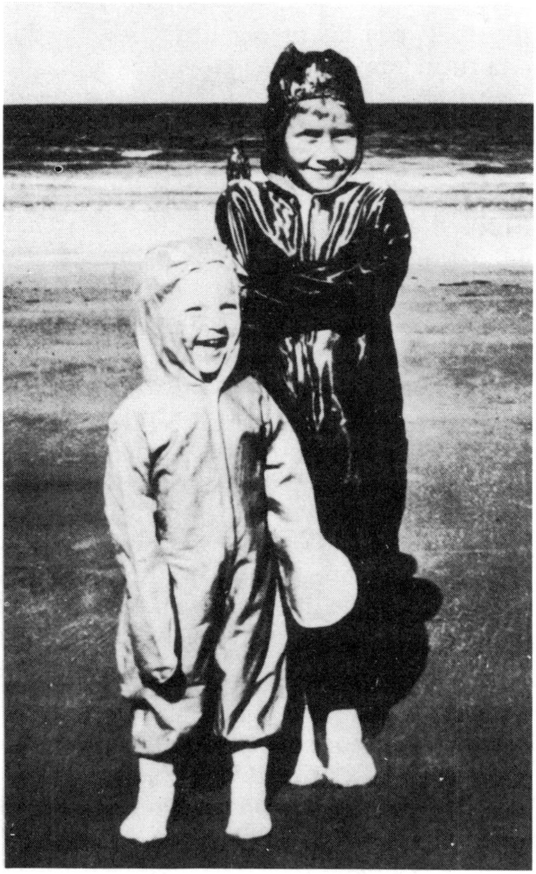

***Figure 19.9:***

***Protective clothing against the box jellyfish Chironex fleckeri, the world's most venomous creature. It is too dangerous to swim in northern waters in the 'stinger season'. Children comprise a large proportion of box jellyfish victims. This illustration shows the protection necessary prior to the era when pantyhose protection, or the later 'stinger suits' were introduced.***

***Nicholas Barnes, at right.***

***Photo, Palm Beach, Cairns, circa 1960.***

powers of observation, together with an excellent memory, allowed him to make associations between his clinical observations and what he saw in the field. His interest in things mechanical or electrical came to the fore in many aspects of his research work. His genius for adaptation and for being able to foresee where difficulties could arise and how to overcome them, was his forte. Whenever there was a problem needing thought he retreated to work alone in his garden. He possessed great intellectual honesty and cared not that some of his findings were not popularly held views at the time. This lonely stance has been the lot also, of several of his successors to this day.

As the momentum of his research gathered, Jack was often torn between his medical practice and his research. He had built up a faithful core of patients who liked his down-to-earth, commonsense approach. It was due to their unfailing support that he could give so much time to the research he considered so important. On the recommendation of local and Shire Councillors, he was awarded an M.B.E. for his contributions to the welfare of their communities. From the earliest times in his research he recognised the need for education to lessen the incidence of stings, and public warnings to alert tourists and visitors to the dangers of swimming at certain times of the year. The Cairns City Council has paid tribute to him by naming its Mangrove Environmental Park 'The Jack Barnes Bicentennial Mangrove Boardwalk'.

As he realised his health was failing, Jack gave his consent for Barbara Kinsey of the Sir George Fisher Centre for Tropical Marine Studies at James Cook University to collate and record his findings of many years. Her two volumes on his work with box jellyfish are the product of this association.[11,12] Jack Barnes passed away on August 11, 1985.

While this biographical sketch recalls Jack Barnes the scientist, and Jack Barnes the physician, Jack Barnes the man emerged through the words of his close friend Graham Cossins whose eulogy records that Jack was –

> *... irritable and belligerent as many short men can be, demanding and critical, unsociable and rude, scathing of politicians and uncooperative with authority ... but under that gruff exterior was a kindly and compassionate associate ... his deeds gave him away and his many faithful patients and his fellow medicos all knew that he practised medicine with skill and honesty and a proper compassion for the sick and frightened ... .*

Of such are the true medical pioneers made.

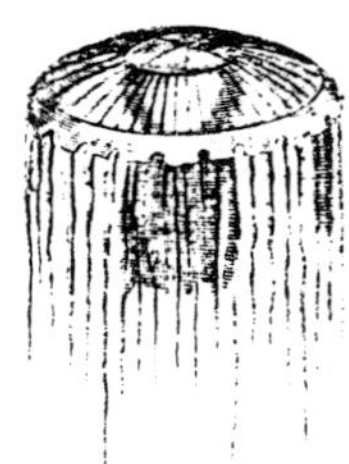

# PIONEER MEDICINE IN AUSTRALIA 20

## *H.J. WILKINSON - THE TRAVAIL OF A PIONEER WITH MUSCLE*

**Geoffrey Kenny**

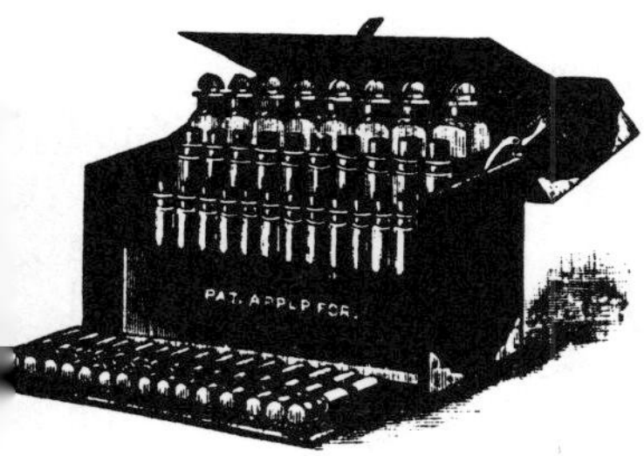

*PIONEERS* in medicine have made contributions to clinical practice, to research, to teaching, and to the encouragement of scholarship. Some have pioneered in several fields. Professor H.J. Wilkinson was such a one, and holds a special place in the history of Australian biomedical science.

Born in Adelaide in 1891, Herbert John Wilkinson entered the medical course of the University of Sydney in 1920 as a mature age student. He graduated with honours in 1925 and immediately joined the staff of its Anatomy Department. After two years overseas experience following the award of a Rockefeller Fellowship in 1928, he returned in 1930 to the city of his birth as Elder Professor of Anatomy and Histology within the University of Adelaide. Subsequently, in 1936, he became Foundation Dean of the Faculty of Medicine in the University of Queensland and the first Professor of Anatomy in its Medical School founded that year. This was the first medical school to be created in Australia for over fifty years and the first to be established since the federation of the Australian colonies and the formation of the Commonwealth of Australia in 1901. In both positions he was breaking new ground in more ways

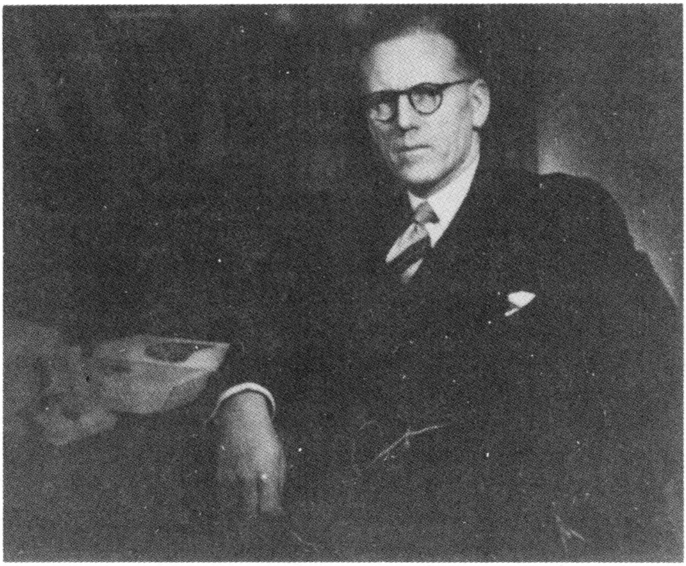

***Figure 20.1:***

***H.J. Wilkinson***

***Lesley M. Williams Collection***

than one. He was the first native-born Australian to be regarded as the Foundation Professor of an Australian anatomy department and to become the Foundation Dean of an Australian medical faculty.

In Australia's retreat from colonialism, H.J. Wilkinson was a significant figure (*Figure 20.1*). His claim to distinction is enhanced by recalling his contribution to scientific knowledge, especially his work (with that of other Australians) in solving the problem of the nature of the motor supply of skeletal muscle fibres. In this connection, the Anatomy Department of the University of Sydney played a leading part.

In 1920, the year in which Wilkinson began his medical course, J.T. Wilson, a graduate of Edinburgh University, ended thirty years in the Challis Chair of Anatomy at the University of Sydney and returned to Britain as Regius Professor of Anatomy at Cambridge University. Wilson is regarded as a 'key figure' in the origin of Australian neuroscience.[1] Although Wilkinson's initial personal contact with Wilson was brief, its impact upon him was lifelong. Shortly after his return to Britain, Wilson reviewed the evidence supporting the case being made at that time for the double innervation of striated muscle fibres.[2] According to the supporters of this concept, both non-myelinated sympathetic nerve fibres and myelinated somatic (cerebro-spinal) nerve fibres supplied skeletal muscle fibres. The principal advocate of this view was the Dutch histologist Boeke (*Figure 20.2*).

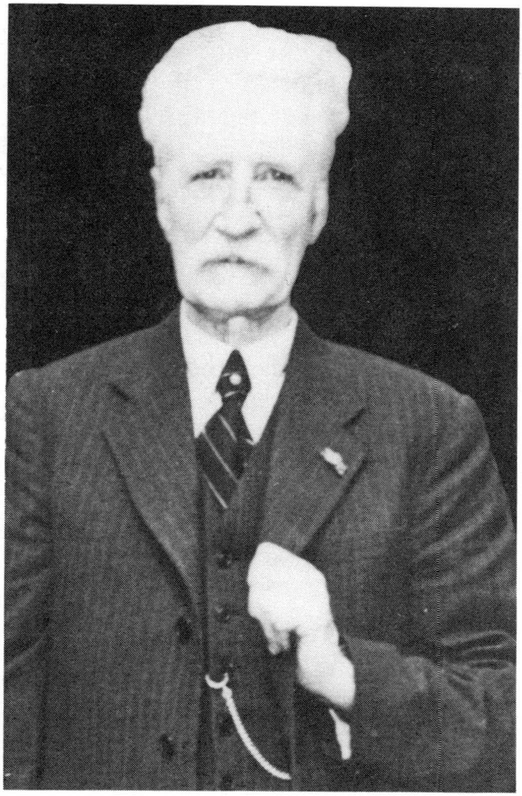

***Figure 20.2: J. Boeke***
***Sydney Sunderland Collection***

In 1921 the attention of Norman Royle (*Figure 20.3*), a Sydney orthopaedic surgeon, was drawn to the existence in skeletal muscle of the non-myelinated nerves considered to belong to the sympathetic nervous system.[3] Royle, who graduated from the University of Sydney in Medicine in 1914, had previously been a Demonstrator in Anatomy during Wilson's tenure of the Challis Chair. During this time he had become associated with a young medical undergraduate, John Irvine Hunter (*Figure 20.4*) who graduated from the University of Sydney in 1920. Shortly after graduation Hunter had been appointed Associate Professor of Anatomy at his *alma mater*. In August 1921 Hunter left Sydney to spend eighteen months abroad, part of which he spent with his former teacher, J.T. Wilson.[4] It may be that it was from Hunter and Wilson that Royle learned of the 'double innervation' of skeletal muscle fibres. Be that as it may, shortly after Hunter returned to the University of Sydney as the second Challis Professor of Anatomy early in 1923, he commenced to collaborate with Royle in further study of the nerve supply to skeletal muscle.

For some time Royle had been treating patients with spastic

paraplegia. With the ultimate aim of enhancing their treatment, he was interested in discovering the details of the mechanism responsible for increase in skeletal muscle tone. Royle accepted the view that each skeletal muscle fibre received a sympathetic nerve fibre. He set out with Hunter to establish the role of this fibre by experimental means. This involved studying the effect of removal on one side of the abdominal sympathetic trunk upon spasticity of the lower limbs in experimental animals. Royle felt satisfied that sympathectomy reduced spasticity in these animals. Subsequently, on 1 September 1923 in a human volunteer with spasticity of the right upper limb and both lower limbs, the right lower limb being more affected, he divided the white ramus communicans of the right second lumbar nerve and avulsed the grey ramus communicans of this nerve together with those of the third and fourth right lumbar nerves; the right sympathetic trunk was divided below the fourth lumbar sympathetic ganglion. He stated that 54 days after operation the limb on the operated side could be relaxed 'almost in a normal manner when walking'.[5]

A similar operation involving avulsion of the grey rami passing from the right sympathetic trunk to the nerves concerned with the formation of the right brachial plexus was performed on another volunteer. This patient suffered from a right spastic hemiplegia and the operation was done in the hope of providing relief from this condition as far as the badly affected upper limb was concerned. The result was similarly encouraging. No time was wasted in communicating these exciting results. The report was made at a meeting of the New South Wales Branch of the British Medical Association on 26 October 1923.

At the same meeting Hunter spoke on the influence of the intramuscular sympathetic nerve fibres upon posture. At this time the tone of skeletal muscle was considered to be composed of two elements, namely, contractile and plastic. The contractile component, 'contractile tonus', was held to be responsible for the assumption of a particular posture and the plastic component, 'plastic tonus', for maintaining this posture. Hunter concluded that Royle's work showed that the sympathetic nerve fibres were responsible for the production of the plastic component and the improvement seen in the two patients was due to the removal of the relevant grey rami communicantes.[6]

In July 1924 delegates, who included Dr William J. Mayo, from the American College of Surgeons, visited the University of Sydney. These delegates were so impressed by the endeavours of Royle and Hunter that they were invited to speak of their work by jointly delivering the prestigious John B. Murphy Oration in Surgery at the Presidential Meeting of the Clinical Congress of the delegates' College. This they did in New York on 20 October 1924. Unfortunately, Hunter died in December on his way back to Australia; Royle fared little better as he became a victim of *encephalitis lethargica* while in the United States and subsequently developed Parkinsonism, which led within a few years to a decline in his activities.[7] It is now thought that Hunter was also a victim of the same disease.[8]

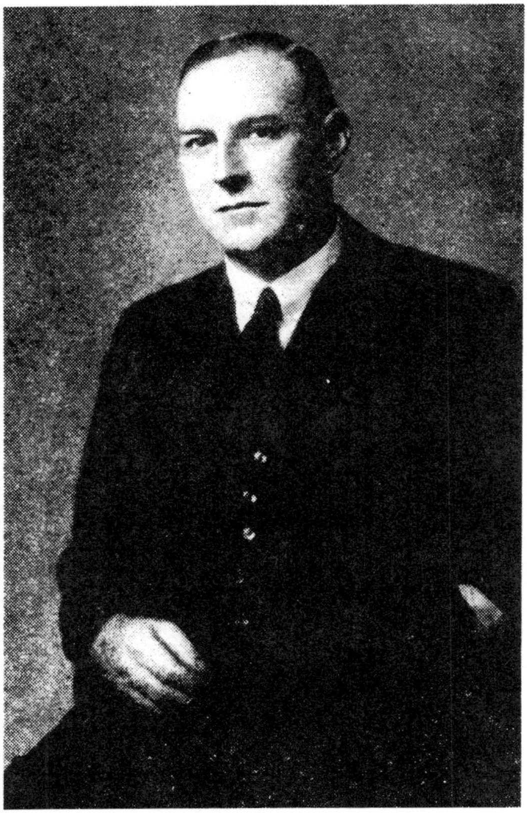

*Figure 20.3: Dr Norman D. Royle Orthopaedic Surgeon, of Sydney.*

It seems likely that Wilkinson's wish to investigate the innervation of skeletal muscle began at about this time. In 1924 while still an undergraduate medical student, he acted as a teacher in histology.[9] The present author was informed by him that this desire arose as a result of a question concerning 'double innervation' that he put to Hunter during the course of a practical class. He was not convinced by the answer and when the opportunity came he decided to look into the matter.

During 1925 and for much of 1926 it appears Wilkinson was

responsible for the teaching of histology within the Anatomy Department of the University of Sydney.[9] In 1926 one of his colleagues in the department was Oliver Latham,[9] a distinguished neuropathologist. Latham had previously collaborated with Hunter in an histological investigation of the innervation of skeletal muscle. The results of this study were published in January 1925.[10] The authors concluded:

> *We have been able to satisfy ourselves by using the gold impregnation method that, quite apart from their vascular supply, the striated muscle fibres of the hen and goat, animals used in experimental researches on the nervous mechanism subserving plastic tonus, have a rich supply of peculiar nerve endings* [*terminations en grappes*] *derived from mixed nerves and plexuses of non-medullated nucleated sympathetic nerves, quite distinct from the end-plates* [*terminations en plaques*] *derived from myelinated somatic motor nerves, that as far as our work goes these two types of nerve terminations en grappes and en plaques do not exist in the same muscle fibres, but each supply separate groups and that we have found little evidence incompatible with the theory that these striped musculatures are divided into alternate groups of muscle fibres served respectively by branches from the somatic and sympathetic nervous systems, the former subserving contractile and the latter plastic tonus.*

This was the situation in his department when Wilkinson began his enquiry concerning the 'double innervation of striated muscle fibres' and related aspects of the innervation of skeletal muscle.

By 1927 Wilkinson was ready to communicate some of his findings. These were summarized by Latham at the Australasian Medical Congress in Dunedin, New Zealand, on 9 February 1927.[11] Earlier findings reported in the paper by Latham were the outcome of work that he and Wilkinson had done in collaboration; the later findings were those of Wilkinson working on his own. Latham reported that Wilkinson had found every striated muscle fibre was supplied by a somatic nerve fibre and that the sympathetic nerve fibres described by Boeke ending in relation to skeletal muscle fibres came from fibres about blood – or lymph – vessels. Wilkinson had also concluded that the *terminations en grappe* in the extrinsic muscles of the eye were sensory nerve endings.

In November 1928 Wilkinson submitted a paper of his own on

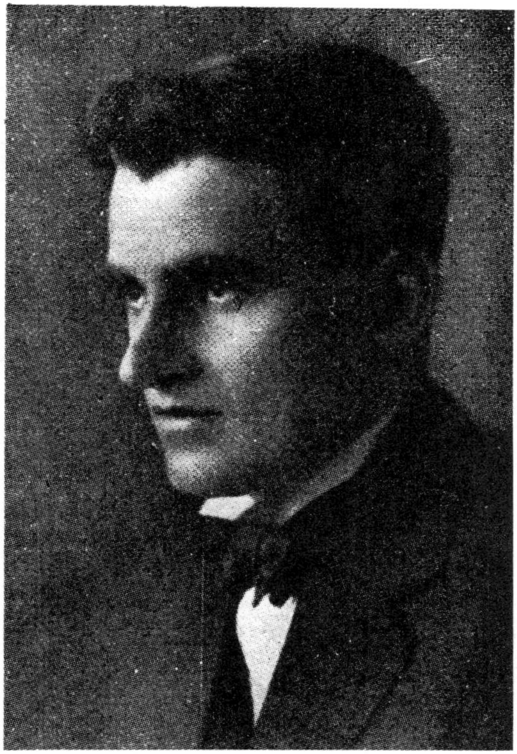

*Figure 20.4:* ***Associate Professor John Irvine Hunter, anatomist, of Sydney.***

the innervation of striated muscle. The paper was accepted for publication and the printer's proofs of it were received by him while he was travelling overseas on his Rockefeller Fellowship. By this time he had been able to examine the preparations on which Boeke had based his concept of the 'double innervation of striated muscle'. As a consequence, he amended the original article and resubmitted the paper. The paper is now regarded as a classic in its field, but its publication in 1929[12] immersed Wilkinson in controversy. He concluded that *all* striated muscle fibres are supplied *solely* by somatic nerves. He had now not only refuted the view of Hunter and Latham but that of Boeke as well. He included in his paper a criticism of Boeke's original preparations and and advanced the view that 'in striated muscle tissue sympathetic nerves supply only the blood vessels and are concerned only with the regulation of the circulation'. Boeke was not pleased and even less pleased when shortly afterwards in a second paper Wilkinson criticized his description of the motor plate of striated muscle.[13] Within four months Boeke had replied with feeling to the statements made by Wilkinson in these two articles.[14] He evidently was unaware at the time of writing that a third paper, prepared by Wilkinson during his stay at the Institute of Neurology of Northwestern University, Chicago, before his return to Australia, was in the press. This paper appeared in the same volume as Boeke's reply and preceded its

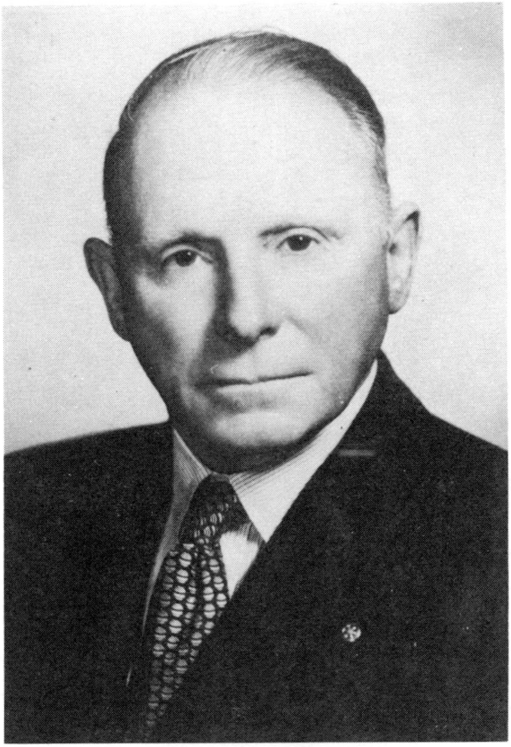

***Figure 20.5: Sir Albert Coates***
***Rowan Webb Collection***

publication by two months. This third paper was to be the first article of two to be published by Wilkinson as the result of repeating the experimental work of Boeke and others who supported the concept of 'double innervation'. However, before Wilkinson learned of Boeke's reaction he had returned to Australia as Elder Professor of Anatomy and Histology at the University of Adelaide.

The controversy surrounding his work did not provide a happy start for Wilkinson in his new position. The third paper had done nothing to assuage wounded feelings. Wilkinson wrote in it 'New evidence is submitted which substantiates the author's recently published criticism ...' and claimed there was now no histological evidence for 'the hypothesis concerning the sympathetic innervation of skeletal muscle.' From personal knowledge the present author is aware of the disillusionment the experience gave Wilkinson. However, with quiet determination he completed his experimental work in Adelaide four years later and concluded:

> *The sympathetic nerves were found only in relation to the blood vessels and no evidence was found to support the hypothesis that striated muscle fibers are innervated by both somatic and sympathetic nerves.*[16]

Wilkinson rested his case with this paper.

It was to be many years before his opinion regarding the role of the sympathetic nerves in striated muscle came to be accepted as fact. He received valuable support for this view in 1931 from three fellow Australians, Albert Coates (later Sir Albert) and Oscar Tiegs working together in Melbourne[17] and Gilbert Phillips working in his previous department in Sydney[18] (*Figures 20.5, 20.6 and 20.7*). Their findings were consonant with his own. Nevertheless, there was no reference to the Australians' work in the book *Problems of Nervous Anatomy* which Boeke published in 1940. Indeed he continued to associate sympathetic and somatic nerve fibres with the innervation of striated muscle fibres.[19]

However, it was referred to by Kuntz in 1945. He had the following comment to make concerning the work of Wilkinson:

> *In view of Boeke's extensive experience with histologic technic and in the interpretation of histologic preparations, his criticism of Wilkinson's work does not inspire confidence in the latter's findings.*[20]

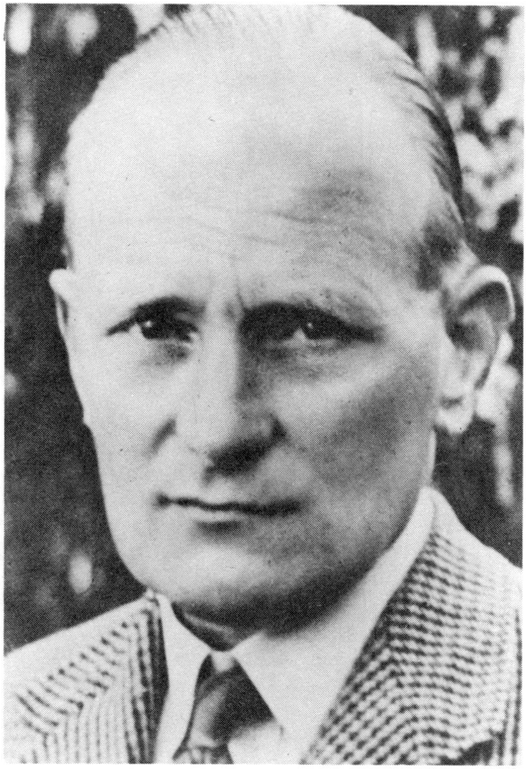

***Figure 20.6: O. W. Tiegs Zoology Department, The University of Melbourne Collection.***

Some ten years later Wilkinson had the satisfaction of realising his conclusions concerning the innervation of skeletal muscle fibres and the role of the intramuscular sympathetic nerve fibres outlined here had been accepted. It cannot be claimed that the elucidation of the innervation of striated muscle was a wholly Australian contribution to knowledge. This is patently not so. However, it can be fairly claimed that Australian scientists played a pioneering role in it and none more so than H.J. Wilkinson who throughout his career remained grateful to colleagues overseas who had helped him in his work especially those in S.W. Ranson's group in Northwestern University, Chicago.

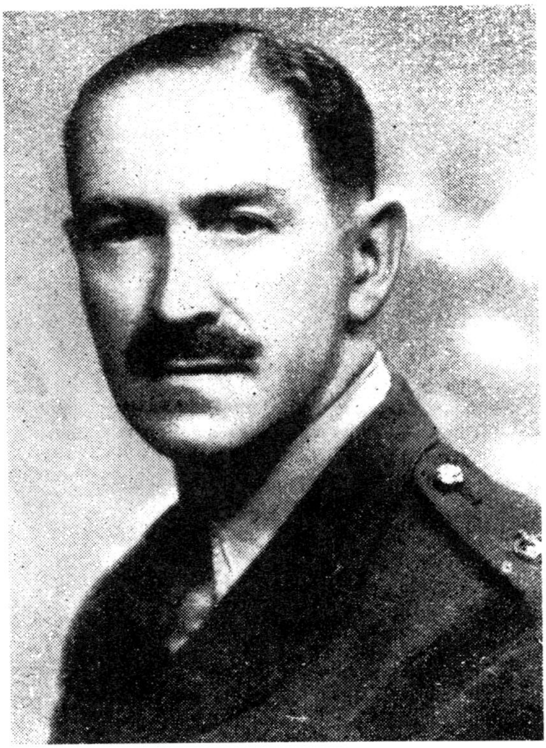

*Figure 20.7: Gilbert Phillips*

Wilkinson's travail with muscle was not limited to his scientific investigations. In 1936 his career took a change in direction with his move to Queensland. Not long after his arrival he found himself involved in another contentious matter, this time with many of his new medical colleagues for providing,as Dean of the Medical Faculty, the foreword to the controversial book written by Sister Elizabeth Kenny (*see Chapter 18*). This dealt with her methods used for the restoration of function in patients with infantile paralysis and cerebral diplegia. Wilkinson stated in his foreword:

> *... as Bacon says: 'Truth is the daughter of Time and not of authority' and we shall not know exactly whether Sister Kenny can obtain results when orthodox treatment fails until the two methods are tried out under similarly favourable conditions.*[21]

Before Professor Wilkinson's retirement in March 1959, it was generally recognized that Sister Kenny had on balance done good and her methods had gained much approval. He had at last the satisfaction of knowing his travail with muscle had not been in vain. Might we apply to his endeavours not the words of Bacon but of Galileo as expressed in Brecht's play:

*Truth is the child of Time, not of authority.*[22]

# *REFERENCES AND NOTES*


## CHAPTER 1

1. 1 **Gardner-Thorpe C.** *James Parkinson 1755–1824: with a Reprint of The Shaking Palsy.* Exeter (Printed by A. Wheaton and Co. Ltd), Dept of Neurology (Royal Devon and Exeter Hospital, Devon), 1987. An account of the life and contributions of "James Parkinson, Physician and Geologist"; his contributions to neurology, and to other branches of clinical medicine and to pharmacy, and to natural history.


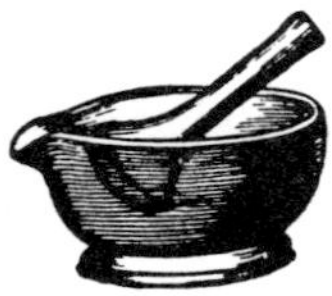


## CHAPTER 2

2. 1 **Public Records Office, London.** Colonial Office PRO CO 201/2

2. 2 **Collins D.** *An Account of the English Colony in New South Wales.* Sydney AH. & Reed AW. 1975:1

2. 3 **George MD.** *London Life in the Eighteenth Century.* London, Kegan Paul, Trench, Trubner & Co. Ltd., 1925

2. 4 **Ibid** p.21

2. 5 **Clark CMH.** *A History of Australia I.* Melbourne, Melbourne University Press, 1962:61

2. 6 **Ibid** p.61

2. 7 **Public Records Office, London.** Colonial Office PRO CO 201/2

2. 8 **Howe to Sydney**, 3rd September, 1786, HRNSW, I, ii, 22-23

2. 9 **Frost A.** *Arthur Phillip 1738-1814; His Voyaging.* Melbourne, Oxford University Press, 1987

2.10 **Public Records Office, London.** Colonial Office 201/1

2.11 **White J.** *Journal of a Voyage to New South Wales.* Sydney, Angus & Robertson, 1962

2.12 **Lloyd C. and Coulter JLS.** *Medicine and the Navy 1200-1900.* Vol III. London, E. & S. Livingston, 1961

2.13 **Ibid** p.10

2.14 **Cobley J.** Thomas Arndell Surgeon, Magistrate and Farmer. *Med J. Aust* 1969; 2:1125-1131

2.15 **Davidson GR.** *Medicine Through the Ages.* London, Methuen & Co. Ltd. 1968:46

**CHAPTER 2 (contd)**


2.16 **Power, Sir DA.** Some Bygone Operations in Surgery. *Brit J. Surg* 1931, 19:171-175

2.17 **Cobley J.** Lesser Known Surgeons of the First Fleet. *Bull Post-Grad* Comm Uni. Syd. 1967 23:291-305

2.18 **White J.** *Op. cit.* p.167

2.19 **Ibid** p.49

2.20 **Ibid** p.50

2.21 **Lloyd C and Coulter JLS.** *Op. cit.* p.41-42

2.22 **Ibid** p.302

2.23 **White J.** *Op. cit.* p.52

2.24 **Ibid** p.56

2.25 **Ibid** p.58

2.26 **Ibid** p.85

2.27 **Ibid** p.89

2.28 **Ibid** p.98

2.29 **Ibid** p.99

2.30 **Ibid** p.102


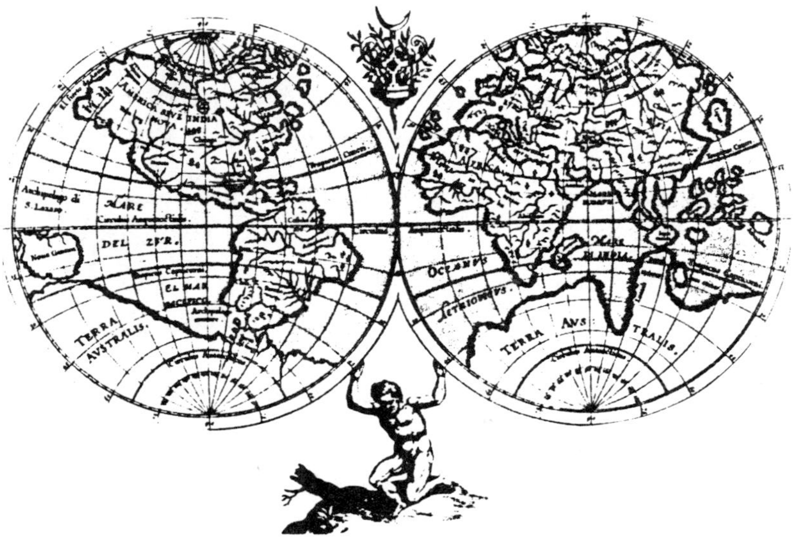

## CHAPTER 3

3. 1 **Raven M.** *Assistant Surgeon Thomas Arndell. The Man he was not.* Sydney, privately published by the author, 1986. (ISBN 0 7316 0464 4).

3. 2 **Raven M.** *Assistant Surgeon Thomas Arndell. The Man he was.* Sydney, privately published by the author, 1988. (ISBN 0 7316 2277 4).

3. 3 **Richards D.** Transported to New South Wales: medical convicts 1788–1850. *Brit Med J* 1987;295:1609-1612

3. 4 **Dan N.** The medical men of the First Fleet. **In** *Australia's Quest for Colonial Health.* Ed. JH Pearn and C O'Carrigan. Brisbane, Department of Child Health, 1983. Chapter 1:3

3. 5 **White J.** *Journal of a Voyage to New South Wales; with sixty-five plates of Non-descript Animals, Birds, Lizards, Serpents, curious cones of trees and other natural Productions.* London, printed for J. Debrett, 1790. Reprint Ed. 1962. Ed AH Chisholm, Sydney, Angus and Robertson.

3. 6 **Anderson D.** John White, Surgeon-General to the First Fleet. *Med J Aust* 1933;1:183

3. 7 **Ford E.** Medical Practice in early Sydney: with special reference to the work and influence of John White, William Redfern and William Bland. *Med J Aust* 1955;2:41-54

3. 8 **Rienits R. White, John (*c.* 1756-1832).** *Aust Dict Biograph.* Melbourne, Melbourne University Press, 1983 (Reprint). Ed AGC Shaw, CMH Clark. Vol 2 1788-1850:594-595

3. 9 **Parsons V. Jamison, Thomas (1745-1811).** *Aust Dict Biograph.* Melbourne University Press, 1983 (Reprint). Ed AGC Shaw, CMH Clark. Vol 1 1788-1850:12-13

3.10 **MacPherson J.** Thomas Jamison. *Univ Syd Med J* 1933:27

3.11 **Ford E.** Thomas Jamison and the beginning of medical journalism in Australia. *Med J Aust* 1954;2:264-266

3.12 **Cobley J.** Worgan, George Bouchier (1757-1838). *Aust Dict Biograph.* Melbourne, Melbourne University Press, 1983 (Reprint). Ed AGL Shaw, CMH Clark. Vol 1. 1788-1850:623

3.13 **Raven M.** *Op. cit.* See Ref 2:15

3.14 **Gray AJ.** John Irving: the first Australian emancipist. *J Roy Aust Hist Soc* 1954;40:316-331

3.15 **Cohen BC.** *A History of Medicine in Western Australia.* Perth, Paterson Brokensha Pty Ltd, 1965:87

3.16 **Smyth AB.** Journal 1787-1789. Reprinted as "The Journal of Arthur Bowes Smyth: Surgeon, *Lady Penrhyn* 1787-1789." Ed PG Fidlow and RJ Ryan. Sydney, Australian Documents Library, 1979:11

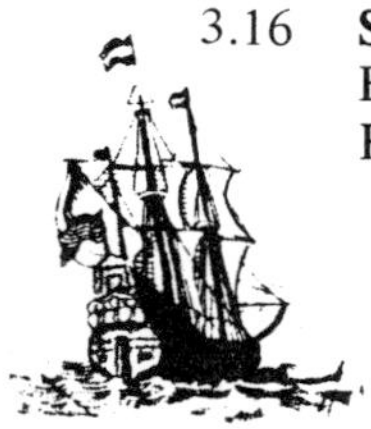

## CHAPTER 3 (contd)

3.17 **Ibid**:18

3.18 **Pearn J.** Ring the bell and win a cigar. Some early experiments on the measurement of human strength in Port Jackson and Van Diemen's Land. *Med J Aust* 1978;2:167-169

3.19 **Pearn J.** French doctors at Sydney Cove. Gallic contact in the second decade after Phillip. **In**: *Australia's Quest for Colonial Health.* Brisbane, Dept of Child Health (U of Q), 1983. Chapter 5:45-61

3.20 **Fletcher BH.** Arndell, Thomas (1753-1821). **In**: *Australian Dictionary of Biography.* Vol 1:1788-1850: A-H. Ed AG Shaw and CM Clark. Melbourne, Melbourne University Press, 1983 (corrigenda):27,28

3.21 **Raven, Marjorie (Mrs).** Great-great-great-grand-daughter of Surgeon Thomas Arndell, formerly Arundell (of 7 Griffin Avenue, Bexley, Sydney, 2207). Personal communication. Mrs Raven notes that Thomas Arndell left his first wife (Esther, née Foscari, of the Jewish faith) following a family difficulty and spent a year with the East India Company. When he left for Australia in the *Friendship*, he had already fathered eight children. In Sydney, he had a further seven children by his convict consort (Elizabeth Burley, alias Dalton) and (after 1807) his wife. Of his fifteen children, eight survived to adult life.

3.22 **Pearn JH.** The enchanted herb. The work of early medical botanists in Australia. *Med J Aust* 1987;147:568-572

3.23 **Whitley GP.** Naturalists of the First Fleet. *Aust Mus Mag* 1938;6:291-304

3.24 **Smyth AB.** See Ref 16:61

3.25 **Ibid**:58

3.26 **Ibid**:80

3.27 **Arndell RM.** *Pioneers of Portland Head.* Brisbane, WR Smith and Paterson, 1976. (1st Printing) (ISBN 0 85881 019 0):32-70.

3.28 **Tench, Captain W.** A complete account of the Settlement at Port Jackson, in New South Wales. Taken on the spot, by Captain Watkin Tench, of the Marines. London, sold by G Nicol, Pall Mall, 1793. Reprinted, with introduction by Lt Fitzhardinge, as part of *Sydney's First Four Years.* Sydney, Library of Australian History (Assoc Roy Aust Hist Soc), 1979:153. (See also pages 37, 97, 146, 148, 176, 211, 215.)

This note of Lowes, in Tench's account, is the first evidence that legitimized Lowes inclusion in the medical history of Australia. His first name is not recorded, and his does not appear on the *Sirius* manifest of 1787. Whether he was a surgeon, or a first aid or sick-berth attendant is unknown; it is possible he joined the *Sirius* crew sometime after Jan 1788, possibly at Cape Town on the resupply voyage.

**CHAPTER 3 (contd)**

3.28 (contd)

This resupply run is described by John Hunter, the Captain of the *Sirius* in his "An Historical Journal of the Transactions at Port Jackson and Norfolk Island" (Aust Facsim Ed 1968; Adelaide, Libraries Board of South Australia:89,116,125). *Sirius* arrived back to the starving colony on 9 May 1789, and it was in June 1789 that the first record of Lowes (in Tench's *Account*) is noted.

Lowes is not listed in Chapman's *1788. The People of the First Fleet* (Sydney, Doubleday Australia Pty Ltd, 1986); but is listed in Fidlow *The First Fleeters* (Sydney, Australian Documents Library, 1981:47). This latter entry however, appears to requote Tench, the latter entry not being 1788 but 26 June 1789.

3.29 **Lowes.** Letter published in the *Dublin Chronicle*; secondarily reported in Historical Records of New South Wales Vol II, Grose and Paterson 1793-1795. Ed FM Bladen (Barrister-at-law). Sydney, Charles Potter, Government Printer 1893:770-771. Letter "State of the Colony 1790" in issue of 13 January 1791 of the *Dublin Chronicle.*

Lowes, probably John Lowes, is known to have been Surgeon's Mate of the *Sirius*. His authorship of the *Dublin Chronicle* letter of 1791 is known from indirect but compelling evidence in Tench's *Narrative.* The only expedition answering to this description in the Letter was that undertaken by Captain Tench, Assistant-Surgeon Arndell, and Mr Lowes, Surgeon's Mate of the *Sirius*, on 26 June 1789. (See Tench's *Complete Account*, p.27). It is evident from this that the above letter was written by Mr Lowes. It is doubtful whether, in the absence of the imprimatur given by Tench's *Narrative*, and *Account,*[28] Lowes would have been known to medical historians.

3.30 **Tench, Capt W.** *Op. cit.* See Ref 28):154:308

3.31 **Ibid**:158

3.32 **King, Jon, King, John.** *Philip Gidley King.* A Biography of the Third Governor of New South Wales. Sydney, Methuen, 1981:54

3.33 **Note:** Bowes Smyth's father was an Overseer of the Poor at the Village of Tolleshurst D'Arcy in Suffolk. For an account of the English Poor Law and its administration by such Overseers, see Cummins CJ. The Development of the Benevolent (Sydney) Asylum 1788-1855. Sydney, Department of Health Internal Publication, 1971:3

3.34 **Fidlow PG, Ryan RJ.** Editor's Preface to "The Journal of Arthur Bowes Smyth: Surgeon, *Lady Penrhyn* 1787-1789". *Op. cit.* (See Ref 16):v

3.35 **Smyth AB.** See Ref 16:51

3.36 **Ibid**:66

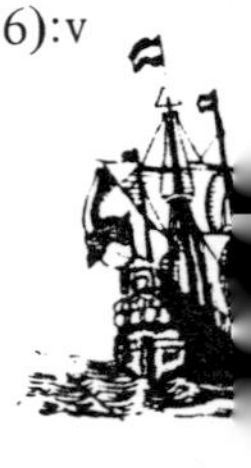

**CHAPTER 3 (contd)**

3.37 **Fletcher BH.** Balmain, William (1762-1803). *Aust Dict Biograph.* Melbourne, Melbourne Univ Press, 1983 (Reprint). Ed AGL Shaw, CMH Clark. Vol I. 1788-1850:51-52

3.38 **Napier SE.** Balmain: the man and the suburb. *J Roy Aust Hist Soc* 1928; 14(5):245-281

3.39 **Gilbert LA.** Considen, Dennis (d. 1815). *Aust Dict Biograph.* Melbourne, Melbourne Univ Press, 1983 (Reprint). Ed AGC Shaw, CMH Clark. Vol I. 1788-1850:242-243

3.40 **MacPherson J.** Dennis Considen, Assistant Surgeon of the first fleet. *Med J Aust* 1927;2:770-773

3.41 **Worgan GB.** Journal of a First Fleet Surgeon. Original held in the Mitchell Library, Sydney (C830). Reprinted: Sydney, Library of Australian History (for the William Dixson Foundation), 1978.

3.42 **An Officer (Anon).** An authentic and interesting narrative of the late expedition to Botany Bay. Aberdeen, Printed for Alexander Keith, 1789. Reprinted by the Library of Australian History (Facsimile Series Number 12), Sydney, 1978:17

3.43 **Smyth AB.** *Op. cit.* (See Ref 26):53

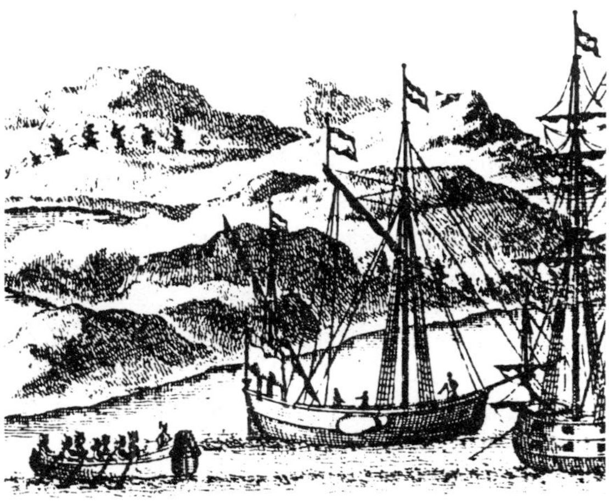

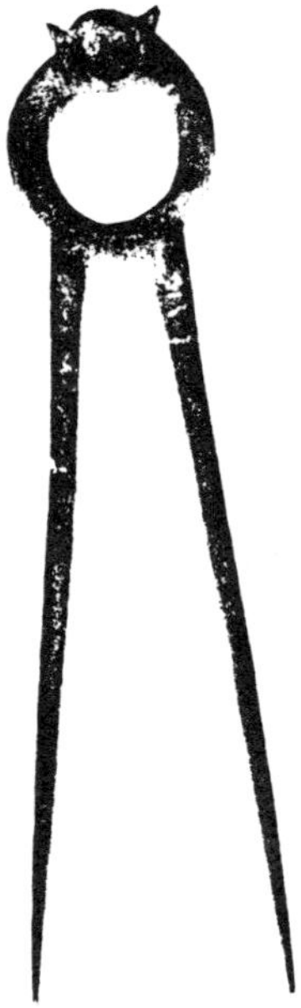

## CHAPTER 4

4. 1 Examination Book of the Company of Surgeons. Archives of the Royal College of Surgeons of England.

4. 2 **Hamilton G.** *A Voyage Round the World.* Berwick, 1793.

4. 3 **Barrow, Sir John.** The Eventful History of the Mutiny and Piratical Seizure of HMS *Bounty*, its causes and consequences. London 1831.

4. 4 **Carpenter J, Pigott L, Whitwell H.** A watch from HMS *Pandora. Antiquarian Horology* 1985;15:560-601.

## CHAPTER 5

5. 1 **Harry Hayter Ramsdale**, 'Diary', MS 5324, Wellcome Institute for the History of Medicine, London. Ramsdale, a former militiaman, had served with an English Brigade supporting Garibaldi in 1860. He returned to England hoping to become a professional soldier, but when rejected, decided to emigrate to Queensland. I am grateful to Dr Richard Palmer of the Wellcome Institute for drawing my attention to this diary.

5. 2 **COL/A6**: 60-1472, Queensland State Archives, Brisbane.

5. 3 *Votes and Proceedings of the Legislative Assembly of Queensland*, 1860: 635-38

5. 4 **O. MacDonagh's**, *A Pattern of Government Growth. The Passenger Acts and their Enforcement* (London: MacGibbon & Kee, 1961) details of the British legislation.

5. 5 **H.R. Woolcock**, *Rights of Passage. Emigration to Australia in the Nineteenth Century* (London: Tavistock, 1986), pp.115-17.

5. 6 *Queensland Government Gazette*, 1861 (2):15-17.

5. 7 Sections 59 to 61 of the 1855 Act.

5. 8 Fares quoted for the *Saldanha* which sailed in October 1861 were £45 for first cabin, £25 for second, £20 for intermediate and £18 for stterage, with children half price.

5. 9 'Jordan's Lambs', By One of Them, Immigration File, Royal Queensland Historical Society Records.

5.10 The passenger and crew lists include details relating to age, sex and occupation. See microfilm Z31, Q.S.A., Brisbane.

5.11 The ration scale varied according to the class, but was sufficient in quantity, being enough for 140 days, and nutritional value, although this would have suffered in the cooking. See Woolcock, *op. cit.*, pp.95-97.

**CHAPTER 5 (contd)**

5.12 Full details of George Young's training, qualifications and experience are listed in the *British Medical Directory* (1861).

5.13 **Ramsdale**, *op. cit*., pp.14 and 41. He was possibly an assistant surgeon during his military service in Italy.

5.14 **Ibid**., pp.13-14.

5.15 *British Medical Directory* (1846 and 1861).

5.16 Voyage time was computed from the *last* port of embarkation to the day a vessel dropped anchor in Queensland waters.

5.17 **COL/A29**: 62-1365, Q.S.A., Brisbane.

5.18 Every ship in pre-refrigeration days carried a farmyard to provide fresh meat, eggs and milk for the saloon table.

5.19 **Ramsdale**, *op. cit.*, p.36.

5.20 The daily quota for each adult was three quarts. The *Clifton* did not carry apparatus for distilling fresh from salt water.

5.21 Teething was classified as a cause of death until 1920.

5.22 **Ramsdale**, *op. cit.*, p.39.

5.23 **Ibid.**, p.35.

5.24 **COL/A28**: 62-1243, Q.S.A., Brisbane.

5.25 **COL/A29**: 62-1365, Q.S.A., Brisbane.

5.26 **COL/A28**: 62-1243, Q.S.A., Brisbane.

5.27 Select Committee Evidence, *Votes and Proceedings*, 1863, 2:440.

5.28 **Ibid.**, 436.

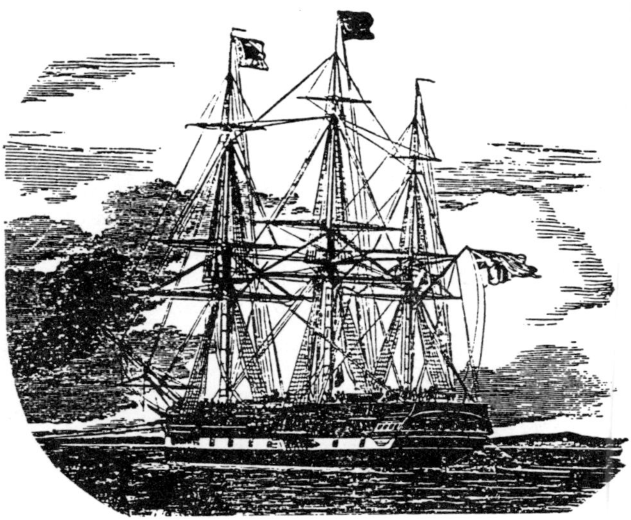

## CHAPTER 6


6. 1 **Turner AJ**. The prevention of parasitic anaemia. *Aust Med Gaz* 1909;**28**: 350.

6. 2 **Editorial.** Ankylostomiasis in Puerto Rico. *Brit Med J* 1906;**2**:386.

6. 3 **Scott HH.** *A History of Tropical Medicine*, based on the Fitzpatrick Lectures delivered before the Royal College of Physicians of London, 1937-1938, Vol. I. London: Arnold, 1938:840.

6. 4 **Schenk ET, McMasters JH.** *Procedure in Taxonomy.* Third Edition enlarged by Keen AM, Muller SW. Stanford, California: Stanford University Press, 1956:54.

6. 5 For an account of the history of hookworm see Kean BH, Mott KE, Russell AJ. *Tropical Medicine and Parasitology.* Classic Investigations Vol. II. New York: Cornell University Press, 1978:287-324.

6. 6 **Hogg JB**. A case of death from anaemia due to Ancylostoma duodenale. *Aust Med Gaz* 1889;**8**:133. This paper was summarised in *Lancet* 1889; **1**:750-751 and *Brit Med J* 1889;**1**:792.

6. 7 Minutes of General Meeting of Medical Society of Queensland (MSQ), 12 April 1892, Archives of the Australian Medical Association, Queensland Branch (ArchAMAQldBr).

6. 8 **Gibson JL, Turner AJ**. Notes on the occurrence of *Ancylostomum duodenale* in Queensland. *Trans Intercol Med Cong Aust* 3rd Sess. September 1892. 1893; 134-137.

6. 9 Exhibit of case of anaemia due to Ancylostoma duodenale by J L Gibson. Report of General Meeting of MSQ, 8 November 1892. *Aust Med Gaz* 1892;**11**:440-441;
**Bacot W**. Cases of earth-eating in north Queensland. *Aust Med Gaz* 1892; **11**:430;
**Bancroft TL**. Entozoal parasites. *Aust Med Gaz* 1893;**12**:258-260;
**Lawes CHE**. Anaemia due to Anchylostomum duodenale – notes of two cases. *Aust Med Gaz* 1895;**14**:445-447;
Exhibition of Ancylostoma duodenale worms by A J Turner. Report of General Meeting of MSQ 8 October 1895. *Aust Med Gaz* 1895;**15**:456.

6.10 **Turner AJ**. A parasitic scourge of warm climates. *Proc R Soc Qld* 1896; **11**:99-102.

6.11 **Ashworth LN**. A case of Anchylostomiasis complicated by the presence of another small worm. *Aust Med Gaz* 1896;**15**:482-484.


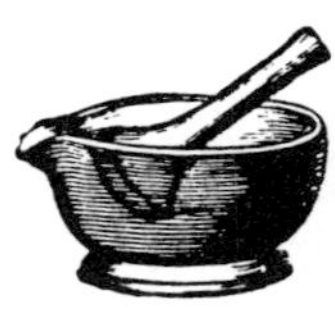

**CHAPTER 6 (contd)**

6.12 **O'Doherty EH.** Presidential Address, Annual General Meeting of Queensland Branch of the British Medical Association (BMA) *Aust Med Gaz* 1898;**18**:47.

6.13 **Bancroft TL.** On a probable way by which the young Ankylostomum duodenale enters the human subject. *Aust Med Gaz* 1902;**21**:66.

6.14 **Scott HH.** *op. cit.*, 508.

6.15 **Kean BH, Mott KE, Russell AJ.** *op. cit.*, 312.

6.16 **McDonald TF.** The earth-eating disease. Letter to Editor *Brisbane Courier,* 23 May 1903.

6.17 Queensland Parliament, Debates (QPD) LXXXIV, 1900, 140.

6.18 **Editorial.** The earth-eating disease. *Brisbane Courier*, 26 May 1903.

6.19 **Turner AJ.** "Earth-eating" disease. The Ankylostoma or "Leech-worm". Letter to Editor *Brisbane Courier*, 30 May 1903.

6.20 Report of the Commissioner of Public Health. Brisbane: Queensland Government Printer, 1904, 5.

6.21 **Hamilton-Kenny F.** Five cases of Ankylostomiasis *Aust Med Gaz* 1906; **25**:399-400.

6.22 Report of the Commissioner of Public Health. Brisbane: Queensland Government Printer, 1909, 3.

6.23 **McDonald TF.** Experiences of Ankylostomiasis in Australia. *J Trop Med* 1908;**11**:25-29.

6.24 **Ibid.**:26

6.25 **Turner AJ.** 1909. *op. cit.*, 350-352.

6.26 **Salter AG.** Ankylostomiasis amongst Queensland children. *Aust Med Gaz* 1909;**28**:352-356.

6.27 Minutes of General Meeting of Queensland Branch of BMA, 2 July 1909, ArchAMAQldBr.

6.28 Report of the Commissioner of Public Health. Queensland Parliament, Papers (QPP) **2**, 1910, 856.

6.29 **Ibid.**:857.

6.30 **Douglas RA.** A Breinl and. the Australian Institute of Tropical Medicine. *Med J Aust* 1977;**1**:713, 748, 784.

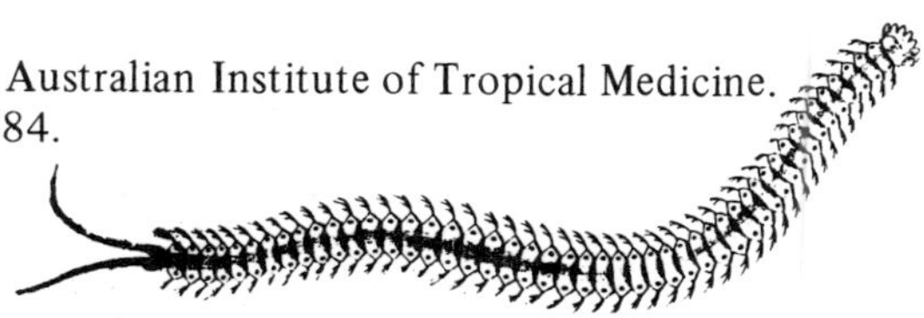

**CHAPTER 6 (contd)**


6.31 **Breinl A.** On the results of journey to northern ports of Queensland, July 1910. Tropical Diseases Research Fund. Report of the Advisory Committee, 1910. London: n.p., 1911, 126-128.

6.32 **Scott HH.** *op. cit*., 844-847.

6.33 **Cilento R.** *Tropical diseases in Australia.* Brisbane. Smith and Paterson, 1940, 223.

6.34 **Breinl A.** Ankylostomiasis. *Trans Aust Med Cong,* 9th Sess. Sydney 1911;**1**:536-542.

6.35 BMA News, Queensland Branch. *Aust Med Gaz* 1911;**36**:87-89.

6.36 **Bocaccio M.** Ground itch and dew poison. The Rockefeller Sanitary Commission, 1909-1914. *J Hist Med & Allied Sciences* 1972;**27**:30-53.

6.37 Final Report of the Australian Hookworm Campaign, Part I 1 October 1919 to 30 September 1924, 5-7.

6.38 **Ibid**.:17-25.

6.39 **Ibid**.:36-38.

6.40 **Ibid.**:94-100.

6.41 Final Report of the Australian Hookworm Campaign, Part II. 1 October 1919 to 30 September 1924, 1.

6.42 **Patrick R.** *A History of Health and Medicine in Queensland, 1824-1960.* St Lucia: University of Queensland Press, 1987, 251.

6.43 **Watson DS, Tozer RA.** Anaemia in Yirrkala. In special supplement on Aboriginal health. *Med J Aust* 1986;**144**:S15;
and interview, 1 October 1986, with Dr D S Watson, Regional Medical Officer (Central), Aboriginal Health, Queensland State Health Department;

6.44 **Turner AJ.** The Jackson Lecture. Preventive medicine. *Med J Aust* 1938; **2**:807.


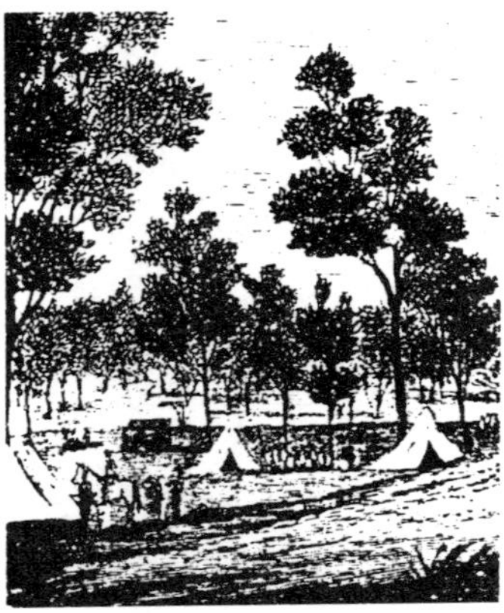

## CHAPTER 7

7. 1 **Thompson G.** Surgeon's Journal "England" 1826. Mitchell Library Sydney PRO 3195.

7. 2 **Thompson G.** Letter to James Wardrop Esq. Sydney 9th October, 1826.

7. 3 **Paissinen TM.** George Combe and Samuel George Morton. *Trans Stud Coll Physns* Philadelphia 1976;**43**:413-5.

7. 4 **Morton SG.** *Crania Americana,* Philadelphia John Pennington 1839.

7. 5 **Sprod D.** *Alexander Pearce of Macquarie Harbour.* Hobart, Cat and Fiddle Press 1977,128.

7. 6 **Parker N.** *Griffin's skull* (awaiting publication).

7. 7 **Morton SG.** Observations on the size of the brain in various races and families of man. *Proc Acad Natural Sciences* Philadelphia 1849;**4**:221-224.

7. 8 **Gould SJ.** *The Mismeasure of man.* Middlesex Penguin Books 1981:54.

7. 9 **Morton SG.** *Catalogue of the skulls of man and the inferior animals.* University of Pennsylvania 1840.

7.10 **Gall FJ.** *Les Fonctions du Cerveau.* 1823 Vol 5 as translated and quoted by Williams WM. *A Vindication of Phrenology.* London Chetto and Windus 1894:26.

7.11 **Gall FJ.** quoted by Williams WM (*ibid*).46

7.12 **Mackenzie C.** Frederick Bailey Deeming. *Mankind* 1934:221-223

7.13 **Mackenzie C.** Explanatory note beside Deeming's skull when displayed in the Museum of the Institute of Anatomy, Canberra.

7.14 **Lombroso C. In** Ferrero GL. *Criminal Man According to the Classification of Cesare Lombroso,* 1911. New York, Putnam IV

7.15 **Goring C.** *The English Convict: A statistical study,* His Majesty's Stationery Office, London 1913.

7.16 **Hooton EA.** *The American Criminal: An Anthropological Study,* Harvard University Press 1939 Vol. 1 309.

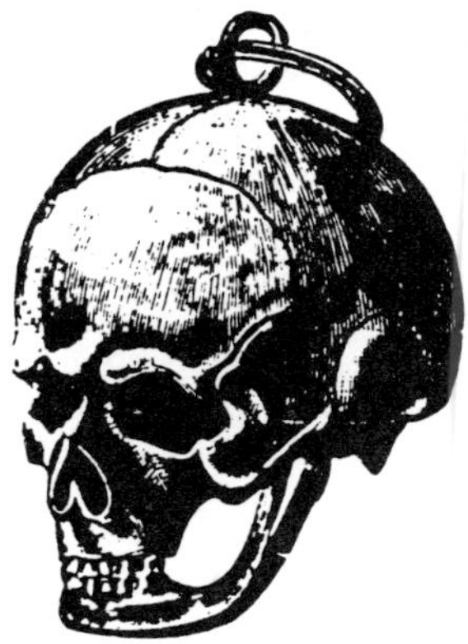

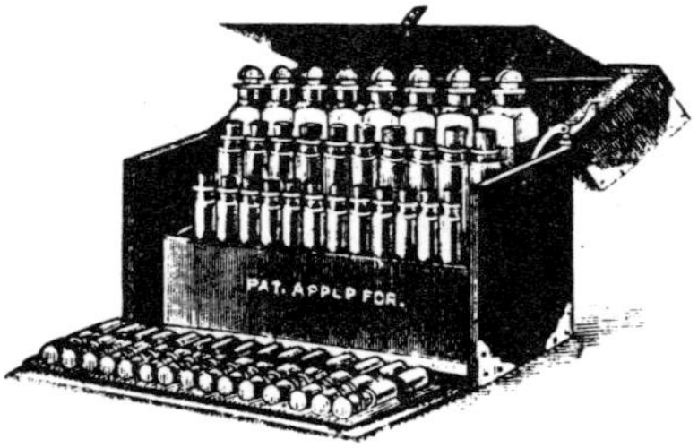


## CHAPTER 8


8. 1 **Wood, Ronald.** Ophthalmia in nineteenth century Australia **in** *Australia's Quest for Colonial Health.* Dept of Child Health, Brisbane 1983, p245.

8. 2 **Duke Elder S.** *System of Ophthalmology* Vol VIII Part I p260. Henry Kumpton London 1965.

8. 3 **Mann, Ida.** Probable origins of trachoma in Australasia. *Bull Org. Mond. Santé* 1957,16,1165-1187.

8. 4 **Bowen, Aubrey.** On ophthalmia of the industrial schools. Prince's Bridge *Aust Med J* Vol 12 1869 pp258-267.

8. 5 **Barrett, Sir James.** *Trans Ophthal Soc Aust* 1941 p9

8. 6 **Corfield WH.** *Reminiscences of Queensland 1862-1899.* AH Frater Brisbane 1921 p20.

8. 7 **QSA** A16025 Letter to Under Secretary Home Secretary's Department from Commissioner of Public Health 12/5/1908.

8. 8 **QSA** A16025 Report to Home Secretary from Dr WF Taylor 16/12/1907

8. 9 **QSA** A16025 Report to Home Secretary from Dr WF Taylor 26/2/1908

8.10 **Bourne, Eleanor E.** Medical inspection of schools. British Medical Officer 23/9/1922.

8.11 **Rodger, Douglas and Priestly H.** Trachoma and allied eye infections in Western Queensland. *Med J Aust* 1915 Vol 2 pp25-29.

8.12 **QSA** A16029 Various reports to the Department dated 18/3/1929 to September 1930.

8.13 **QSA** A16029 Reports to Director of School Medical Services from EO Marks.

8.14 Report to Chief Medical Officer, School Health Services from EO Marks dated 26/1/1954 (in possession of Dr Elizabeth Marks).

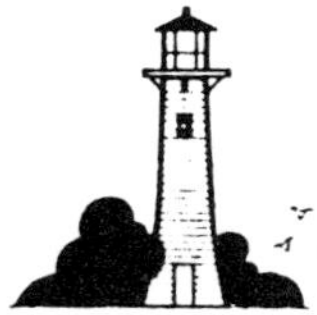

## CHAPTER 9


9. 1 **Pliny, the Elder.** *Historia Naturalis,* Book 9, Chapter 35.

9. 2 **The Bible.** *Matthew* 7:6.

9. 3 **Smith G.** *Gemstones.* London: Chapman and Halley, 1971;473.

9. 4 **Kornitzer** *L. The Pearl Trader.* New York: Sheridan House. 1937;16,45.

9. 5 **Wilson H.** *Cyclone Coasts.* Melbourne: Rigby, 1980; 17.

9. 6 **Mulvaney D. and White J.**, eds. *Australians to 1788.* Sydney: Fairfax. 1987; 94, 263.

9. 7 **Hainsworth D.** *Builders and Adventurers.* Melbourne: Cassell. 1968; 73.

9. 8 **Cobcroft M.** *Brought to this Distress.* Ipswich: Narkos. 1987; 69, 102.

9. 9 **Fanning E.** *Voyages and Discoveries in the South Seas, 1792-1832.* Salem: Marine Research Society. 1924; 329.

9.10 **Coombs H.** Proposals for Re-establishment of the Pearling Industry. *Nth Aust Development Committee.* 1946; 6-8.

9.11 **MacDonald A.** *In The Land of Pearl and Gold.* London: Blackie and Son. 1907, 268, 289.

9.12 **Lack C.** The Taming of the Great Barrier Reef. *J Roy Hist Soc Qld* 1959; 6: 130.

9.13 **Singe J.** *The Torres Strait.* Brisbane: Univ of Qld. 1950; 167-171.

9.14 **Benham C.** *Pearl Diver's Luck.* New York: Norton. 1950; 25, 137.

9.15 **Cobcroft M.** A Dead Whale or a Stove Boat. *Occ Papers Med Hist Aust;* Melbourne: University Press. 1984; 2:65.

9.16 **Bligh A.** *The Golden Quest.* Carlisle (WA): Herperian. 1984.

9.17 **Idriess I.** *Forty Fathoms Deep.* Sydney: Angus and Robertson. 1937; 45, 81, 147, 184, 203, 236, 245, 274.

9.18 **Bartlett N.** *The Pearl Seekers.* London: Melrose. 1954; 62, 82, 138, 170, 208, 223.

9.19 **Jackson P.** Medical Aspects of Diving. *J Postgrad Gen Pract* Oct 1985; 43-53.

9.20 **Clark A.** *The Coast of Coral.* London: Shakespeare Head. 1956, 119-131.

9.21 **Banfield E.** *Tropic Days.* London: Fisher Unwin. 1918; 219.

9.22 **Coppleson V.** *Shark Attack.* Sydney: Angus and Robertson. 1962: 102.

9.23 (Author not given). Sharks. Sydney: *Readers' Digest. 1986; 87.*

9.24 **Berge V. and Lanier H.** *Pearl Diver.* London: Heinemann. 1930; 158.

9.25 **Covacevich J, Davie P, and Pearn J.** Eds *Toxic Plants and Animals.* Brisbane: Qld Museum. 1987; 73-214.

## CHAPTER 10

10. 1 **Douglas RA.** Dr Anton Breinl and the Australian Institute of Tropical Medicine. Part 2. *Med J Aust* 1977;1:748-751.

10. 2 **Harloe LJ.** White Man in Tropical Australia: Anton Breinl and the Australian Institute of Tropical Medicine [B.A. (Hon) Thesis] James Cook University of North Queensland, 1987;42-45.

10. 3 **Breinl, Anton.** *Australian Diction of Biography* Vol 7; 1891-1939.

10. 4 **Dale HH.** Advances in Medical Therapeutics. *Br Med J* 1950; Special Issue 1:4.

10. 5 **Jaumees K.** A Century of Service 1881-1981. Townsville 1981.

10. 6 **Fielding JW.** The Australian Institute of Tropical Medicine. Townsville North Queensland. Reminiscences Staff and Work 1910-1930. Hand written manuscript of 126 pages. Undated, probably 1953.

10. 7 **Gibney HJ, Smith AG.** Eds. *A Biographical Register 1788-1939.*

10. 8 **Crowther, Sir William.** Personal communication. June 1977.

10. 9 **Nicoll W.** Conditions of Life in Tropical Australia. *J Hyg* (Lond.) 1918. 16:69.

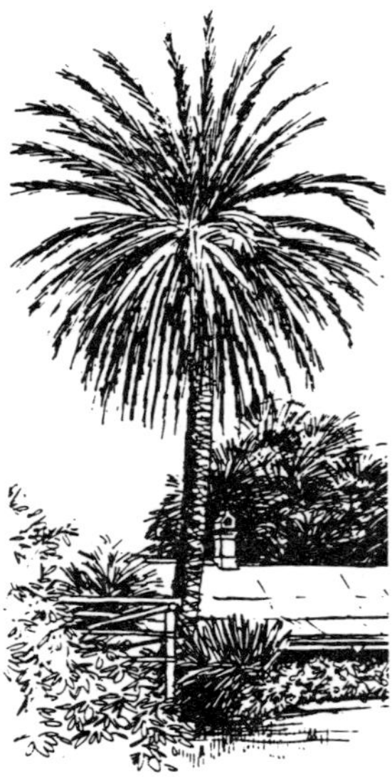

10.10 **Obituary.** Professor W.J. Young, *Aust Jour Sc* 1942;4:191.

10.11 **Obituary.** Henry Priestley, *Med J Aust.* 1961;1:876.

10.12 **Slater EC.** Townsville-Home of Australian Biochemistry. Trends in Biochemical Sciences. February 1979. N30.

10.13 **Obituary.** Thomas Peter Anderson Stuart. *Med J Aust* 1920;1:244.

10.14 **Love WWR.** *Australian Dictionary of Biography* Vol 10; 1891-1939.

## CHAPTER 11

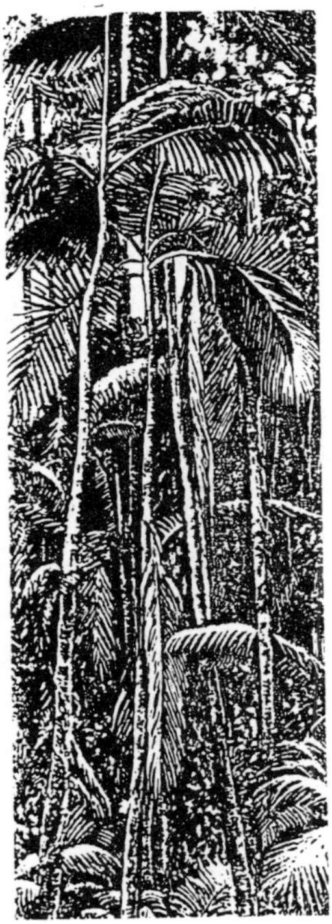

11. 1 **Butcher BW.** Science and the Imperial Vision: The Imperial Geophysical Experimental Survey 1928-1930. *Historical Records of Australian Science* 1984: Vol. 6, No. 1: 31.

11. 2 **MacLeod R.** On Visiting the 'Moving Metropolis': Reflections on the Architecture of Imperial Science. *Historical Records of Australian Science* 1981: Vol. 5, No. 3: 1-16.
See **Ileto RC.** Outlines of a Non-linear Employment of Philippine History in *Reflections on Development in Southeast Asia.* Singapore: Institute of Southeast Asian Studies, 1988 (forthcoming) for a discussion of "the nineteenth-century rise of the medical profession – a sign of progress – based on the actual intersection of medicine, politics, and society during the cholera epidemics that swept the colony from 1820 to 1902."

11. 3 Since the late 1960s some notable works on Australian women (understandably by women) in history have appeared. See **Dixon M.** *The Real Matilda: Woman and Identity in Australia 1799 to the Present.* Ringwood: Penguin, 1984; **Kingston B.** *My Wife, My Daughter, and Poor Mary Ann.* Melbourne: Nelson, 1980; Windschuttle E. ed. *Women, Class and History: Feminist Perspectives on Australia 1788-1978.* Melbourne: Fontana Collins, 1980.

11. 4 Henry Reynolds has been inordinately successful in changing attitudes towards the Australian Aboriginals. See **Reynolds H.** *Race Relations in Queensland.* Townsville: James Cook University, 1978; Reynolds H. *The Other Side of the Frontier: Aboriginal Resistance to the European Invasion of Australia.* Ringwood: Penguin, 1984.

11. 5 An early exception is **Bolton GC.** *A Thousand Miles Away: A History of North Queensland to 1920.* Canberra: Australian National University Press, 1970.

11. 6 **Breinl A, Young WJ.** Tropical Australia and Its Settlement. *Med J Aust,* Vol. I, 2, 10 and 17 May 1919: 253-259, 375-382, 395-404.

11. 7 **Douglas RA.** Dr Anton Breinl and The Australian Institute of Tropical Medicine. *Med J Aust* 1977; 64, 19: 715.

**CHAPTER 11 (contd)**

11. 8 *Townsville Bulletin* April 18 1907. **Frodsham G.** Speech to the Townsville Chamber of Commerce.

11. 9 **Australian Archives CP78/5 item 2.** Governor-General's Office: 'Correspondence relating mainly to the Tropical Diseases Research Fund and a proposal for an Australian Institute of Tropical Medicine, 1901-1911: Tropical Diseases Institute Townsville', 1909-1911.
"Memorandum from the Bishop of North Queensland containing a scheme for the furthering of the scientific study of the diseases of Tropical Australia".
*The Queenslander*, June 11 1910: 23 & 29. There is no dispute that Frodsham displayed, in his ecclesiastical sphere, concern for all in Northern Australia who were subjected to the tyranny of tropical diseases. Travels on horseback through his extensive diocese acquainted him with the situation of both European and indigenous people. The fate of half-castes in particular worried the Bishop, who was reported in *The Queenslander* as having observed that they were living "no better than dogs".

11.10 **Ramsay Smith,** *Townsville Bulletin* 6 March 1907.

11.11 **Atherton Young J, Jervie Sefton A, Webb N.** *Centenary Book of the University of Sydney Faculty of Medicine.* Sydney: University Press, 1984: 238-243.

11.12 **Australian Archives CP78/5 item 2.** Anderson Stuart to Frodsham 11 May 1907 c/f the attitude of Henry Allen of the University of Melbourne who was Frodsham's "only hope" as so many Australian medical men were in constant opposition to Frodsham's plans for the Townsville centre.

11.13 **Barclay E.** Fevers and Stinks: Some Problems of Public Health in the 1870s and 1880s. *Queensland Heritage* 1971; Vol 2 No. 4: 3.

11.14 **Australian Archives CP78/5 item 2.** Frodsham to Anderson Stuart undated.

11.15 **Sax S.** *A Strife of Interests: Politics and policies in Australian health services.* Sydney: Allen & Unwin, 1984: 14-19.

11.16 *The Immigration Restriction Act* (No. 17 1901) was legislation under which the 'White Australia Policy' operated. Some legislation such as the *Aboriginals Protection and Restriction of the Sale of Opium Act* (No. 1 1901) did not so much attempt to protect the aborigines but discriminate against the Chinese.

11.17 **Evans R.** Charitable Institutions of the Queensland Government to 1919 [MA Thesis]. Brisbane: University of Queensland: December 1979.

**CHAPTER 11 (contd)**


11.18 **Cilento RW, Lack C.** *Triumph in the Tropics.* Brisbane: WR Smith & Paterson, 1959: 433.

11.19 **Australian Archives CP78/5 item 2. Dr** TG Ross to Governor-General "Consideration of an Institute for the study of tropical diseases from a medical standpoint", May 1907.

11.20 **Breinl papers,** Breinl to Hunt 6 October 1912.

11.21 **Elkington JSC.** *Tropical Australia: Is It Suitable for a Working White Race.* Melbourne: Government Printer, 1905.
**Goldsmith J.** The Necessity for the Study of Tropical Medicine in Australia. *Intercolonial Medical Congress of Australia Hobart 1902.* Melbourne: Government Printer, 1903: 178-179.
**Arthur R.** The Colonisation of Tropical Australia. *Medical Congress Transactions:* Vol 2. Melbourne, Government Printer, 1923: 93-97.

11.22 **Yarwood AT.** The White Australia Policy. A Re-interpretation of its Development in the Late Colonial Period. *Historical Studies* 1962; 10, 39: 257-269; see also **Markus A.** *Fear and Hatred: Purifying Australia and California 1850-1901.* Sydney: Hale & Iremonger, 1978; **McQueen H.** *A New Britannia: An argument concerning the social origins of Australian radicalism and nationalism* (Rev ed). Ringwood: Penguin, 1986: 29.

11.23 **Macfie M.** How Can Tropical and Sub-Tropical Australia Be Effectively Developed? (Read at the Australian Association of the advancement of Science, Adelaide, 1907). Adelaide: Government Printer, 1907.

11.24 **Australian Archives CRSA 1920 item 575/28.** Atlee Hunt story of establishment. Government funding started in 1911 and by the outbreak of the first world war amounted to over £4000 per annum.

11.25 **Colthart L.** "Australia Misère": The Northern Territory in the Nineteenth Century [PhD Thesis]. Brisbane: University of Queensland Press, 1984: viii.

11.26 **Roe M.** *Nine Australian Progressives: Vitalism in Bourgeois Social Thought.* Brisbane: University of Queensland Press, 1984.

11.27 **Ibid**: 12.

11.28 *Australian Medical Congress Transactions of the Eleventh Session held in Brisbane 21-28 August 1920.* Brisbane: WF Taylor (Gov. Printer), 1921: 39-69.

11.29 **Roe:** *Nine Australian Progressives...:* 130-131.

11.30 **Lowe DM.** *History of Bourgeois Perception.* Chicago: The University of Chicago, 1982: 17.

**CHAPTER 11 (contd)**


11.31 **Cumpston JHL.** *The Health of the People: A Study in Federalism.* Canberra: Roebuck Society, 1978: 44.

11.32 **Mozley, Moyal A.** Medical Research in Australia: A Historical Perspective. *Search:* Vol 12 No 9 September 1981: 303.

11.33 In North Queensland, separation has been a perennial problem since the 1880s, see **Doran C.** *Separatism in Townsville 1884 to 1894: "We should govern ourselves".* Townsville: James Cook University, 1981.

11.34 **McQueen H.** Queensland: A State of Mind. *Meanjin:* Vol 38 No 1, 1979: 41-51.

11.35 **Coltheart.** "Australian Misère ...": vii-viii.

11.36 **Ibid**: 38

11.37 **Australian Archives CP78/5 item 2** Samuel J. Way to G. Frodsham 10 May 1907.

11.38 **Fielding J.** A History of the Australian Institute of Tropical Medicine 1909-1930. Manuscript, *c.*1953: 24-34.

11.39 **Black RH.** Dr Bellamy of Papua. *Med J Aust* Vol II No 6, 10, 17 & 24 August 1957: 180-197, 232-233, 279-284.

11.40 *Report of the Royal Commission on Health.* Melbourne: MJ Green (Gov Printer) 1926: 452.

11.41 **Ibid**: 542.

11.42 **Ibid**: 455.

11.43 *Townsville Bulletin* 4 October 1927.

11.44 **Australian Archives SP1061** Hunt to Breinl 10 December 1919.

11.45 **Australian Archives SP1061** 'Hookworm Campaign'. Minutes of meeting of the Committee of Management of the A.I.T.M. 18 & 19 January 1921: 3.

11.46 **Australian Archives SP1061/1** Mapleston to Editor *Med J Aust* copy of letter February 1922: 2.
He recommended the Institute be upgraded: Townsville was not the ideal site for the study of obscure and perplexing conditions which could best be investigated in their own localities. A couple of movable laboratories were his answer to the question of location.

11.47 **Australian Archives SP1061/1**, 209 Cilento to Cumpston 11 February 1923.

11.48 **Fielding J**. A History of the Australian Institute ...: 47.

11.49 *Courier Mail* Research Work, Townsville Institute, 31 May 1928.

11.50 **Ibid.**

**CHAPTER 11 (contd)**

11.51 *The Courier* 5 June 1928. The Townsville Institute, Dr Cilento in Reply.

11.52 **Fisher FG.** Raphael West Cilento: Medical Administrator, Legislator, and Visionary 1893-1945. [MA Thesis] Brisbane: University of Queensland: 41-42.

11.53 *North Queensland Register* 12 January 1914.

11.54 **Bolton.** *A Thousand Miles...;* 177.

11.55 **May C.** *Topsawyers: The Chinese in Cairns 1870 to 1920.* Townsville: James Cook University, 1984.

11.56 *Queensland Parliamentary Papers* 1922 Vol 1: 1155.

11.57 **Australian Archives SP1061/1** Breinl to Hunt 27 September 1919: 8. Breinl's recommendations were enacted by Cilento.

**CHAPTER 12**

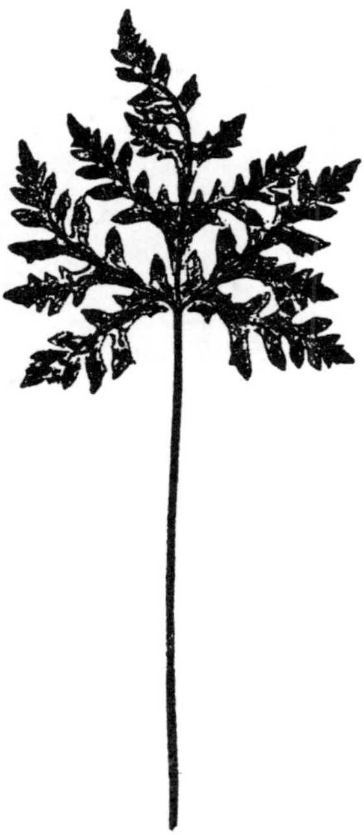

12. 1 Rainforest Conservation Society of Queensland 1986. Tropical Rainforests of north Queensland. Australian Heritage Commission Special Australian Heritage Publication number 3.(Australian Government Publishing Service: Canberra).

12. 2 1972. The Dyirbal Language of north Queensland. (Cambridge University Press: Cambridge).

12. 3 **Horsfall N.** 1987. Personal communication.

12. 4 **Harris DR.** 1978. Adaptation to a tropical rainforest environment: Aboriginal substance in northeastern Queensland in Blurton-Jones, NG and Reynolds V (eds) *Human Behaviour and Adaptation* (Taylor and Francis: London).

12. 5 **Dixon RMW.** 1976. Tribes and Boundaries in Australia. **In** Peterson N. ed. *Tribes and Boundaries in Australia* Social Anthropology Series No 10. (Australian Institute of Aboriginal Studies: Canberra).

**CHAPTER 12 (contd)**


12. 6 **Dixon RMW.** 1977. *A Grammar of Yidinj.* (Cambridge University Press: Cambridge).

12. 7 **Tindale NB. 1940.** Results of the Harvard-Adelaide Universities Anthropological Expedition 1938-1939: Distribution of Australian Aboriginal Tribes: A field survey. *Trans Roy Soc SA.* 64(1):140-231.

12. 8 **Tindale NB and Birdsell JB.** 1941. Results of the Harvard-Adelaide Universities Anthropological Expedition 1938-39: Tasmanoid tribes in north Queensland. *Rec S.A. Mus* 7:1-9.

12. 9 **Horsfall N.** 1983. The prehistoric occupation of Australian rainforests. (Conference Paper, Griffith University, "The Future of the Australian Rainforests", Dec. 1983).

12.10 **Horsfall N.** 1984. Theorising about northeast Queensland prehistory. *Qd Archaeological Research* 1:

12.11 1986. Aborigines and toxic northeastern Queensland rainforest plants. **In** Covacevich J, Davie P and Pearn J, eds. *Toxic Plants and Animals.* A Guide for Australia. (Queensland Museum: Brisbane).

12.12 **Lumholtz C.** 1889 (facsimile reprint 1980). Among Cannibals: Account of four Years Travels in Australia, and of Camp Life with the Aborigines of Queensland (Australian National University Press: Canberra).

12.13 **Webb LJ.** 1960. Some new records of medicinal plants used by the Aborigines of tropical Queensland and New Guinea. *Proc Roy Soc Qd* 71(6): 103-110.

12.14 1969. The use of plant medicines and poisons by Australian Aborigines. *Mankind* 7: 137-46.

12.15 **Isaacs J.** 1987. Bush Food. Aboriginal Food and Herbal Medicine. (Wheldons Pty Ltd: 43 Victoria Street, McMahons Point 2060, NSW).

12.16 **Farnsworth NR.** 1966. Biological and phytochemical screening of plants. *J Pharm Sci* **55**: 225-76.

12.17 **Reid E.** 1979. The records of Western Australian plants used by Aboriginals as medicinal agents. (School of Pharmacy, Western Australian Institute of Technology: Perth).

12.18 **Roth WE.** 1903. North Queensland Ethnography: Bulletin No 5. Superstition, Magic, and Medicine. (Government Printer: Brisbane).

12.19 Personal communication, Mrs Bessie Jerry.

12.20 **Flecker H, Stephens GB, and Stephens SE.** 1948. Edible plants in north Queensland. *N Q Nat* 4: 4-19.

**CHAPTER 12 (contd)**

12.21 **Davis G and Covacevich J**. 1984. Aboriginal Walkway. *Wildlife Australia* Winter: 8-10.

12.22 **Dowling R and Kleinschmidt H.** 1987. Toxic native and garden plants in subtropical Queensland, **in** Covacevich J, Davie P and Pearn J. (eds) *Toxic Plants and Animals.* A Guide for Australia (Queensland Museum: Brisbane).

12.23 **Harris J and Pearn J.** 1987. Bullrout Stings **In** Covacevich J, Davie P, and Pearn J. (eds) *Toxic Plants and Animals.* A Guide for Australia (Queensland Museum: Brisbane).

12.24 **MacPherson J.** The Eucalyptus in the daily life and medical practice of the Australian Aborigines. *Mankind* 2(6): 175-180.

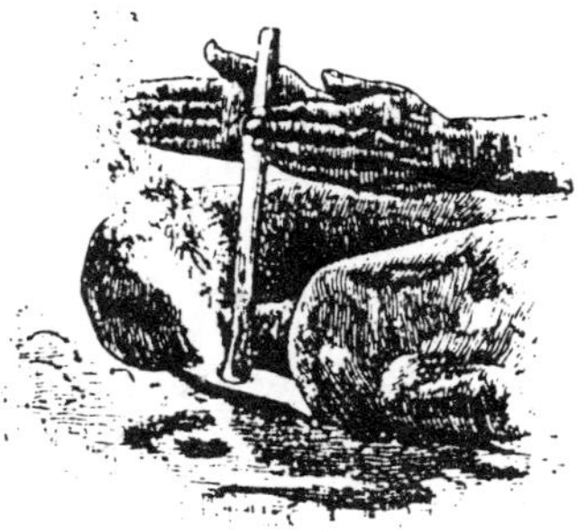

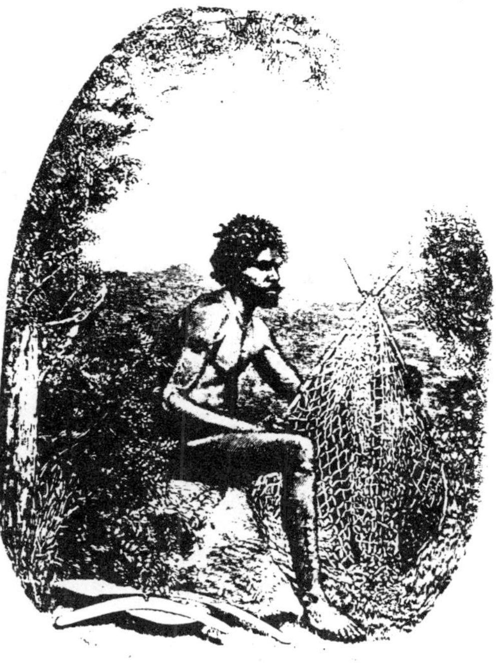

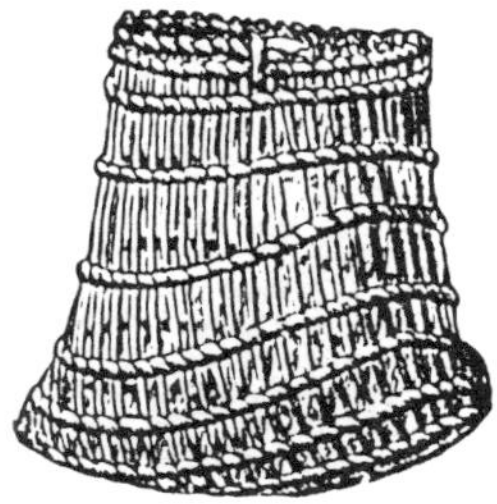

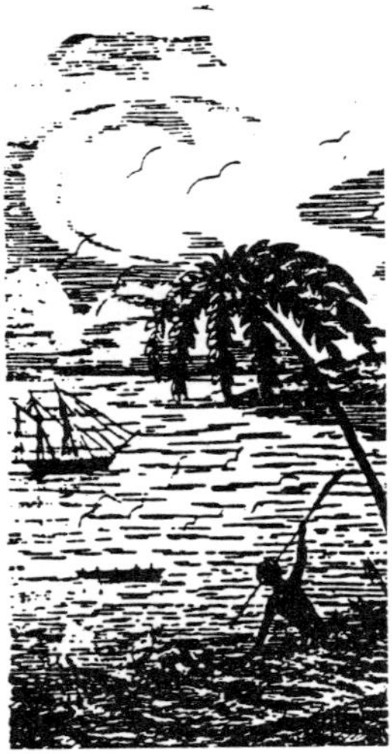

## CHAPTER 13

13. 1 **May D.** An Historical Account of the Health of Aborigines on North Queensland Cattle Stations in R MacLeod and D Denoon (eds) (forthcoming).

13. 2 **Nathan P and Leichleitner Japanangka D.** *Health Business.* Richmond: Heinemann Educational. 1983.

13. 3 **Mayman J.** Why Joan Winch Needs $650,000. *Aust Society* 1988:7:22-3, 49.

13. 4 **Queensland State Archives:** Special Batch on Medical and Inspectorial: Director Generals' Report: Sixth Session of National Health and Medical Research Council: A31756.

13. 5 **Australian National Library:** Aust. Inland Mission Records MS5574: Dunbar Hospital Box 78.

13. 6 **QSA:** HOS 14/C/D1 Normanton Hospital Minute Book. 1 May 1934-24 October 1936.

13. 7 **A.R. Aboriginals Department 1920.** Queensland Parliamentary Papers 1921:2: 559.

13. 8 Cited in A.R. Aboriginals Dept 1933. Queensland Parliamentary Papers 1934:1: 883.

13. 9 **A.R. Aboriginals Department 1928.** Queensland Parliamentary Papers 1929:1: 1214.

13.10 **QSA:** A/29545 Special Branch. Burketown Hospital to Home Sec. Office. 11 July 1934.

13.11 **Ibid.**

13.12 **A.R. Northern Protector of Aboriginals 1900.** *Queensland Votes and Proceedings* 1901:4: 1335.

13.13 **QSA:** A/29545 Special Batch. Rules of Normanton Hospital. When the rules were revised in 1916 this clause remained unchanged.

13.14 At Normanton charge was 10 shillings.

13.15 **A.R. Northern Protector of Aboriginals 1901.** Queensland Parliamentary Papers 1902:1: 1140.

13.16 **Ibid.**

13.17 **Lorraine Station Letterbook:** J Kirkaldy to Secretary, Burketown Hospital. 27 November 1913. The manager had earlier indicated that the station would be responsible for hospital fees.

**CHAPTER 13 (contd)**

13.18 **QSA**: HOM/J454. Georgetown Aboriginal Protector to Home Sec. 23/834.

13.19 **QSA**: Special Batch Hospital Board – Normanton. A/29545.

13.20 **QSA**: Special Batches Hospital Boards Burketown/Normanton/Croydon. A/29546.

13.21 **ANL**: Aust. Inland Mission Records MS5574: Dunbar Hospital. Box 79. Folder 3.

13.22 Cited in QSA: Special Batch Hospital Boards Burketown/Normanton/ Croydon. A/29546. CPA to Under Sec. Dept HHA, 10 August 1937. In 1939 the Committee agreed to treat Aborigines in the operating theatre providing the Department constructed a new Aboriginal ward.

13.23 **Ibid.**

13.24 **Moodie PM.** The Health Disadvantages of Aborigines, **in** FS Stevens (ed) *Racism: the Aust. Experience.* Vol 2, Sydney: ANZ Book Co. 1972.

13.25 **QSA**: Special Batch A/29545. RW Wehrle to Under Secretary, Home Office 3 February 1923.

13.26 **QSA**: HHA Bundles, A/4035. Dr Burke Gaffney to CPA. 24 January 1939.

13.27 **Ibid.**

13.28 **Ford M.** *End of a Beginning.* Melbourne: Hodder and Stoughton. 1973: 36.

13.29 **ANL**: Australian Inland Mission Records MS5574: Dunbar Hospital: Box 79, Folder 1. Payne to Hughes. 20 February 1940.

13.30 **QSA**: Special Branch. A/29546. JR Hulbert to Minister for HHA. 18 May 1939.

13.31 **Nathan P and Leichleitner Japanangka D.** *Health Business.* Richmond: Heinemann Educational. 1983: 68-93.

13.32 In 1927 eight Aborigines formerly from Coen, Ingham and Cardwell areas were charged with the attempted murder of Toby Burketown on Palm Island. In what appeared to be a tribal matter, the men had cut out a large piece of flesh from their victim. (*North Queensland Register.* 12 December 1927: 98).

13.33 **O'Conner E.** *Spirit Man,* Sydney: Angus & Robertson. 1980: 7.

13.34 **Ibid.**, p100. Elizabeth O'Conner was well qualified to write such a book. She spent many years on a Gulf cattle station which had a large Aboriginal staff.

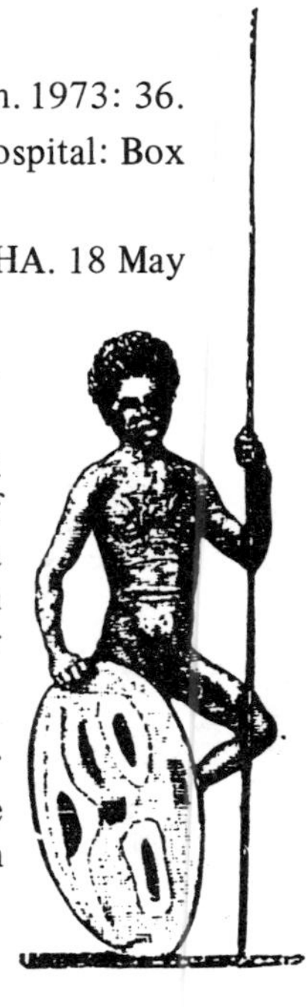

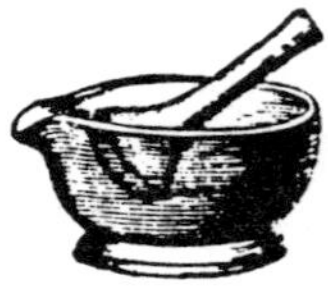

## CHAPTER 14


14. 1 **de Vidas, Jack.** *Med J Aust* 1947 2: 394.

14. 2 **Hackett, Earle.** *Lady Bones* Collins/ABC 1984. 119 *et seq*.

14. 3 **Pearn, John.** *In the Capacity of a Surgeon* 1988 University of Queensland.

14. 4 **Patrick, Ross.** *Horsewhip the Doctor* U.Q. Press, Brisbane 1985, 1-6.

14. 5 *Chamber's Encyclopaedia.* Vol. 10. 1880:276.

14. 6 **Patrick, Ross.** *A History of Health and Medicine in Queensland 1824-1960* U.Q. Press Brisbane 1987. 75 and elsewhere.

14. 7 **Patrick, Ross.** *The Royal Women's Hopsital, Brisbane – The First Fifty Years*. Boolarong Pub. Brisbane 1988. 10th *et seq*.

14. 8 **Thearle MJ, Gregory H.** Choices for Childbirth: Midwifery in nineteenth and early twentieth century Queensland. *Queensland Heritage* (new series) Vol 1. 1988.

14. 9 **Forster, Frank MC.** *Walter Lindsay Richardson – an Obstetrician.* Privately printed.

14.10 **Hopkins, Paul.** *Med J Aust* 1955 1: 752.

14.11 **Forster, Frank MC.** *Progress in Obstetrics and Gynaecology in Australia* John Sands, Sydney 1967.


## CHAPTER 15


15. 1 *Encyclopaedia Britannica,* Capetown, 15th Ed. 1985; Vol 15, 570.

15. 2 **Boyce PJ,** J.S. Hampton, The Governor, **in** *Westralian Portraits,* ed. L. Hunt, UWA Press, 1979: 45-51.

15. 3 **Bateson C.** *The Convict Ships, 1787-1868,* A.H. & A.W. Reed, 1974.

15. 4 *Australian Dictionary of Biography,* Vol. 1, 1788-1850, ed. D. Pike, Melbourne University Press, 1966: 508-509.


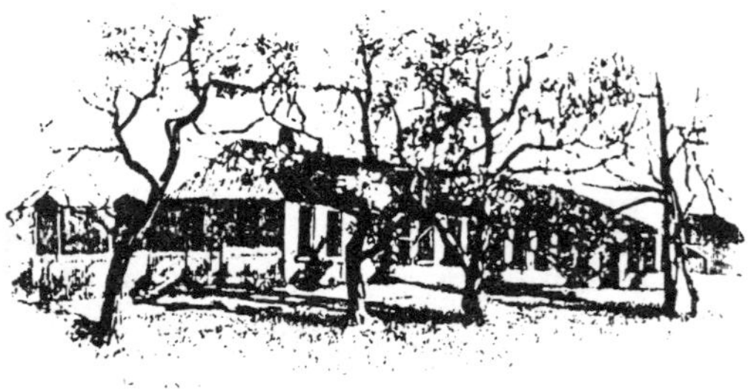


15. 5 **Morison MP.** *Western Towns and Buildings,* ed. M.P. Morison & J. White, University of Western Australia Press, 1979; Ch 1, 34.

15. 6 **Trollope A.** *Australia and New Zealand,* London, 1873 Vol II: 79-150.

**CHAPTER 15 (contd)**

15. 7 **Crowley FK.** *Australia's Western Third,* Macmillan, London, 1960: 35-37.

15. 8 **Cohen B.** *A History of Medicine in Western Australia,* Paterson Brokensha, Perth W.A., 1965: 69.

15. 9 **Boyce PJ.** The Governors of Western Australia under Representative Government 1870-1890, University Studies in History, 1961-62; UWA Press 4: 1, 101-143.

15.10 **Boyce PJ.** The Role of the Governor in the Crown Colony of Western Australia, 1829-1890; MA Thesis, UWA, 1961: 163-187.

15.11 **Battye JS.** *Western Australia* Clarendon Press, Oxford 1924. 10: 243-257

15.12 *Australian Dictionary of Biography* Vol 4, 1851-1890, ed. D Pike, Melbourne University Press, 1972: 278.

15.13 *Australian Dictionary of Biography* Vol 4, 1851-1890 ed. D Pike, Melbourne University Press, 1972: 280.

15.14 **Joyce RB.** *Sir William MacGregor* Oxford University Press 1971: 306, 367.

15.15 **Thomis MI.** *A Place of Light and Learning* University of Queensland Press, 1985.

15.16 Government House, Darwin, Northern Territory Information Service, 1980: 8.

15.17 **Holthouse H.** *Illustrated History of Queensland* Rigby, 1978: 230.

15.18 **Clark CMH.** *A History of Australia,* Melbourne University Press, 1987: 6, 269.

15.19 **Fysh H.** *Taming of the North* Angus & Robertson, 1933: 107.

15.20 *Australian Dictionary of Biography,* Vol 9, 1891-1939 Eds. B Nairn & G Serle, Melbourne University Press, 1983: 49-50.

15.21 **Patrick RK.** *A History of Medicine in Queensland,* University of Queensland Press, 1986.

15.22 *Who's Who in Australia* 1988, 26th Edition, Ed. KA Cadman, The Herald and Weekly Times Ltd, Melbourne.

15.23 **Rowland HE, Sir James.** March 1988, personal communication.

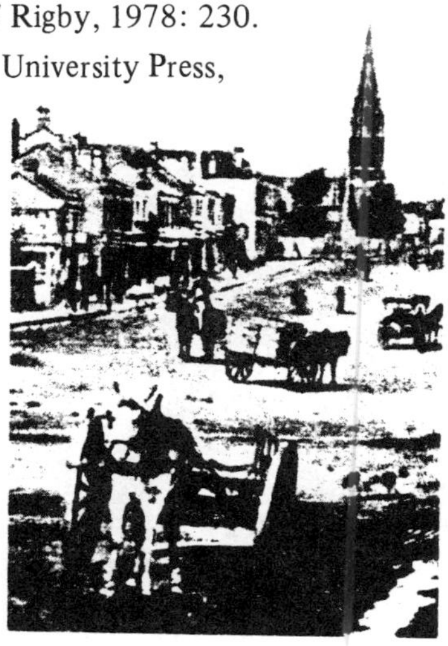

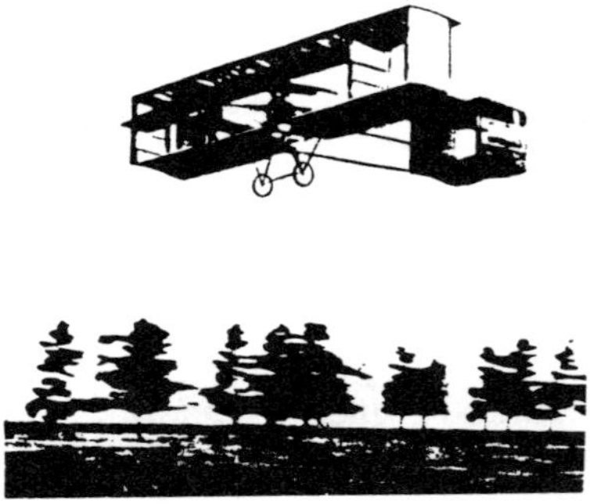

## CHAPTER 16

16. 1 **O'Leary TJ.** *North and Aloft.* A personal memoir of service and adventure with the Royal Flying Doctor Service in far northern Australia. Ed. JH Pearn and G Anderson. Brisbane, Amphion Press (Dept Child Health, University of Queensland Publishing Unit), 1988.

16. 2 **O'Leary TJ.** *Western Wings of Care.* A Personal Memoir of Aviation Development and Clinical Life with the Royal Flying Doctor Service in Outback Australia. Ed. JH Pearn and G Anderson. Brisbane, Amphion Press (Dept Child Health, University of Queensland Publishing Unit), 1988.

## CHAPTER 17

17. 1 "The Australasian Trained Nurses' Association Register of Members", 1910, Websdale, Shoosmith Ltd, Sydney, p.7 – Rule (xviii).

17. 2 **Cohn V.** 1975 *Sister Kenny: The Woman Who Challenged the Doctors*, The University of Minnesota Press, Minneapolis, p.36.

17. 3 **Kenny E and Ostenso M.** 1944, *And They Shall Walk*, Dodd, Mead & Co., New York, p.18.

17. 4 Photograph (Fig.1) in the possession of Mrs F. Mohr. Also personal communication.

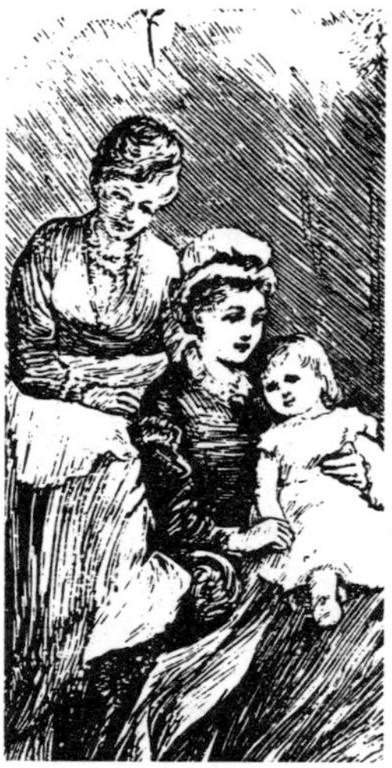

17. 5 **Cohn V.** 1975, *op. cit.*

17. 6 "The Australasian Trained Nurses' Association Register of Members", *op. cit.* p. 145 – Rules for Obstetric Nurses.

17. 7 **Morten H.** 1897, *The Midwives' Pocket Book*, The Burdett Series, Scientific Press Ltd., Southampton, London.

17. 8 "The Australasian Trained Nurses' Association Register of Members", *op. cit.* p. 194-5 – Obstetrics Register.

17. 9 **Cohn V.** *op. cit.*, p.37.

17.10 "The Australasian Trained Nurses' Association Register of Members", *op. cit.*, p.9 – Regulations of State Branches.

17.11 **Holloway K.** 1982, Personal Communication.

**CHAPTER 17 (contd)**


17.12 *Welcome's Professional Nurse's Diary*, 1915-1916, Australian Edition, p.54 – General Principles of Nursing.

17.13 **Abel-Smith B.** *A History of the Nursing Profession*, Heinemann, London, p.96.

17.14 **Duhig J.**, 1960, The Fabulous Sister Kenny, *Nation,* April 23, p.9.

17.15 **Knox E.** 1935, *Medical Directory for Australia*, Knox, Sydney, p.206.

17.16 "The Australasian Nurses' Association Register of Members", *op. cit.* p.194-195.

17.17 Australian Army Records Office Letter.

17.18 The Lancet Commission on Nursing, 1932, *The Lancet*, London, p.29.

17.19 **Lawton Roberts R.** 1892, *Illustrated Lectures on Nursing and Hygiene*, H.K. Lewis, London, p.15.

17.20 **Pearn J.** 1988 The Sylvia Stretcher: A perspective of Sister Elizabeth Kenny's contribution to first aid management of the injured, *Med J Aust* 1988 (in press).

17.21 *Illustrated Catalogue of Surgical Instruments and Appliances*, 1938, Taylor and Elliott Surgical Company, Brisbane, p.B/297.

17.22 **Kenny E.** 1936. Evidence given to Queensland Royal Commission, Kenny Collection.

17.23 **Kenny E.** 1942, *Treatment of Infantile Paralysis in the Acute Stage*, Bruce Publishing Co., St Paul.

17.24 **Dungan R.** 1934, "Report of Observation on Work Done by Sister Kenny at the Muscle Re-Education Clinic, Townsville", 24th August.

17.25 **Kenny E.** 1944, *op. cit.* p.94.

17.26 **Duhig J.** 1936. Evidence given to Queensland Royal Commission, Kenny Collection.

17.27 **Kenny E.** 1934 "Report on the Muscle Re-Education Clinic, Townsville", Appendix A, p.2.

17.28 **Kenny E.** 1937 *Infantile Paralysis and Cerebral Diplegia*, Angus and Robertson, Sydney, p.3.

17.29 **Teece L.** 1937, Review of Miss Kenny's Text Book, Appendix to "Report of the Royal Commission on the Investigation of Infantile Paralysis", Queensland, December.

17.30 **Hertz M.** 1937 "Sister Kenny Mystery Report: Exclusive Review by Famous Specialist", *Smith's Weekly,* November 27th.

**CHAPTER 17 (contd)**


17.31 **Kenny E.** 1936 *op. cit.*

17.32 **Hansen J.** 1983, Personal Communication.

17.33 **Cilento R.** 1936, Evidence given to the Queensland Royal Commission, Kenny Collection.

17.34 **Starr K.** 1939 "A Report to the Minister for Health, NSW, on Sister Kenny's Method", Morris Printers, Newcastle, May.

17.35 **Kenny E.** 1936 *op. cit.*

17.36 **Kenny E.** 1939 "Summary of lectures given at the Brisbane General Hospital", October 17th.

17.37 **Kenny E.** 1936 *op. cit.*

17.38 **Kenny E.** 1950 "The Kenny Therapist in the Fight Against Polio", Kenny Collection.

17.39 **Rountree J.** 1935, Letter to Mr Hanlon, November 1st.

17.40 **Wilkinson H.** 1937, Foreword to Sister Kenny's Text Book *Infantile Paralysis and Cerebral Diplegia*, p.xvi.

17.41 **Wilkinson et al.**, 1940, Letter to Mr Forgan Smith, Kenny Files, Queensland Archives.

17.42 **Little N. et al.**, 1940, Letter to *The Brisbane Courier Mail*, March 15th.

17.43 **Kenny E.** 1952, "Doctors, I Salute You", *The American Weekly*, March 2nd, p.8.

17.44 **Cilento R.** 1934, "Report on the Muscle Re-Education Clinic in Townsville", August 24th, p.24, Kenny Collection.

17.45 **Kenny E.** 1951, "Why I Left America", *The Digest of World Reading*, July 2nd, p.84.

17.46 **Elizabeth Kenny Obituary**, 1953, *Med J Aust* January 17th, p.85.

17.47 **Knapp M.** 1955, "The Contribution of Sister Elizabeth Kenny to the Treatment of Poliomyelitis", Archives of Physical Medicine and Rehabilitation, August, p.510.

17.48 **Benjamin S.** 1985, Letter to Mr Jack Kenny from Director of Public Relations and Marketing, Sister Kenny Institute, March 29th.

17.49 **Albertson D.** 1978, "Sister Kenny's Legacy", Hennepin County Historical Society, Hennepin County.

17.50 **Wilson J.** 1986, "The Sister Kenny Clinics: What Endures"? *The Australian Journal of Advanced Nursing*, Vol 3, No.2.


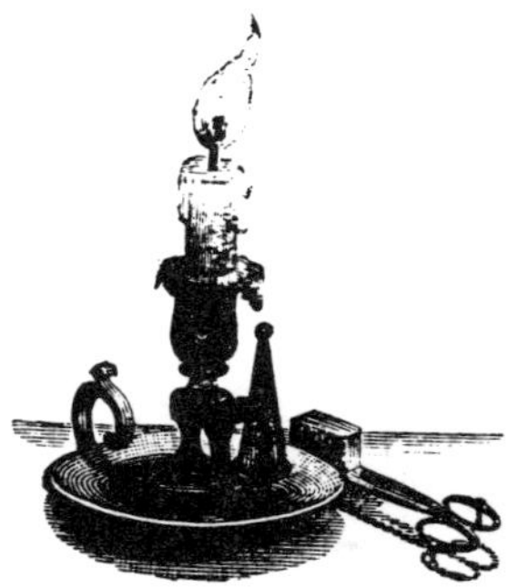

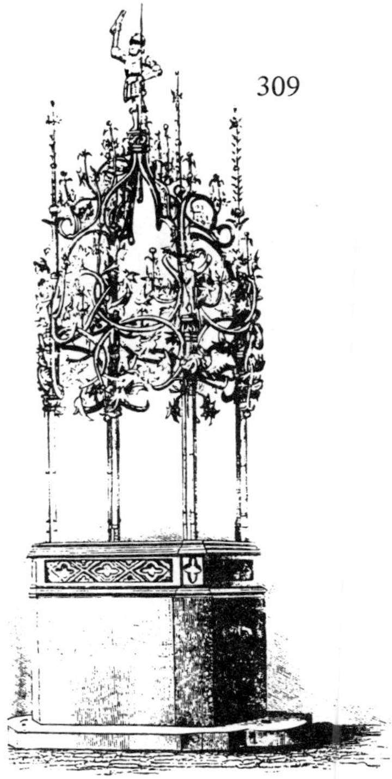

## CHAPTER 18

18. 1 **Bompas GC.** 1885. *Life of Frank Buckland by his Brother-in-law, George C Bompas with a portrait.* 3rd Edition. Smith Elder and Co, London.

18. 2 **Burgess GHO.** 1967. *The Curious World of Frank Buckland.* John Pinker, Royal Opera Arcade, London.

18. 3 **Cooke A.** 1986. A note on Dr Frank Buckland. *Journal of The Royal College of Physicians of London* **20**, 145.

18. 4 **Roughley TC.** 1951. *Fish and Fisheries in Australia.* Angus and Robertson, Sydney.

## CHAPTER 19

19. 1 **Flecker H.** Injuries by Unknown Agents to Bathers in North Queensland. *Med J Aust* 1945;**1**:98.

19. 2 **Southcott RV.** Irukandji Sting to North Queensland Bathers without Production of Weals but with Severe General Symptoms. *Med J Aust* 1952;**1**:272.

19. 3 **Barnes JH.** Cause and Effect in Irukandji Stingings. *Med J Aust* 1964, **1**:897.

19. 4 **Barnes JH.** Observations on Jellyfish Stingings in North Queensland. *Med J Aust* 1960;**2**:993.

19. 5 **Barnes JH.** *Chironex fleckeri* and *Chiropsalmus quadrigatus* – Morphological Distinctions. *The North Queensland Naturalist* 1965;**32**:137.

19. 6 **Barnes JH and Endean R.** A Dangerous Starfish – *Acanthaster planci* (Linne). *Med J Aust* 1964;**1**:592.

19. 7 **Barnes JH.** The Crown of Thorns Starfish as a Destroyer of Coral. *Australian Natural History* December 1966.

19. 8 **Barnes JH.** Siphonophores, Part I of a Series. *The North Queensland Naturalist* 1962;**30**:131.

19. 9 **Barnes JH.** Siphonophores, Part 2 of a Series. *The North Queensland Naturalist* 1964;**32**:135.

19.10 **Kinsey B.** Barnes on Box Jellyfish. James Cook University of North Queensland (Pub. 1986).

19.11 **Kinsey B.** More Barnes on Box Jellyfish. James Cook University of North Queensland (Pub. 1988).

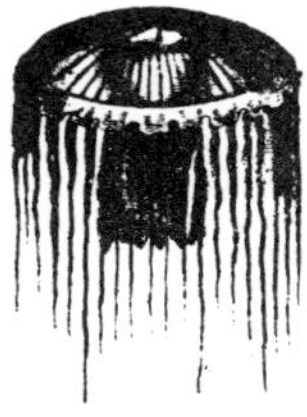

## CHAPTER 20


20. 1 **McIntyre AK.** Origins of Australasian neuroscience: a personal view. *Proc Aust Physiol Pharmacol Soc* 1983;40-7.

20. 2 **Wilson JT.** The double innervation of striated muscle. *Brain* 1921; **44**:234-47.

20. 3 **Royle ND.** The treatment of spastic paralysis by sympathetic ramisection. *Surg Gyn Obstet* 1924;**39**:701-20.

20. 4 **Anonymous.** John Irvine Hunter. [Obituary] *Med J Aust* 1924;**2**:669-72.

20. 5 **Royle ND.** A new operative procedure in the treatment of spastic paralysis and its experimental basis. *Med J Aust* 1924;**1**:77-86.

20. 6 **Hunter JI.** The postural influence of the sympathetic innervation of voluntary muscle. *Med J Aust* 1924;**1**:86-9.

20. 7 **Burkitt AN.** Norman Dawson Royle [Obituary]. *Med J Aust* 1944;**1**: 570-1.

20. 8 **Cleland KW.** Anatomy. **In**: Young JA, Sefton AJ, Webb N. Eds. *Centenary Book of the University of Sydney Faculty of Medicine.* Sydney University Press, 1984:266-02.

20. 9 **Cleland KW.** Histology and Embryology. **In**: Young JA, Sefton AJ, Webb N, Eds. *Centenary Book of the University of Sydney Faculty of Medicine.* Sydney University Press, 1984: 303-319.

20.10 **Hunter JI, Latham O.** A contribution to the discussion of the histological problems involved in the conception of a somatic and sympathetic innervation of voluntary muscle. *Med J Aust* 1925;**1**:27-36.

20.11 **Latham O.** The histological evidence for the sympathetic innervation of striated muscle fibres [Abstract]. *Med J Aust* 1927;**1**:485.

20.12 **Wilkinson HJ.** The innervation of striated muscle. *Med J Aust* 1929; **2**:768-93.

20.13 **Wilkinson HJ.** Observations on the sole-plates of motor end-organs. *J Comp Neurol* 1930; **50**:133-36.

20.14 **Boeke J.** Some remarks on the papers by HJ Wilkinson on the innervation of striped muscle-fibers. *J Comp Neurol* 1930;**51**:299-309.

20.15 **Wilkinson HJ.** Experimental studies on the innervation of striated muscle. *J Comp Neurol* 1930;**51**:129-51.

20.16 **Wilkinson HJ.** Further experimental studies on the innervation of striated muscle. *J Comp Neurol.* 1934;**59**:221-38.

**CHAPTER 20 (contd)**


20.17 **Coates AE, Tiegs OW.** Are the skeletal muscles of the extremities directly innervated by sympathetic nerves? *Aust J Exp Biol Med Sci* 1931;**8**: 99-106.

20.18 **Phillips G.** On the apparent diminution in skeletal muscle tonus following removal of the lumbar sympathetic trunk. *Med J Aust* 1931;**1**:628-32.

20.19 **Boeke J.** The sympathetic ground-plexus in the glands, muscles and connective tissues of the body. **In**: *Problems in Nervous Anatomy.* London: Oxford University Press, 1940;45-81.

20.20 **Kuntz A.** Sympathetic nerves in relation to skeletal muscle. **In**: *The Autonomic Nervous System.* Philadelphia: Lea and Febiger, 1945: 357-82.

20.21 **Wilkinson HJ.** Foreword. **In**: Kenny E. *Infantile Paralysis and Cerebral Diplegia : Methods Used for the Restoration of Function.* Sydney: Angus and Robertson, 1937; i-xvii.

20.22 **Brecht B.** *The life of Galileo.* tr. by H. Brenton. London: Eyre Methuen, 1980: 31.


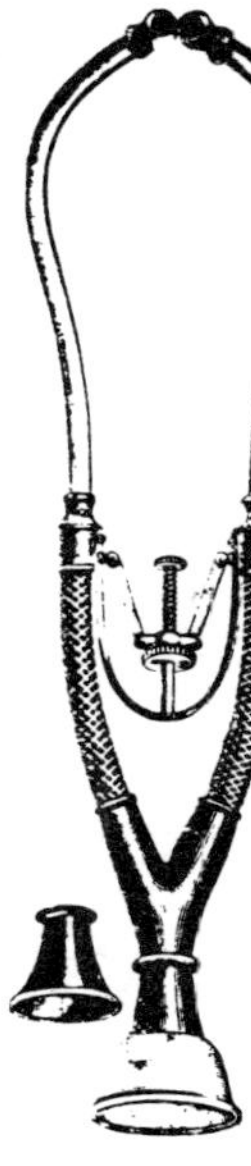

# INDEX

References to Figures are in **bold face.**

**B (contd)**



**C**

## C (contd)



## C (contd)



## D

## D (contd)

## D (contd)



## D (contd)



## E



## F

**Q**



**R**



**R (contd)**



**S**

## S (contd)



## S (contd)

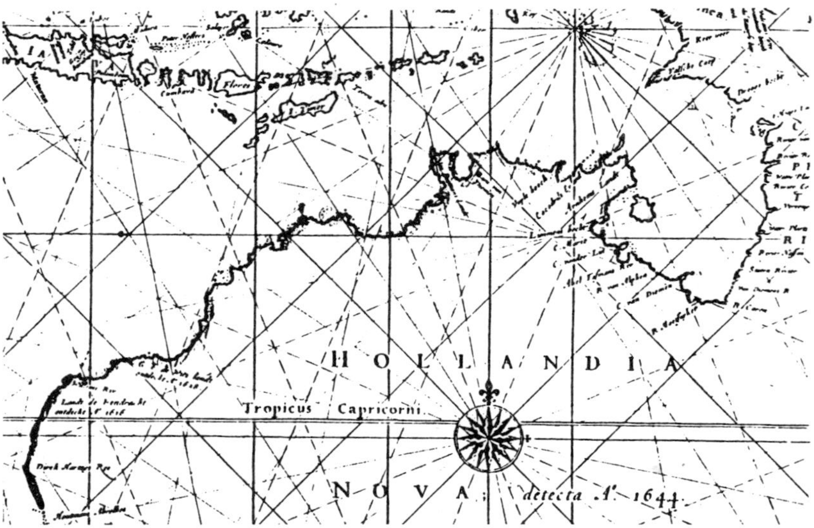
H O L L A N D I A
Tropicus Capricorni
N O V A detecta A° 1644

## *THE COVER*

Progress towards better health, for all Australians, has advanced on many fronts. Pioneers in disparate fields have contributed to the reduction of disease and to the promotion of better health, and to the practice of high quality medicine which helps to achieve this. The cover of this book illustrates some of the many themes inherent in pioneering medicine in Australia.

Portrayed are Dr Alfred Jefferis Turner, Queensland's first paediatrician, who did so much to reduce infant mortality, to eradicate hookworm, and to reduce the dangers of lead paint for children in all Australia. Dr Turner is portrayed working at his hobby, the study of moths and butterflies, of which branch of science he is also a founding father in this country. Shown also is Sister Elizabeth Kenny, pioneering nurse, whose campaigns for poliomyelitis therapy spread throughout the world; and whose influence leading to the professional independence of nurses has been most significant.

Illustrated also is a ship of the First Fleet, with its symbolism of naval medicine, the health of convicts, the prevention of scurvy, and the role of the surgeons who were the first pioneers of European medicine. The rainforest plants symbolise the Aboriginal pharmacopoeia which existed for twenty millennia before the arrival of the First Fleet.

Other themes relate to public health and tropical medicine, aboriginal health, surgery and preventive medicine, the health of Emigrants, and of medical research itself.

This cover was the concept of Mr Paul Ramsden; the artistry has been executed by Mr Robert Allen (both of the Queensland Museum) whose skills have done so much to promote an awareness of the rich fabric of Australian medical history.

JHP